CARDIOVASCULAR DISEASE IN THE OCTOGENARIAN AND BEYOND

Cardiovascular Disease in the Octogenarian and Beyond

Edited by

Nanette K Wenger MD, FACC, MACP, FACCP, FSGC
Professor of Medicine (Cardiology)
Emory University School of Medicine
Atlanta, Georgia
USA

MARTIN DUNITZ

First published in the United Kingdom in 1999 by
Martin Dunitz Ltd
The Livery House
7–9 Pratt Street
London NW1 0AE

A CIP catalogue record for this book is available from the British Library.

ISBN 1–85317–581–1

Distributed in the United States by:
Blackwell Science Inc.
Commerce Place, 350 Main Street
Malden, MA 02148, USA
Tel: 1–800–215–1000

Distributed in Canada by:
Login Brothers Book Company
324 Salteaux Crescent
Winnipeg, Manitoba, R3J 3T2
Canada
Tel: 204–224–4068

Distributed in Brazil by:
Ernesto Reichmann Distribuidora de Livros, Ltda
Rua Coronel Marques 335, Tatuape 03440–000
Sao Paulo,
Brazil

Composition by Wearset, Boldon, Tyne and Wear.
Printed and bound in Great Britain by Cambridge University Press, Cambridge, UK.

CONTENTS

Contributors

Joseph S Alpert, MD
University of Arizona Health Sciences Center
Department of Medicine
1501 North Campbell Avenue
Tuscon, AZ 85724-5035
USA

Hossein Amirani, MD
Medical College of Wisconsin
2030 North Lake Drive
Milwaukee, WI 53202
USA

Sary F Aranki, MD
Division of Cardiac Surgery
Brigham & Women's Hospital
75 Francis Street
Boston, MA 02115-6195
USA

Melvin D Cheitlin, MD
San Francisco General Hospital
1001 Potrero Avenue, Room 5G1
San Francisco, CA 94110
USA

Lawrence H Cohn, MD
Division of Cardiac Surgery
Brigham & Women's Hospital
75 Francis Street
Boston, MA 02115-6195
USA

Philippe Delfaut, MD
Cardiac Medicine & Electrophysiology
55 Essex Street
Suite 3-2
Millburn, NJ 07041
USA

Douglas G Ebersole, MD
The Watson Clinic
1600 Lakeland Hills Boulevard
PO Box 95000
Lakeland, FL 33804-5000
USA

Eric L Eisenstein, DBA
Department of Medicine
Cardiology Division
Box 3865
Duke University Medical Center
Durham, NC 27710-7510
USA

Walter H Ettinger Jr, MD, MBA
J Paul Sticht Center on Aging
Bowman Gray School of Medicine
Medical Center Blvd
Winston-Salem, NC 27157
USA

Jane C Evans, MPH
Framingham Study
5 Thurber Street
Framingham, MA 01701
USA

Jerome L Fleg, MD
Human Cardiovascular Studies Unit
Laboratory of Cardiovascular Science
Gerontology Research Center
National Institute on Aging, NIH
5600 Nathan Shock Drive
Baltimore, MD 21224-6823
USA

Joseph Francis, MD, MPH
Vanderbilt Medical Center
Division of Cardiology
Room 315 MRB II
2220 Pierce Avenue
Nashville, TN 37232-6300
USA

Linda P Fried
The Johns Hopkins Medical Institutions
Baltimore, MD 21205
USA

Gottlieb C Friesinger, MD
Vanderbilt Medical Center
Division of Cardiology
Room 315 MRB II
2220 Pierce Avenue
Nashville, TN 37232-6300
USA

Gary Gerstenblith, MD
The Johns Hopkins Hospital
591 Carnegie Building
600 N. Wolfe Street
Baltimore, MD 21287
USA

Kathryn A Glatter, MD
Division of Cardiovascular Medicine
University of California at San Francisco
Medical Center
505 Parnassus Ave
San Francisco, CA 94143-0124
USA

Claudia F Gravina Taddei, MD
Dante Pazzanese Institute of Cardiology
Sao Paulo, Brazil
and
Division of Cardiology
Emory University School of Medicine
1364 Clifton Road N.E.
Atlanta, GA 30322
USA

Gabriel Gregoratos, MD
Division of Cardiovascular Medicine
University of California at San Francisco
Medical Center
505 Parnassus Ave
San Francisco, CA 94143-0124
USA

Joseph A Guzzo, MD
Division of Cardiology
The University of North Carolina at Chapel Hill
CB# 7075
Burnett-Womack Building
Chapel Hill, SC 27599-7075
USA

W Dallas Hall, MD
Emory University School of Medicine
Atlanta, GA
USA

William R Hazzard, MD
J Paul Sticht Center on Aging
Department of Internal Medicine
Section on Gerontology and Geriatrics
Bowman Gray Medical Center
Medical Center Blvd
Winston-Salem, NC 27157
USA

David R Holmes Jr, MD
Division of Cardiovascular Diseases
Mayo Clinic
Rochester, MN 55905
USA

William B Kannel, MD
Framingham Study
5 Thurber Street
Framingham, MA 01701
USA

Andrzej S Kosinski, PhD
Division of Cardiology
Emory University School of Medicine
1364 Clifton Road N.E.
Atlanta, GA 30322
USA

Ryszard B Krol, MD
Cardiac Medicine & Electrophysiology
55 Essex Street
Suite 3-2
Millburn, NJ 07041
USA

Richard A Kronmal, PhD
CHS Century Square
1501 4th Avenue
Suite 2105
Seattle, WA 98101
USA

Lewis H Kuller, MD, DrPH
University of Pittsburgh
Graduate School of Public Health
130 De Soto St
Pittsburgh, PA 15261-0001
USA

Martin G Larson, ScD
Framingham Study
5 Thurber Street
Framingham, MA 01701
USA

Carl J Lavie, MD
Ochsner Clinic
1514 Jefferson Highway
New Orleans, LA 70121-4135
USA

Lorraine L Mackstaller, MD
University of Arizona Health Sciences Center
Department of Medicine
1501 North Campbell Avenue
Tuscon, AZ 85724-5035
USA

Paul E McGann, SM, MD
J Paul Sticht Center on Aging
Section on Gerontology and Geriatrics
Bowman Gray Medical Center
Medical Center Blvd
Winston-Salem, NC 27157, USA

Richard V Milani, MD
Ochsner Clinic
1514 Jefferson Highway
New Orleans, LA 70121-4135
USA

Douglas C Morris, MD
Emory Heart Center
Emory University School of Medicine
Building A, Room 2100
1365 Clifton Road NE
Atlanta, GA 30322
USA

Charles J Mullany, MB, MS
Mayo Medical School/Foundation
Division of Thoracic & Cardiovascular Surgery
Rochester, MN 55905-0001
USA

Meena Nathan, MD
Division of Cardiac Surgery
Brigham & Women's Hospital
75 Francis Street
Boston, MA 02115-6195
USA

Eric D Peterson, MD, MPH
Department of Medicine
Cardiology Division
Box 3236
Duke University Medical Center
Durham, NC 27710-7510
USA

Paula M Podrazik, MD
Clinical Pharmacology & Geriatrics
Northwestern University Medical School
303 East Superior, Jennings 209
Chicago, IL 60611-3042
USA

Atul Prakash, MD
Cardiac Medicine & Electrophysiology
55 Essex Street
Suite 3-2
Millburn, NJ 07041, USA

Michael W Rich, MD
Geriatric Cardiology Program
Cardiovascular Division
Department of Internal Medicine
Barnes-Jewish Hospital (North Campus) at
Washington University Medical Center
216 South Kingshighway Boulevard
St Louis, MO 63110
USA

William C Roberts, MD
Baylor Cardiovascular Institute
Baylor University Medical Center
3500 Gaston Avenue
Dallas, TX 75246
USA

Sanjeev Saksena, MD
Cardiac Medicine & Electrophysiology
55 Essex Street
Suite 3-2
Millburn, NJ 07041
USA

Stephen F Schaal, MD
Ohio State University
1655 Upham Drive
669 Means Hall
Columbus, OH 43210-1251
USA

Janice B Schwartz, MD
Professor of Medicine
Chief, Clinical Pharmacology & Geriatrics
Northwestern University Medical School
303 East Superior, Jennings 209
Chicago, IL 60611-3042
USA

Leslee Shaw, PhD
Division of Cardiology
Emory University School of Medicine
1364 Clifton Road N.E.
Atlanta, GA 30322
USA

Sidney C Smith Jr, MD
The University of North Carolina at Chapel Hill
CB# 7075
Burnett-Womack Building
Chapel Hill, SC 27599-7075
USA

John A Spittell Jr, MD
Mayo Medical School
614 Memorial Parkway
Rochester, MN 55902
USA

David H Spodick, MD, DSc
University of Massachusetts Medical School
Saint Vincent Hospital
Cardiology Divison
Worcester, MA 01604
USA

Donald D Tresch, MD
Medical College of Wisconsin
2030 North Lake Drive
Milwaukee, WI 53202
USA

Ronald E Vlietstra, MD, ChB
The Watson Clinic
1600 Lakeland Hills Boulevard
PO Box 95000
Lakeland, FL 33804-5000
USA

Betty Wang, RN
Cardiac Medicine & Electrophysiology
55 Essex Street
Suite 3-2
Millburn, NJ 07041
USA

Jeanne Y Wei, MD, PhD
Beth Israel Hospital
330 Brookline Avenue
Boston, MA 02215
USA

William S Weintraub, MD
Division of Cardiology
Emory University School of Medicine
1364 Clifton Road N.E.
Atlanta, GA 30322
USA

Nanette K Wenger, MD
Division of Cardiology
Emory University School of Medicine
Thomas K Glenn Memorial Building
69 Butler Street SE
Atlanta, GA, 30303
USA

Jeff D Williamson, MD, MHS
J Paul Sticht Center on Aging
Bowman Gray School of Medicine
Medical Center Blvd
Winston-Salem, NC 27157
USA

Peter W F Wilson, MD
Framingham Study
5 Thurber Street
Framingham, MA 01701
USA

Susan J Zieman, MD
The Johns Hopkins Hospital
591 Carnegie Building
600 N. Wolfe Street
Baltimore, MD 21287
USA

This volume is dedicated to our grandsons

Kevin Scott Wiatrak
Jesse David Wiatrak

with hope that they will age successfully in a knowledgeable and caring world

Introduction

Nanette K Wenger

Changes in the demography of the worldwide population, including that of the United States, provided the impetus for this monograph. Since the mid 19th century, there has been an almost doubling of life expectancy at birth in the United States, from about 40 years to about 80 years. Life-expectancy for men and women has increased even more dramatically during the past few generations. Not only has the elderly population increased in both developed and developing nations, but the aged population itself has become older as more people survive to very advanced age. During the past half century, the aging of the US population has been most pronounced among the oldest old.[1,2] Favorable health-related behavioral changes may further accentuate this trend. The population over 85 years is anticipated to triple in the half century between 1980 and 2030. As early as 2010, there will be more than 12 million octogenarians and older in the USA, increasing to 18 million by 2030. The number of centenarians is increasing at a rate of 8% annually; healthy centenarians often have a brief period of illness before death, typically succumbing to an acute rather than a chronic disease. The World Health Organization cites that the largest elderly populations (aged 75 years and older) currently reside in Brazil, China, the European Union, India, Japan, Russia and the USA, totalling 54 million women and 33 million men. By 2025, this aged population will increase by 140% to encompass 122 million women and 86 million men.

Concomitantly, the prevalence of cardiovascular disease has increased dramatically with aging. Since cardiovascular disease is the most prevalent illness in the elderly population, it is the major determinant of survival at very elderly age. It constitutes the major cause of death and disability in elderly persons, with a likelihood of these adverse outcomes of as much as 58% at ages 85 years and older. Although some reports describe altered expectations of the outcome of an illness in elderly patients, it remains controversial whether these expectations reflect aging per se or whether they relate to medical care systems in specific countries where options for the care available for elderly patients differ from those for a younger population. In a health care delivery system where age influences health policy, elderly patients may have different expectations of the outcomes of management of a specific illness.

Almost half of all octogenarians have some clinical manifestation of cardiovascular illness: coronary heart disease, cerebrovascular accident, peripheral arterial disease or heart failure. Cardiovascular disease exerts an enormous impact on the need for hospital, ambulatory and custodial care as well. The socioeconomic impact of the burgeoning octogenarian population and their high prevalence of cardiovascular illness continues to escalate. A pivotal goal of the medical care system in an era of upwardly spiralling health care costs should be to provide an increased duration of active life expectancy, rather than an expanded period of frailty and dependency.[3] A major challenge is the ascertainment of whether the current allocation of health care resources constitutes a cost-effective approach to attaining a meaningful quality of life for the 40–50% of the now almost 8 million US octogenarians and beyond with symptomatic heart disease. When a treatment is undertaken, issues that mandate evaluation relate to the alleviation or limitation of the patient's symptoms; maintenance of a sense of well-being; restoration or preservation of physical and mental functional abilities that permit relative self-sufficiency and independence; and retardation of the progression of the underlying disease if feasible.[4] The dominant cardiovascular disease burden at elderly age is due to coronary heart disease, followed by hypertensive cardiovascular disease. About 20% of octogenarians have clinical evidence of coronary heart disease, with the numbers of elderly patients with coronary disease steadily increasing. Although octogenarians currently comprise less than 5% of the US population, they account for over 20% of hospital admissions for acute myocardial infarction and 30% of myocardial infarction deaths.[5] Hypertension is present in more than half of the US population aged 65 years and older. The estimated prevalence of heart failure is 10% for those older than 75 years. Heart failure is the most frequent hospital discharge diagnosis for patients in the Medicare population; 50% of all hospitalizations for heart failure occur in patients aged 75 years and older. Societal problems reflect the escalating costs of the long-term care characteristic of chronic cardiovascular illness at elderly age as well as for its episodic and often highly symptomatic exacerbations. The latter may require expensive and invasive high technology interventions. An increasing use and disproportionate share of health care resources is characteristic at advanced age.[6] Given the considerable cost of contemporary high-technology cardiovascular interventions,

what is required is determination of the resultant functional state of the aged patient. What are the resources that must be expended relative to the health benefits obtained? Specific focus should be on the resultant independence and life satisfaction. The relative roles of improved expectations of very elderly persons regarding their cardiovascular health status and those of their healthcare providers have been incompletely explored.

The heterogeneity of the elderly population poses major challenges, in that the varience of any variable is likely to increase with increasing age, particularly among the oldest old. Among the important factors contributing to this heterogeneity are the variable changes of aging in multiple organ systems, varying concomitant disease states, multiple drug therapies that increase not only the potential for drug toxicity but for drug interactions, and the varying social settings in which an illness occurs. There may be major variability between custodial and independent living settings and with differing degrees of social support. Women in the octogenarian age group are likely to be widowed, with frequent resultant lowered socioeconomic status, decreased social support, and less access to medical care. Although stereotypes of elderly patients with cardiac illness have often characterized them as having prominent disability and dependency, many contemporary elderly cardiac patients appear and behave younger than their chronological age and anticipate an extended and active retirement. Although current improvements in cardiac care appear to have postponed mortality, it remains uncertain whether there has been a comparable delay in the onset of morbidity and disability. An important concern of care is limiting the frailty of elderly patients with chronic illness, i.e., lessening the adverse effects of nonfatal but highly disabling conditions.[7]

Today the life expectancy of an 80-year-old man in the USA is 7 years and that of an 80-year-old woman 9.1 years. These individuals can anticipate functioning independently for at least half of this time frame. This aging of the population is a social phenomenon without historical precedent. As a result, neither components of government nor other social institutions are knowledgeable about appropriate actions or responses to the burgeoning health, medical, psychosocial, and other needs of the oldest old. Contemporary governmental health insurance systems fail to reimburse for the multidisciplinary supportive services that could enable continued maintenance of a home-based lifestyle for aged persons with cardiovascular illness. There remains uncertainty as to how to reform and revise public and private institutional structures and policies that continue to cater to population characteristics of earlier years. At the same time, physicians and scientists have inadequate information to guide their provision of advice for and to craft solutions to these dilemmas. Few scientific studies of the evaluation and therapies of cardiovascular diseases involve elderly patients, and the scarcity of clinical studies involving octogenarians and older is striking. The limited information that is available addresses predominantly the outcome of mortality, with little attention to morbidity and functional status and even less to meaningful quality of life attributes. The compelling issue is typically whether postponement of severe or debilitating disease is likely to occur as the result of an intervention. Equally lacking is information about the health values of the oldest old as a basis to guide their cardiovascular care and interventions.

Physicians are charged to act in the best interest of their patients. Clinicians must appreciate the elderly patient's personal value systems, health beliefs, and their desired outcomes of cardiovascular therapies in delineating treatment options and in making recommendations among them.

This monograph is designed to review the database for cardiovascular disease and its recognition and management in the octogenarian and beyond. In addition, it highlights relevant gaps in our knowledge, information that must be accrued to guide the cardiovascular care of our oldest old in the next millennium.

With appreciation to the chapter authors for their thoughtful and scholarly contributions; to my secretaries Julia Wright and Jeanette Zahler for their expert and meticulous attention to review of the manuscript; and to Alan Burgess and his colleagues at Martin Dunitz for their enthusiastic and professional nurturing of the monograph from its developmental phase through publication.

Nanette Kass Wenger

References

1. National Center for Health Statistics. Vital Statistics of the United States, 1998, Vol 11, Section 6, Washington, DC.

2. US Bureau of the Census. *Major Improvement in Life Expectancy: 1989*. Statistical Bulletin. July–September 1990. Washington, DC: US Bureau of the Census, US Government Printing Office, 1990.

3. Olshansky FJ, Carnes BA, Cassel C. In search of Methuselah. Estimating the upper limits of human longevity. *Science* (1990) **250**:634–40.

4. Deyo RA. The quality of life, research, and care. *Ann Intern Med* (1991) **114**:695–7.

5. Roper WL, Koplan JP, Speers MA et al. Cardiovascular disease surveillance, ischemic heart disease, 1980–1989. Center for Disease Control and Prevention, 1993.

6. Manton KG, Vaupel JW. Survival after the age of 80 in the United States, Sweden, France, England, and Japan. *N Engl J Med* (1985) **333**:1232–5.

7. Lawton MP. A multidimensional view of the quality of life in frail elders. In: Birren JE, Lubben JE, Rowe JC, Deutchman DE (eds). *The Concept and Measurement of Quality of Life in the Frail Elderly*, (Academic Press, San Diego, 1991) 3–27.

1

The landscape of cardiovascular illness in the next millennium: challenges and opportunities for the care of the oldest old

Nanette K Wenger

Changes in demography

The current average life expectancy of an 80 year old individual in the USA is 8 years, with the subset of the population older than 85 years of age constituting the fastest growing segment of US society.[1] Whereas the number of Americans over the age of 85 years increased from 0.6 million in 1950 to 2.7 million in 1985, the number of individuals over 65 years of age only doubled during this time period. As this oldest old portion of the population is anticipated to continue to increase in size, it is essential to get a better understanding of the parameters and value systems of these individuals and the characteristics of cardiovascular diseases that are so highly prevalent among the very elderly. By the year 2000 the US population older than 75 years of age will have grown to 16 million, a quarter of whom will be older than 85 years.[2,3] There will be more than 100 000 people aged 100 and older. By the year 2025, 5–9% of the population of developed nations is estimated to be at least 80 years of age.[4] In the USA, the population aged 80 years and older will increase from 2.7% in 1990 to 4.5% in 2025.[4] This unprecedented and accelerating growth of the very aged population has challenged the ability of governmental and nongovernmental health-care agencies and services to evolve and adapt to the changing demography. The compelling need to create new paradigms for public health policy is hampered by limitations of scientific knowledge and by critical uncertainties about prudent individual and societal strategies that are likely to effect favorable health outcomes for this population at risk, the oldest old.

The oldest of the elderly patients constitute a highly heterogeneous group, with widely differing severities of illness, functional and cognitive status, psychosocial needs, and expectations of medical care, to name a few. None of these relates significantly either to each other or to chronological age.

Changes in functional status and disability

The US population today is not only older but healthier. Most elderly individuals in the United States are generally in good health, alert and functional, and live independently at home well into their eighth and ninth decades. Nonetheless, information from the Cardiovascular Health Study[5] suggests that the functional status of community-dwelling elderly individuals declines substantially between ages 75 and 84 years and older than 85 years of age. Confirmatory data identify that although

85% of men and 78% of women older than 65 years of age live independently at home, at age 85 years and older, 46% of men and 62% of women require either assistance at home or nursing-home care.[6] Additional relevant gender differences are that 52% of women older than 85 years of age live alone, compared with only 29% of similarly aged men. Coronary disease, however, contributes little to the disability of elderly age that requires personal assistance for activities of daily living.

Important new information derives from the Center for the Demography of Aging at Duke University.[7] Age-standardized current disability rates for older Americans are lower than was the case 15 years ago, 21.3% in 1994 versus 24.9% in 1982. Not only have the disability rates fallen dramatically, but the reduction appears to be accelerating, with the decline in disability prevalence from 1989–1994 being significantly larger than that from 1982–1989. In absolute terms, there are an estimated 1.2 million fewer older disabled persons in 1994 than would have been the case if 1982 prevalence rates had not changed. These declines were evident even among those aged 95 years and older, and for the highest levels as well as for all levels of disability. Potential contributors to this more favorable landscape include improved nutrition, better public health measures, favorable lifestyle changes including a decrease in cigarette smoking, higher levels of education, improved economic status and an array of medical advances.

As increased numbers of reasonably healthy and active individuals attain very elderly age, more precise assessment of their functional capabilities will be indicated to determine suitable recreational and leisure activities, and, for a minority of these people, vocational activities. The overriding concern of these seniors is and will be maintenance of an independent and self-sufficient lifestyle, which requires maintenance of functional capabilities. This aged population, as well, can be anticipated to have a continuing interest in and requirement for preventive care, including preventive cardiovascular care. The major challenge is to develop cost-effective preventive strategies that can extend years of health and vigor and lessen years of disability.

By contrast, some elderly individuals consider illness and disability an inevitable consequence of aging. Such negative attitudes can inappropriately lower expectations of outcomes of preventive and medical therapies, of functional capabilities and of recovery after illness. Public education is required to dispel this myth, as societal attitudes often affect the beliefs of individual elderly persons and of their families as well.

A recent study of health values in very old (80–98 years) hospitalized patients suggests that most would prefer increased quantity of life in their current state of health to less time in excellent health.[8] This negates previous assumptions that elderly individuals value quality over quantity of life. Owing to the widespread interindividual variations evident in this study, health values should be ascertained directly from individual aged cardiac patients by health-care providers as a basis for advising and guiding their clinical care. As well, specific guidelines for cardiovascular care at advanced elderly age and basic constructs for general health policy for this growing segment of the population must encompass consideration of the wide variation in individual health preferences of the very old.

The USA is the only nation in the world with a politically vigorous organization of aged individuals, the American Association of Retired Persons (AARP). This group represents a powerful asset for determining the advocacy posture regarding cardiovascular care in the upper age ranges.

Prevalence of cardiovascular illness

Planning for cardiovascular care in the twenty-first century must address the converging issues of an increasing size of the elderly population and, in particular, the high proportion of very elderly patients; and the high prevalence of cardiovascular disease, often requiring costly high technology diagnostic and therapeutic modalities. Information from the National Center for Health Statistics identifies that in 1990 one-third of persons older than 75 years of age had been diagnosed by a physician as having heart disease.[9] The prevalence of cardiovascular disease at ages 75–84 years in the Framingham cohort was 44% in men and 28% in women; in the age group 85–94 years, the prevalence increased to 48% in men and 43% in women. Heart disease is the major predictor both of mortality and health-care use at elderly age and cardiovascular disease is responsible for the majority of deaths in octogenarians. The prognosis of cardiac illness is influenced substantially by access to diagnostic and therapeutic interventions. These are influenced, in turn, by elderly patients' and their physicians' perceptions about the value and indications for such care, by governmental and private allocation of health-care resources, and by societal attitudes about the importance of cardiac care at advanced age. The current use of health services at very elderly age may only partially reflect the need for such services, as statistics regarding use are determined by the access to care and the availability of such care. Furthermore, community surveys underestimate both disability and disease prevalence in the oldest

old as they fail to include the individuals residing in nursing homes.

Diagnostic challenges

Both limitations in obtaining information from the clinical history and confounding features in the interpretation of the physical examination render noninvasive diagnostic tests of greater value at elderly than at younger age. As an example, many classic manifestations of cardiovascular disease may be masked by the sedentary lifestyle currently characteristic of progressive aging. Altered mental acuity, cognitive disturbances related to medications, and/or depression may obscure or complicate the clinical history. The typical chest pain of myocardial infarction is reported by only one-third of patients older than 85 years. Because of the poor representation of elderly patients in many studies, the limitations of diagnostic tests in an elderly population have been inadequately explored, that is, which of the test abnormalities are unique to the aging process and which reflect occult or undetected cardiovascular disease. The resting electrocardiogram, for example, is abnormal in about half of all elderly individuals, with abnormalities evident even in those without a history of heart disease or hypertension. The specific ECG evidence of myocardial infarction is also far more frequent than anticipated based on the clinical history, particularly in elderly women.[10] As well, arrhythmias are highly prevalent at 24-hour ambulatory electrocardiography, even in the absence of recognized cardiovascular disease,[11] rendering it challenging to distinguish the signal of serious arrhythmia from the background arrhythmic 'noise'.

Coronary heart disease

Clinical evidence of coronary heart disease is present in approximately 20% of both men and women by age 80 years. The 5% of octogenarians in the current US population account for more than 20% of all hospitalizations for acute myocardial infarction, as well as 30% of myocardial infarction hospital deaths.[12] Not only is coronary heart disease highly lethal at elderly age, but disability among survivors is excessively prominent among the oldest old. The likelihood of disability or death from cardiovascular disease approaches 58% in the population aged 85 years and older. Activity limitation is present in 50% of men and 20% of women with coronary disease at ages 55–64 years, in contrast to 85% and 55%, respectively, at age 75 years and older.

Myocardial infarction mortality in the Myocardial Infarction Triage and Intervention Registry[13] increased 10-fold at elderly age. Mortality rates were 2% below age 55 years compared with 17.8% at 75 years of age and older. Confounding these data are major differences in the application of beneficial therapies at elderly versus younger age. For patients older than 75 years compared with those younger than 75 years: 5% versus 39% for coronary thrombolysis, 7% versus 29% for percutaneous transluminal coronary angioplasty, 5% versus 11% for coronary artery bypass graft surgery, and 57% versus 82% for a therapy as simple and inexpensive as aspirin use.[14] Older age adversely affects post-hospital survival after myocardial infarction as well. A three- to four-fold greater mortality is described after age 75 than below 55 years of age.[15] As such, benefits of medical and revascularization therapies shown to improve survival when delivered at elderly age may exceed those for younger persons, owing to the high risk status of elderly patients.

Despite the increased hospital mortality rates and excess of postoperative complications and resultant costs of coronary artery bypass graft surgery in octogenarians, survivors typically are pain free, often with restored functional status and have comparable 5-year survival to the 80–85 year old US population.[16–19]

Other cardiovascular problems

The median age of pacemaker implantation is currently 70 years in the United States; thus the geriatric population is a major beneficiary of such therapy. Pacemaker implantation can improve both symptoms and the quantity and quality of life.[20]

Calcific aortic stenosis is the dominant valvular disease for which surgery is performed in old age; after age 80 calcific aortic stenosis is more common among women than men. Aortic valve replacement can be performed with acceptable mortality and morbidity even in octogenarians and increases survival, improves symptomatic and hemodynamic status, and substantially enhances quality of life.[21]

Although nearly 10% of persons older than age 80 have a history of atrial fibrillation,[22] optimal therapeutic strategies have not been adequately defined for this population.

The prevalence of heart failure increases with increasing age, at least in part as a consequence of improved outcomes of cardiovascular illness in younger years. Although precise data on hospitalization rates for heart failure are unavailable for octogenarians, more than 50% of all heart failure hospital admissions involve individuals older than 75 years of age; it appears that as much as a third of these hospitalizations are for patients over the age of 80 years.[23] Mortality rates for heart failure increase with advancing age;[24] the annual mortality rate is more than 150/100 000 patients among octogenarians. This represents an area of expanding morbidity and disability as well.

Components of clinical and societal decision-making at very elderly age

There has been a striking increase in the use of cardiovascular procedures in octogenarians; for example, from 1987 to 1990 use of coronary bypass graft surgery at age 80 years and older increased 67% and that of percutaneous transluminal coronary angioplasty 129%.[25] The consequences of these changes in clinical practice are pivotal because the octogenarian population in the US is anticipated to quadruple over the next half century.[26,27] Although not specifically addressing octogenarians but all patients older than age 65, the increase in the US versus the Canadian use of cardiac procedures did not translate into improved 1-year survival after acute myocardial infarction; the mean age of US patients was 76.3 years and Canadian patients 75.4 years, with 15% and 12% respectively aged at least 85 years.[28] The escalation of procedural interventions at very elderly age has demonstrated the feasibility of invasive advanced technology approaches to care. Far less well documented is the global benefit and procedure- and population-specific value of this category of care as regards health outcomes. Which are appropriate, which are of inconstant benefit, which are detrimental?

The costs associated with caring for elderly cardiac patients have already risen dramatically; as a result many health-care decision-makers have begun to question the value of aggressive interventions in those nearing the chronological end of life.[29,30] This challenges society to determine what health care can and should be offered to the very aged to attain a favorable health prospect. The cardiac care of frail elderly persons involves decisions that weigh the risks and benefits of medical and surgical therapeutic modalities in patients with limited life-expectancy; these risks and benefits remain poorly delineated. As a result there is currently a high degree of individualization of care in the very elderly population, without a robust scientific basis. Clearly, a priority is to identify those characteristics of very elderly patients that predict favorable outcomes from specific interventions; as well as those specific interventions most likely not only to enhance survival but to lessen morbidity and disability and improve quality of life. Because of the comorbidities characteristic at elderly age, the effect of competing risks may constrain the ability to assess specific interventions.[31] Undocumented assumptions currently encourage an aggressive approach to cardiovascular diagnosis and treatment, even at younger elderly age, but place emphasis solely on the primacy of physical comfort for the octogenarian and beyond. Research efforts must ascertain the appropriateness of these divergent approaches, particularly for vigorous octogenarians and older.

Data from a variety of sources suggest that both medical and public health interventions contribute importantly to survival at older age. The survival of octogenarians and older is greater in the United States than in Sweden, France, England or Japan;[32] this is at least in part because elderly US patients receive more prompt and effective medical care. The oldest age groups do not necessarily incur disproportionately high medical care expenditures. For example, the 1989–1990 Medicare costs for those dying at age 70 averaged $22 590 in the last 2 years of life; this contrasts with $8296 for those surviving to age 101.[33] However, most long-term care costs are not covered under Medicare entitlements and thus are not reflected in these statistics.

Equally important is to characterize the attributes of individuals with successful aging, those who remain active, alert and energetic in their eighties and nineties. We must delineate those lifestyle characteristics such as nutrition, physical activity, psychosocial status, work, retirement, etc. associated with decreased disability and dependency in later life. These data will form the basis for instituting health promotion and health protection interventions that are likely to enhance successful aging.

Given the decrease in the loss of biological fitness with aging and the overwhelming contribution of cardiovascular disease to morbidity at elderly age, how should we encourage or enhance preventive interventions in this population? If the proportion of the life span spent in a functional, nondisabled state at very elderly age continues to increase, how should we approach the application of diagnostic and therapeutic cardiovascular procedures in this population? Age-based decisions about access to care must address these diverging curves of biological and chronological aging. If improved and more aggressive medical care at elderly age has decreased disabling health problems among the very elderly, how should these data regarding the decline in disability rates among elderly Americans affect clinical decision-making for therapeutic services, that is, should cardiovascular interventions vary by physiological rather than by chronological age? Exploration is warranted to accrue credible information about the application of advanced technology and often costly options for the acute cardiovascular care of the very aged population with successful aging.

Societal perceptions, as well as those of physicians, their aged patients, and these patients' families influence public policy and decisions for the care of individual elderly patients. Both evolving contemporary information and the undertaking of new research studies should provide a scientific database to buttress societal decisions about preventive and therapeutic cardiovascular care for the octogenarian and beyond in the next millennium.

References

1. Williams TF. Demographics of aging. *Cardiovasc Clin* (1992) **22**:3–7.
2. United States Bureau of the Census. *Statistical Abstract of the United States: 1996*, 116th edn. (US Government Printing Office: Washington DC, 1996).
3. United States Bureau of the Census. *Projections of the Population of the United States, by Age, Sex, and Race: 1988 to 2080*. Current Population Reports, Series P-25, No. 1018. (US Government Printing Office: Washington DC, 1989).
4. Pollock SR, ed. *Statistical Forecasts of the United States*, 2nd edn (Gale Research: Detroit, MI, 1995) xl–813.
5. Bild DE, Fitzpatrick A, Fried LP et al. Age-related trends in cardiovascular morbidity and physical functioning in the elderly: The Cardiovascular Health Study. *J Am Geriatr Soc* (1993) **41**:1047–56.
6. Schneider EL, Guralnik JM. The aging of America. Impact on health care costs. *JAMA* (1990) **263**:2335–40.
7. Manton KG, Corder L, Stallard E. Chronic disability trends in elderly United States populations: 1982–1994. *Proc Natl Acad Sci USA* (1997) **94**:2593–8.
8. Tsevat J, Dawson NV, Wu AW et al for the HELP Investigators. Health values of hospitalized patients 80 years or older. *JAMA* (1998) **279**:371–5.
9. National Center for Health Statistics. *Current Estimates from the National Health Interview Survey, 1989*. Vital and Health Statistics Series 10. Data from the National Health Survey No. 176. DHHS, PHS. (Hyattsville, MD: Centers for Disease Control, 1990).
10. Furberg CD, Manolio TA, Psaty BM et al for the Cardiovascular Health Study Collaborative Research Group. Major electrocardiographic abnormalities in persons aged 65 years and older (the Cardiovascular Health Study). *Am J Cardiol* (1992) **69**:1329–35.
11. Ingerslev J, Bjerregaard P. Prevalence and prognostic significance of cardiac arrhythmias detected by ambulatory electrocardiography in subjects 85 years of age. *Eur Heart J* (1986) **7**:570–5.
12. Centers for Disease Control and Prevention. *Cardiovascular Disease Surveillance, Ischemic Heart Disease, 1980–1989*. Division of Chronic Disease Control and Community Intervention. DHSS, PHS. (CDC: Atlanta, Georgia, 1993).
13. Weaver WD, Litwin PE, Martin JS et al for the MITI Project Group. Effect of age on use of thrombolytic therapy and mortality in acute myocardial infarction. *J Am Coll Cardiol* (1991) **18**:657–62.
14. Rogers WJ, Bowlby LJ, Chandra NC et al for the Participants in the National Registry of Myocardial Infarction. Treatment of myocardial infarction in the United States (1990 to 1993). Observations from the National Registry of Myocardial Infarction. *Circulation* (1994) **90**:2103–14.
15. Goldberg RJ, Gore JM, Gurwitz JH et al. The impact of age on the incidence and prognosis of initial acute myocardial infarction: the Worcester Heart Attack Study. *Am Heart J* (1989) **117**:543–9.
16. Weintraub WS, Clements SD, Ware J et al. Coronary artery surgery in octogenarians. *Am J Cardiol* (1991) **68**:1530–4.
17. Tsai TP, Denton TA, Chaux A et al. Results of coronary artery bypass grafting and/or aortic or mitral valve operation in patients ≥ 90 years of age. *Am J Cardiol* (1994) **74**:960–2.
18. Jaeger AA, Hlatky MA, Paul SM et al. Functional capacity after cardiac surgery in elderly patients. *J Am Coll Cardiol* (1994) **24**:104–8.
19. Peterson ED, Cowper PA, Jollis JG et al. Outcomes of coronary artery bypass graft surgery in 24 461 patients aged 80 years or older. *Circulation* (1995) **92**(Supplement II):II-85–91.
20. Shen W-K, Hammill SC, Hayes DL et al. Long-term survival after pacemaker implantation for heart block in patients >65 years. *Am J Cardiol* (1994) **74**:560–4.
21. Levinson JR, Akins CW, Buckley MJ et al.

Octogenarians with aortic stenosis. Outcome after aortic valve replacement. *Circulation* (1989) 80(Supplement I):I-49–56.

22. Wolf PA, Benjamin EJ, Belanger AJ et al. Secular trends in the prevalence of atrial fibrillation: the Framingham Study. *Am Heart J* (1996)131:790–5.

23. Graves EJ. *Vital and Health Statistics. National Hospital Discharge Survey: Annual Summary, 1990.* National Center for Health Statistics. Series 13: Data from the National Health Survey, No. 112. (DHHS publication No. (PHS) 92-1773: Hyattsville, MD, 1992).

24. Gillum RF. Epidemiology of heart failure in the United States. *Am Heart J* (1993) 126:1042–7.

25. Peterson ED, Jollis JG, Bebchuk JD et al. Changes in mortality after myocardial revascularization in the elderly. The National Medicare Experience. *Ann Intern Med* (1994) 121:919–27.

26. US Department of Commerce. *Current Population Reports Special Studies, P23-178, in sixty-five Plus in America.* (US Government Printing Office: Washington DC, 1992).

27. US Congress, Senate, Special Committee on Aging. Aging America: Trends and projections/prepared by U.S. Senate Special Committee on Aging in conjunction with American Association of Retired Persons, the Federal Council on the Aging and the Administration on Aging. (DHHS Publication: Washington DC, 1991).

28. Tu JV, Pashos CL, Naylor CD et al. Use of cardiac procedures and outcomes in elderly patients with myocardial infarction in the United States and Canada. *N Engl J Med* (1997) 336:1500–5.

29. Callahan D. Must the old and young compete for health care resources? *Neurosurgery* (1990) 27:160–4.

30. Chelluri L, Grenvik A, Silverman M. Intensive care for critically ill elderly: mortality, costs, and quality of life. Review of the literature. *Arch Intern Med* (1995) 155:1013–22.

31. Welch HG, Albertsen PC, Nease RF et al. Estimating treatment benefits for the elderly: the effect of competing risks. *Ann Intern Med* (1996) 124:577–84.

32. Manton KG, Vaupel JW. Survival after the age of 80 in the United States, Sweden, France, England, and Japan. *N Engl J Med* (1995) 333:1232–5.

33. Lubitz J, Beebe J, Baker C. Longevity and Medicare expenditures. *N Engl J Med* (1995) 332:999–1003.

2

Advanced aging and the cardiovascular system

Jeanne Y Wei

Introduction

Although mortality rates due to heart disease have declined during the past 25 years, cardiovascular disease remains the largest single cause of death in women and men over age 70 years.[1,2] It represents a leading cause of morbidity in older persons and comprises a major and growing portion of hospitalization and health-care costs.[1–3] It would be important, therefore, to consider those age-associated morphological and physiological changes that may influence cardiac diagnosis and treatment in older individuals, as well as those aspects of the medical evaluation and management of cardiovascular disease that are usually different for older compared with younger adults.[4–30]

Morphological Differences

The aging vasculature

Arteries tend to stiffen with age. In younger adults, there are elastin fibers in the subintima and media that confer a mechanical advantage which enables the central arteries to help to propel blood forward into the periphery through elastic recoil during diastole. With advancing age, there is a progressive loss of elastin and a progressive increase in its replacement by tightly cross-linked, nondistensible collagen. There is also a progressive thickening of the smooth muscle layers. Taken

together, these physical changes tend to significantly increase the mechanical burden on the older person's heart, because the heart must now supply virtually all the force that is needed to propel the blood forward into the periphery. In addition, superimposed on this increased mechanical demand on the heart is the increased vascular resistance due to arterial stiffening. More work is therefore required of the heart in the older person to push blood through the stiff, inelastic, nondistensible arteries. With these typical age changes in the arteries, arterial pulse pressures tend to widen. Systolic pressures increase as blood traverses the rigid arteries and diastolic pressures fall since the rigid senescent arteries lack the elasticity that is needed to maintain the intravascular pressures during diastole. These changes often result in the age-associated increase in systolic blood pressure that is so commonly observed.[9–17]

In the central as well as peripheral arteries, the proximal portion of the vessel tends to change first, and eventually these changes tend to involve the entire vessel. In the heart, the left coronary artery usually manifests changes before the right one, with lesions initially appearing during late youth or mid-adulthood, whereas the right and posterior descending coronary arteries do not commonly show change until after the fifth decade. With advancing age, the stiffened arteries become less distensible passively and also have less ability to vasodilate actively so that they are less able to increase blood supply in response to higher demands or physiological stresses.

In the intima of an artery, the endothelial cells become less homogeneous in size, shape and axial orientation, so that intraluminal blood flow may be less laminar and lipid deposition may increase independently of atherosclerosis.[4] The subendothelial layer thickens and its connective tissue, calcium and lipid content increase with age, especially around the internal elastic membrane. In the media, prominent age-associated changes include increased thickness of the smooth muscle layers, progressive elastin fragmentation and increased calcification. A larger percentage of the arterial smooth muscle cells have nuclear tetraploidy or octaploidy and their protein content also tends to increase. These age-related changes contribute to greater stiffness of the vessel walls (including the coronary arteries) and a reduction in the vasodilating capacity. They also probably contribute to the progressive compensatory myocyte loss and hypertrophy in the aging heart.[14,18,19]

The aging myocardium

Until relatively recently, it was thought that congestive heart failure in older persons often developed as a result of the older heart's inability to contract. It is now established that impaired heart muscle relaxation (i.e. diastolic dysfunction), not impaired heart muscle contraction (i.e. systolic dysfunction), is the major cause of heart failure in the older person, especially in women, over the age of 80 years. This is because, with advancing age, it takes much longer for the heart to relax. Although the heart muscle in an older person is able to pump blood as well as it does in the young, it is not able to relax as rapidly, so the heart chamber in the old is not able to fill as effi-

ciently. Contrary to long-prevailing thought, more oxygen and energy are required for relaxation (diastole) than for contraction (systole). It is therefore not surprising that the development of relaxation abnormalities often precedes that of contraction abnormalities. The rate of filling of the heart declines with age, so that by age 70, it may be only half of that value which was present at 30 years. In addition, ventricular filling becomes increasingly dependent upon the atrial contraction with advancing age.

When the left ventricle is not able to relax completely, it will not be able to contract as strongly during the next cycle. The problem of prolonged diastole becomes further exacerbated when the heart beats faster, which occurs for example during physical activity or when the older person becomes ill or develops a fever (normally, when the heart rate rises, diastole becomes shortened). In young persons, a rapid heart rate is usually well tolerated. In older persons, however, even minor exertion can lead to shortness of breath and fatigue. About 50% of persons over age 80 years experience congestive heart failure that is caused primarily by impaired relaxation (diastolic dysfunction).

Because the heart in an older person has reduced early diastolic ventricular filling and depends heavily upon the atrial contraction during late diastole for over half of the ventricular filling, a shortened diastole during increased heart rate could compromise cardiac output (the amount of blood the heart could pump) more in the older than the younger heart. Similarly, a loss of regular atrial contraction, which occurs for example during atrial fibrillation or atrial tachycardia, could also reduce cardiac output far more in the older compared to the younger heart.

Why do muscle abnormalities develop as we get older? There are several reasons. First, as previously discussed, the blood vessels become stiffer with age, so the older heart is required to pump against a greater resistance. This places a greater work load on the heart, which in turn causes a cell loss of heart myocytes and causes the remaining heart muscle cells to enlarge in compensation. The progressive cell loss is associated with increased connective tissue formation and collagen deposition. In addition, there is also increased cross-linking of collagen fibers as well as calcium and amyloid protein deposition between cells within the heart wall. The increased size of heart cells together with the increased connective tissue in which the heart cells are embedded make the heart muscle stiffer and therefore more resistant to changes in shape. More energy is then required to cause the stiffer heart to dilate.

There are alterations inside the cells—characterized by impaired calcium usage and decreased energy turnover—that also cause the heart muscle to take longer to relax. Heart muscle relaxation depends on the dissociation of ionized calcium from the myofilaments and the uptake of the ionized calcium from the cytoplasm into storage sites. The rate of calcium uptake into storage slows down with age. Consequently, there is a decreased rate and capacity for handling of intracellular ionized calcium. In addition to these changes, the decrease in catecholamine content in the heart, the decline in capillary density and reserve blood supply to the heart, and the reduced blood oxygen content all further serve to make the heart more vulnerable to stress-induced decompensation.

How does the heart lose some of its ability to adapt? The answer may lie partly in the heart muscle's DNA and also in the regulation of gene expression. The induction of certain immediate early genes (*c-fos, c-jun*) in the heart is reduced with age.[4] Because the heart cells that are called cardiac myocytes do not usually undergo proliferation after early postnatal life, they are lifelong in their terminally differentiated state. As such, each cell is a living record of cumulative events that have occurred to the organism in general and the heart in particular. If some inefficient cellular repair mechanism occurs as a result of the age-associated accumulation of changes due to exposure to a variety of chemicals, that problem could become significant over time. It is also possible that a number of signaling pathways from the cell surface to the nucleus might be altered with age, and might contribute to the observed functional changes. The heart cells' mitochondria—intracellular bodies that aid in energy synthesis—are more susceptible to oxidative damage than other parts of the cell. It is possible that signaling changes, or damage to mitochondria, might contribute to the development of age-related heart disease.

Functional changes
Blood pressure regulation

The age-associated increase in arterial wall stiffness together with the increase in vessel lumen radius tends to make the elderly more susceptible to modest changes, both increments and decrements, in plasma volume. Decreased arterial distensibility usually also attenuates baroreceptor reflex function. Age-associated increases in plasma norepinephrine concentrations may also contribute to the higher arterial pressures in older persons. With advancing age, plasma renin activity and plasma angiotensin II and aldosterone concentrations often tend to decrease. Plasma vasopressin concentrations may be lower at baseline and may show a smaller increase after a hypovolemic stimulus. Plasma vasopressin levels may tend to increase more after a hyper-osmotic stimulus in older than in younger persons. Plasma atrial natriuretic peptide concentrations may increase with age, while end organ responsiveness to atrial nutriuretic peptide may decrease. Thus, in spite of what seem to be several apparently compensatory hormonal changes that would tend to lower rather than raise blood pressure in older persons, a progressive age-associated rise in systolic arterial pressure none the less still usually occurs.

Cardiac output

With advancing age, cardiac output tends to be decreased, both at rest and during exercise. These changes probably only partly reflect decreases in metabolic demands and in muscle mass. Contributing determinants of cardiac output that may be influenced by age include heart rate, loading conditions (preload and afterload), intrinsic muscle performance and neurohumoral regulation. The maximal heart rate that can be attained during physical exercise decreases progressively, as does the heart rate response to most other physiological stimuli.[4] For ventricular loading, the early diastolic ventricular filling declines such that by age 70 years it is reduced to approximately half the value at age 30 years. Therefore, preload (ventricular filling) becomes increasingly dependent upon atrial contraction.

The afterload (arterial resistance to left ventricular ejection) rises steadily with age, as the ascending aorta becomes progressively stiffer and the total cross-sectional area of the peripheral vascular bed becomes progressively smaller. This change is of substantial clinical importance because of the systolic and diastolic functional consequences of the increased workload on the heart. With regard to intrinsic muscle performance, there tends to be preservation of myocardial contractile

strength, while the relaxation process becomes substantially lengthened. Changes in myocardial excitation–contraction coupling may be present, even in the absence of myocardial hypertrophy. Thus, the aged heart has impaired diastolic performance with prolonged relaxation. The clinical impact of these changes, not surprisingly, is substantial.

Myocardial performance

The increased duration of myocardial relaxation time as well as the increased stiffness of the myocardium, both of which tend to retard ventricular filling, probably contribute to higher left ventricular diastolic pressures at rest and during exercise in older persons. Thus, pulmonary and systemic venous congestion may occur and cause symptoms of heart failure in elderly persons even in the presence of normal systolic function. The presence of increased left ventricular wall thickness, even of mild degree, may further impair ventricular filling. With increased afterload or systolic stress on the ventricle (due to decreased arterial compliance), left ventricular hypertrophy may occur, even in the absence of hypertension. Usually the development of diastolic abnormalities precedes that of systolic abnormalities, and it often antedates the development of measurable hypertrophy.

Age-associated increases in the interstitial fibrosis and cross-linking of collagen in the heart may significantly increase the myocardial stiffness and further contribute to diastolic abnormalities. Myocardial ischemia due to age-related decreases in capillary density and coronary reserve can also cause diastolic abnormalities in the absence of coronary atherosclerotic disease. The diastolic ventricular abnormalities may also be due partly to age-associated decreases in rate and maximal capacity of calcium sequestration by the sarcoplasmic reticulum, an age-associated increase in net transsarcolemmal calcium influx, or both. Decreased oxidative phosphorylation and cumulative mitochondrial peroxidation may further impair myocardial function, especially during periods of increased metabolic demand or cardiovascular stress.

Physiological responses

Resting values

With advancing age, the adjustments in left ventricular end-diastolic and stroke volumes in response to alterations in cardiac preload may decline. Resting systolic arterial pressure tends to rise gradually between the ages of 20 and 60 years (by approximately 20 mmHg) in Americans and then usually steepens, increasing by another 20 mmHg between ages 60 and 80 years. The resting heart rate usually shows less change with advancing age, in the absence of heart disease.

Normal activities

In the very elderly, cardiovascular compensatory mechanisms are often delayed or insufficient, so that dizziness or syncope due to postural change, meal consumption, defecation or urination are common. A modest amount of diuretic-induced sodium depletion, for example serum sodium reduction from 142 to 138 mmol/l, can result in marked postural hypotension even in healthy older persons. These age changes underscore the vulnerability of the elderly to common, relatively mild hemodynamic stresses that are usually well tolerated by younger individuals. After consumption of a moderately sized meal, the elderly tend to have a substantial drop in arterial pressure, whereas younger persons show no change or a slight increase in arterial pressure. Postprandial hypotension can lead to

postprandial syncope or angina. The magnitude of the postprandial or postural blood pressure reduction appears to be directly related to the basal supine blood pressure, indicating that homeostatic mechanisms may be further impaired in elderly hypertensive persons.

Acute exercise stress

During physical exertion, the maximal increase in ejection fraction tends to be less with advancing age. For a given increase in cardiac output, the concomitant rise in systemic and pulmonary arterial pressures is substantially greater in older persons. In addition, exercise-induced increases in cardiac output may depend more on augmented cardiac filling (preload) and less on myocardial beta-adrenergic responsiveness. The ability to accommodate increased venous return is partly hampered in the elderly by reduced vascular and myocardial compliance.

Effects of conditioning

The cardiovascular adaptation to exercise training may be altered with age, but physical training at least partly reverses a number of the age-associated changes in cardiovascular function. These findings suggest that some age-associated cardiovascular changes may reflect a more sedentary lifestyle. In addition to the partial improvement of physiological changes, exercise conditioning may also help to maintain favorable health characteristics and reduce overall morbidity and mortality from disease in the elderly. The age-associated progressive decline in maximal oxygen uptake, which is greater in sedentary persons and is associated with decreased health status, has been shown to be improved with exercise conditioning. Elderly persons who are exercise-conditioned also tend to have higher levels of physical performance, lower body fat and plasma insulin concentrations, and lower resting blood pressure and heart rate, as well as lower rates of development of myocardial infarction and congestive heart failure. Muscle strength training also apparently results in greater functional mobility and has been shown to improve balance and gait in frail elderly persons.[7,8]

Clinical implications
Hypertension

Hypertension (defined as systolic pressure greater than 160 mmHg and diastolic pressure greater than 95 mmHg) rises in prevalence with age and has been reported to occur in over 50% of persons over the age of 70 years. Hypertension is a major risk factor for coronary heart disease, stroke and congestive heart failure, even in very old age. Fortunately, there are many efficacious medications to treat hypertension. In addition, a number of non-pharmacological approaches are effective as well.

Blood pressure response regulation

Compensatory blood pressure and heart rate response mechanisms in the elderly are often delayed or insufficient. These changes explain why fainting is common in older women and men during normal daily activities such as arising from a bed, eating a meal or going to the toilet. These changes also explain why modest decreases in intravascular fluid volume, such as that which occurs during heat prostration, viral illness, diarrhea or decreased oral fluid intake, can often result in large drops in blood pressure that can cause falls or fainting in the elderly.

Older women lose balance and fall more frequently than older men, and women are seven times more likely than men to sustain a hip fracture when they fall.

Congestive heart failure

In older persons, congestive heart failure is a very common problem. The prevalence of heart failure rises extremely steeply with age starting in the fifth decade, doubling every 10 years in men and every 7 years in women. It is six times more common in 65–74 year-old persons compared with those 45–54 years of age. Over 75% of cases of overt congestive heart failure in older persons are associated with hypertension or coronary heart disease. Thus, the high prevalence of congestive heart failure in old persons is partly due to advanced age but also partly due to increased prevalence of disease. Diastolic dysfunction, not systolic dysfunction, is the major cause of heart failure in the elderly patient. Among patients over 80 years old with heart failure, over 50% have normal or near-normal systolic function. Older persons with preserved systolic function and impaired diastolic function are sometimes treated erroneously with aggressive diuretics, vasodilators and digitalis, which may further reduce ventricular filling and/or impair relaxation and actually exacerbate rather than alleviate their cardiac decompensation. It is important, therefore, to be aware of the high prevalence of diastolic dysfunction in old age and to tailor the therapy to the older person's pathophysiology.

Why diastolic dysfunction?

With advancing age, there is an age-associated prolongation in the time required for the myocardium to relax. The process of myocardial relaxation requires more oxygen and energy than contraction; relaxation is therefore more vulnerable than contraction to hypoxia and ischemia. There is decreased coronary artery vasodilating capacity in response to stress with advancing age. Consequently, in an older person, the heart, even without coronary artery disease, may be exposed to lower levels of oxygen and may even be mildly hypoxic during periods of hemodynamic stress. Therefore, the tendency to develop diastolic abnormalities is increased in older persons.

Generally, patients with chronic heart failure due predominantly to nonischemic systolic dysfunction have gradually worsening symptoms and have paroxysmal nocturnal dyspnea, whereas those patients with heart failure due to nonischemic diastolic dysfunction have a more abrupt onset of symptoms and more rapid clinical deterioration. The acute left ventricular dysfunction that occurs in patients with myocardial ischemia or infarction is both systolic and diastolic, presents acutely and may deteriorate abruptly. Older patients with diastolic dysfunction often have underlying hypertension or coronary heart disease, and may present in acute decompensation related to elevated arterial pressure or acute myocardial ischemia. Other causes of heart failure that need to be considered include acute volume overload, valvular disease, pulmonary embolism, hypertrophic cardiomyopathy, pericardial constriction (acute tamponade or chronic pericarditis), restrictive cardiomyopathy and less commonly, high-output states.

The clinical distinction between heart failure due mainly to systolic dysfunction and that due to diastolic dysfunction is often difficult, regardless of the patient's age. In addition, many conditions including ischemic heart disease and valvular disease, result in both systolic and diastolic dysfunction, with possibly one component appearing to dominate at a given time. An objective evaluation of myocardial and valvular function may be helpful for diagnostic as well as therapeutic decisions.

So what can be done about it?

The good news is that, fortunately, it is possible to at least partly reverse many of the observed age-related changes in the heart muscle and vasculature through exercise conditioning and proper nutrition. Muscle strength training, even in frail nonagenarians and centenarians, can result in greater mobility, improved balance and gait, in addition to improved cardiovascular function. It also decreases mental stress and improves emotional well-being.

For those who are not able to exercise regularly, medications are also available that may be helpful in partly reversing the age-related changes. Every drug has negative side-effects, however, and should be used only when the benefits outweigh the risk. Nonpharmacological therapy, including exercise, is much better.

Increased physical activity, reduction of body weight and reduction of sodium, fat and alcohol intake, as well as stress management techniques, are all important for reducing heart disease and hypertension. In addition to exercise and proper nutrition, the use of exogenous estrogen in certain individuals may also be helpful for preventing coronary artery disease.

Exogenous estrogen may also be important for preventing osteoporosis and hip fracture in older women. Before deciding about estrogen therapy, careful inquiry should be made about potential contraindications to estrogen replacement such as breast cancer and/or a family history of breast cancer or endometrial cancer. Likewise, one should be informed about the possible risks of endometrial cancer (low absolute risk), breast cancer (potential risk) and vaginal bleeding (often absent at low doses).

A program of health promotion should include increased physical activity and exercise, proper nutrition, reduced use of tobacco and alcohol, and efforts at improving mental health and reducing adverse effects of stress and mental disorders.

In conclusion, in some situations, age-related changes in the cardiovascular system contribute to the development of disease while at other times, they may mimic disease. Consideration of these age-associated factors is important for the accurate diagnosis and optimal management of elderly patients.

References

1. American Heart Association. *1997 Heart and Stroke Facts (Statistical Supplement)* (American Heart Association Center: Dallas, 1997).
2. Health Care Financing Administration Office of the Actuary. Expenditures and percent of gross national product for national heart expenditures, by private and public funds, hospital care, and physician services, calendar years 1960–87. *Health Care Finance Rev* (1998) **10**:2.
3. Wittels EH, Hay JW, Gotto AM. Medical costs of coronary artery disease in the United States. *Am J Cardiol* (1990) **65**:432–6.
4. Wei JY. Age and the cardiovascular system. *N Engl J Med* (1992) **327**:1735–9.
5. Wenger N. Rehabilitation of the coronary artery disease patient: capturing patients. *Am J Cardiol* (1997) **80**:66–8H.
6. Gheorghiade M, Benatar D, Konstam MA et al. Pharmacotherapy for systolic dysfunction: a review of randomized clinical trials. *Am J Cardiol* (1997) **80**:14–27H.
7. Fiatarone MA, O'Neill EF, Ryan ND et al. Exercise training and nutritional supplementation for physical frailty in very elderly people. *N Engl J Med* (1994) **330**:1769–75.
8. Nelson ME, Fiatarone MA, Morganti CM et al. Effects of high-intensity strength training on multiple risk factors for osteoporotic fractures. A randomized controlled trial. *JAMA* (1994) **272**:1909–14.
9. Strassburger TL, Lee HC, Daly EM et al. Interactive effects of age and hypertension on volumes of brain structures. *Stroke* (1997) **28**:1410–17.
10. Schina MJ Jr, Neumyer MM, Healy DA et al. Influence of age on venous physiologic parameters. *J Vasc Surg* (1993) **18**:749–52.
11. Byrne EA, Fleg JL, Vaitkevicius PV et al. Role of aerobic capacity and body mass index in the age-associated decline in heart rate variability. *J Appl Physiol* (1996) **81**:743–50.
12. Galarza CR, Alfie J, Waisman GD et al. Diastolic pressure underestimates age-related hemodynamic impairment. *Hypertension* (1997) **30**:809–16.
13. Zabalgoitia M, Rahman SN, Haley WE et al. Comparison of left ventricular mass and geometric remodeling in treated and untreated men and women >50 years of age with systemic hypertension. *Am J Cardiol* (1997) **80**:648–51.
14. Czernin J, Muller P, Chan S et al. Influence of age and hemodynamics on myocardial blood flow and flow reserve. *Circulation* (1993) **88**:62–9.
15. Franklin SS, Gustin W 4th, Wong ND et al. Hemodynamic patterns of age-related changes in blood pressure. The Framingham Heart Study. *Circulation* (1997) **96**:308–15.
16. Yu CM, Sanderson JE. Right and left ventricular diastolic function in patients with and without heart failure: effect of age, sex, heart rate, and respiration on Doppler-derived measurements. *Am Heart J* (1997) **134**:426–34.
17. O'Rourke RA, Chatterjee K, Wei JY. Atherosclerotic coronary heart disease in the elderly. *J Am Coll Cardiol* (1987) **10**:52–6A.
18. Olivetti G, Melissari M, Capasso JM, Anversa P. Cardiomyopathy of the aging human heart. *Circ Res* (1991) **68**:1560–8.
19. Lie JT, Hammond PI. Pathology of the senescent heart: anatomic observations on 237 autopsy studies of patients 90 to 105 years old. *Mayo Clin Proc* (1988) **63**:552–64.
20. Feinberg WM, Blackshear JL, Laupacis A et al. Prevalence, age distribution, and gender of patients with atrial fibrillation. Analysis and implications. *Arch Intern Med* (1995) **155**:469–73.
21. Harris TB, Launer LJ, Madans J, Feldman JJ. Cohort study of effect of being overweight and change in weight on risk of coronary heart disease in old age. *BMJ* (1997) **314**:1791–4.
22. Krumholz HM, Wei JY. Acute myocardial infarction: clinical presentations and diagnosis. In: Gersh BJ, Rahimtoola SH, eds, *Acute Myocardial Infarction*, 2nd edn (Chapman & Hall: New York, 1997) 123–35.

23. Wei JY, Markis JE, Malagold M, Grossman W. Time course of serum cardiac enzymes after intracoronary thrombolytic therapy. *Arch Intern Med* (1985) **145**:1596–600.

24. Forman DE, Bernal JLG, Wei JY. Management of acute myocardial infarction in the very elderly. *Am J Med* (1992) **93**:315–26.

25. Forman DE, Berman AD, McCabe CH et al. PTCA in the elderly: the 'young-old' versus the 'old-old'. *J Am Geriatr Soc* (1992) **40**:19–22.

26. Krumholz HM, Forman DE, Kuntz RE et al. Coronary revascularization after myocardial infarction in the very elderly: outcomes and long-term follow-up. *Ann Intern Med* (1993) **119**:1084–90.

27. Mullany CJ, Darling GE, Pluth JR et al. Early and late results after isolated coronary artery bypass surgery in 159 patients aged 80 years and older. *Circulation* (1990) **82**:IV229–36.

28. Reardon M, Malik M. QT interval change with age in an overtly healthy older population. *Clin Cardiol* (1996) **19**:949–52.

29. Swahn E, Wallentin L. Low-molecular weight heparin (Fragmin) during instability in coronary artery disease (FRISC). *Am J Cardiol* (1997) **80**(5A): 25–9E.

30. Tcheng JE. Impact of eptifibatide on early ischemic events in acute ischemic coronary syndromes: a review of the IMPACT II trial. *Am J Cardiol* (1997) 80(4A): 21–8B.

3

The heart in persons over 80 years of age: analysis of 490 necropsy cases

William C Roberts

Introduction

As in any body tissue or organ, changes take place in the cardiovascular system as life progresses. Some of these changes allow easy identification of the very elderly heart when examining autopsy cardiac specimens as unknowns. The 'normal' elderly heart has relatively small ventricular cavities and relatively large atria and great arteries. The ascending aorta and left atrium, in comparison with the relatively small left ventricular cavity, appear particularly large. The coronary arteries increase in both length and width; the former, particularly in association with the decreasing size of the cardiac ventricles, results in arterial tortuosity. (The young river is straight and the old one, winding.) The leaflets of each of the four cardiac valves thicken with age, particularly the atrioventricular valves; these have a smaller area to occupy in the ventricles because of the diminished size of the latter. Histological examination discloses large quantities of lipofuscin pigment in myocardial cells; some contain mucoid deposits ('mucoid degeneration'). These changes appear to affect all population groups of elderly individuals irrespective of where they reside on the earth or their level of serum lipids. An elevated systemic arterial pressure appears to both accelerate and amplify these normal expected cardiac changes of aging. Both the aorta and its branches and the major pulmonary arteries

and their branches enlarge with age. Because the enlargement is in both the longitudinal and the transverse dimensions, the aorta, as the coronary arteries, tends to become tortuous. This process is further amplified as the vertebral bodies become smaller and the height, somewhat shorter. The major pulmonary arteries appear to be too short and have too low a pressure to dilate longitudinally.

The amount of information at necropsy in very elderly persons is relatively sparse. In 1983, Waller and Roberts[1] described some clinical and necropsy findings in 40 American patients aged 90 years and over. In 1988, Lie and Hammond[2] reported findings at necropsy in 237 patients aged 90 and older. In 1991, Gertz and associates[3] described composition of coronary atherosclerotic plaques in 18 persons 90 years of age and over. In 1993, Roberts[4] described cardiac necropsy findings in an additional 53 patients 90 years of age and over. In 1995, Shirani and co-workers[5] described cardiac findings at necropsy in 366 Americans aged 80 to 89 years, and in 1998 Roberts[6] described cardiac findings at necropsy in six centenarians. Also in 1998 Roberts and Shirani[7] compared cardiovascular findings in 490 patients studied at necropsy in three age categories: 80–89, 90–99 and ≥100 years. This chapter expands on that previous comparative study.

Methods

Patients

The files of the Pathology Branch, National Heart, Lung, and Blood Institutes, National Institutes of Health, Bethesda, Maryland, from 1959 to 1993, and those of the Baylor University Medical Center, Dallas, Texas, beginning January 1993, were searched for all accessioned cases of patients aged at least 80 years of age. Of 511 such cases found, adequate clinical information was available in 490 necropsy patients and they are the subject of this chapter. The clinical and cardiac morphological records, photographs and postmortem radiographs of the heart, histological slides of the heart, and the initial gross description of the heart were reviewed. All 490 hearts were originally examined by WCR, who recorded gross morphological abnormalities in each case.

Sources of patients

Of the 490 cases, the hearts in 412 were obtained from 12 Washington, DC, area hospitals, and the hearts in the other 78 cases, from hospitals outside that area, including 25 from Baylor University Medical Center. Of the 490 hearts, 37 (8%) were examined in 1970 or before; 153 (31%), from 1971 through 1980; 244 (50%), from 1981 through 1990; and 56 (11%) were examined from 1991 through 1997.

Definitions

Sudden coronary death was defined as death within 6 hours from the onset of new symptoms of myocardial ischemia in the presence of morphological evidence of significant atherosclerotic coronary artery disease (≥1 major epicardial coronary artery narrowed > 75% in cross-sectional area by atherosclerotic plaque). Most patients who died suddenly did so out-

side a hospital; a few, however, died shortly after admission to an emergency room. Sudden, out-of-hospital death also occurred in some patients with cardiac disease other than atherosclerotic coronary artery disease. In each case, an underlying cardiac disease generally accepted to cause sudden death was present at necropsy. *Acute myocardial infarction* was defined as a grossly visible left ventricular wall lesion confirmed histologically to represent coagulation-type myocardial necrosis. *Ischemic cardiomyopathy* was defined as chronic congestive heart failure associated with a transmural healed myocardial infarct and a dilated left ventricular cavity.

Cardiac morphological data

Hearts were fixed in 10% phosphate-buffered formalin for 3–15 days before examination. They were 'cleaned' of parietal pericardium and postmortem intracavity clot, and the pulmonary trunk and ascending aorta were incised approximately 2 cm cephalad to the sinotubular junction. *Heart weight* was then measured on accurate scales by WCR (Lipsaw scale before 1971, accurate to 10 g, and Mettler P1210 scale after 1971, accurate to 0.1 g). Heart weight was considered increased if it was greater than 350 g in women and over 400 g in men. Most hearts were studied by cutting the ventricles transversely at approximately 1-cm thick intervals from apex to base parallel to the atrioventricular groove posteriorly. In each heart, the sizes of cardiac ventricular cavities (determined by gross inspection), presence of left ventricular necrosis (acute myocardial infarct) and fibrosis (healed myocardial infarct), status of the four cardiac valves, and the maximal degree of cross-sectional luminal narrowing in each of the three major (left anterior descending, left circumflex, and right) epicardial coronary arteries were recorded.

Results

Number of patients in each of the three groups

Certain clinical and necropsy cardiac findings in the 490 cases are summarized in Table 3.1. The 490 patients were divided into three groups: the octogenarians (80–89 years; $N = 391$ (80%)); the nonagenarians (90–99 years; $N = 93$ (19%)); and the centenarians ($\geq$100 years; $N = 6$ (1%)); 248 (51%) were women and 242 (49%) were men.

Clinical findings

The clinical manifestations of the various cardiac disorders probably represent minimal numbers: many patients apparently were unable to provide much clinical information, many came to the hospital from nursing homes, and many had varying degrees of dementia. Nevertheless, angina pectoris was noted in the records of 137 (35%) of the 391 octogenarians, in five (5%) of the 93 nonagenarians, and in none of the six centenarians. A history of a hospitalization for an illness compatible with acute myocardial infarction was present in 78 (20%) of the 391 octogenarians, in 18 (19%) of the 93 nonagenarians, and in none of the six centenarians. Chronic congestive heart failure was present in 36% (140/391) of the octogenarians, in 25% (23/93) of the nonagenarians, and in none of the six centenarians. A history of systemic hypertension was present in 44% (174/391) of the octogenarians, in 54% (50/93) of the nonagenarians, and in none of the centenarians. Diabetes mellitus was present in 14% (56/391) of the octogenarians, in 9% (8/93) of the nonagenarians, and in none of the six centenarians.

Causes of death

The causes of death in the 490 patients are summarized in Table 3.2. A cardiac condition was the cause of death in 51% (198/391) of the octogenarians, in 32% (30/99) of the nonagenarians, and in none of the centenarians. A noncardiac but vascular condition was responsible for death in 13% (52/391) of the octogenarians and in 20% (19/93) of the nonagenarians. A noncardiac and a nonvascular condition was responsible for death in 36% (141/391) of the octogenarians, in 47% (44/93) of the nonagenarians, and in all six of the centenarians.

Cardiac necropsy findings

Cardiac findings at necropsy are tabulated in Table 3.1.

Heart weight

The mean heart weights were largest in the octogenarians and smallest in the centenarians (449 g versus 420 g versus 328 g). Heart weight was increased (>400 g in men; >350 g in women) in 131 (64%) of the 205 men and in 157 (74%) of the women, and the percentage was highest in the octogenarians.

Calcific deposits in the heart

Calcific deposits were present in the heart at necropsy in 444 (91%) of the 490 patients and were most common in the *coronary arteries*—in all cases being located in atherosclerotic plaques and not in the media—81% (398/490); in the *aortic valve cusps* in 47% (228/490)—heavy enough to result in aortic stenosis in 10% (51/490); *mitral valve annulus* in 39% (190/490)—very heavy deposits in 13% (63/490), and in the apices of one or both left ventricular *papillary muscles* in 17% (85/490). The cardiac calcific deposits were

Variable	Age group (years)		
	80–89 (N = 391)	90–99 (N = 93)	≥100 (N = 6)
Mean age (years)	84 ± 4	93 ± 4	102
Male:female	194 (50%):197 (50%)	52 (56%):41 (44%)	2/4
Angina pectoris	137 (35%)	5 (5%)	0
Acute myocardial infarction	78 (20%)	18 (18%)	0
Chronic congestive heart failure	140 (36%)	23 (25%)	0
Systemic hypertension (history)	174 (44%)	50 (54%)	0
Diabetes mellitus	56 (14%)	8 (9%)	0
Atrial fibrillation	57 (15%)	35 (38%)	0
Heart weight (g):range (mean)	185–900 (449)	220–660 (420)	240–410 (328)
Men	230–830 (493)	285–660 (436)	335&410 (372)
Women	185–900 (409)	220–630 (406)	240–385 (306)
Cardiomegaly			
Men >400 g	103/154 (67%)	27/49 (55%)	1/2
Women >350 g	133/165 (81%)	23/42 (55%)	1/4
Cardiac calcific deposits			
None	43 (11%)	3 (3%)	0
Present	348 (89%)	90 (97%)	6 (100%)
Coronary arteries	304 (78%)	89 (96%)	5
Aortic valve cusps	164 (42%)	59 (63%)	5
Heavy (stenosis)	43 (11%)	8 (9%)	0
Mitral annulus	146 (37%)	42 (45%)	2
Heavy	52 (13%)	11 (12%)	0
Papillary muscle	37 (9%)	42 (45%)	6
Numbers of *patients* with 0, 1, 2, or 3 major (right, left anterior descending, left circumflex) coronary arteries ↓ >75% in cross-sectional area			
0	159 (41%)	33 (35%)	2
1	67 ⎫	20 ⎫	2
2	71 ⎬ 232 (59%)	32 ⎬ 60 (65%)	2
3	94 ⎭	8 ⎭	0
Mean	1.7	1.5	1.5
Number of major coronary *arteries* (3/patient) ↓ >75% in cross-sectional area by plaque			
0	0/477	0/99	0/6
1	67/201	20/60	2/6
2	142/213	64/96	4/6
3	282/282	24/24	0
Totals	491/1173 (42%)	108/279 (39%)	6/18 (33%)
Left ventricular necrosis and/or fibrosis			
Necrosis only	54 (14%)	10 (11%)	0
Fibrosis only	101 (26%)	20 (21%)	2
Both	37 (9%)	5 (5%)	0
Ventricular cavity dilatation			
Neither	222 (57%)	58 (62%)	4
One	84 (21%)	4 (4%)	2
Right ventricle	42	2	2
Left ventricle	42	2	2
Both	85 (22%)	31 (34%)	0
Cardiac amyloidosis (massive)	14 (4%)	8 (9%)	0

Table 3.1
Certain clinical and necropsy findings in 490 patients aged 80–103 years

	Age group (years)		
	80–89 (N = 391)	90–99 (N = 93)	≥100 (N = 6)
Cardiac	198 (51%)	30 (32%)	0
Coronary artery disease	129/198 (65%)	12/30 (40%)	0
Acute myocardial infarction	90	12	0
Chronic congestive heart failure	15	3	0
Sudden	19	3	0
Coronary bypass	7	0	0
Valvular heart disease	41/198 (21%)	3/30 (10%)	0
Aortic stenosis	33	3	0
Aortic regurgitation	2	0	0
Mitral regurgitation	5	0	0
Mitral stenosis	1	0	0
Primary cardiomyopathy	7/198 (4%)	1/30 (3%)	0
Hypertrophic	4	0	0
Idiopathic dilated	3	1	0
Secondary cardiomyopathy	16/198 (8%)	8/30 (27%)	0
Amyloidosis	14	8	0
Hemosiderosis	1	0	0
Myocarditis	1	0	0
Pericardial heart disease	3/198 (2%)	0	0
Vascular, noncardiac	52 (13%)	19 (20%)	0
Stroke	17/52 (33%)	6/19 (32%)	0
Abdominal aortic aneurysm	14/52 (27%)	5/19 (26%)	0
Peripheral arterial disease	11/52 (21%)	5/19 (26%)	0
Aortic dissection	4/52 (8%)	0/19 (0)	0
Pulmonary embolism	6*/52 (11%)	3/19* (16%)	0
Noncardiac and nonvascular	141 (36%)	44 (47%)	6 (100%)
Cancer	52/141 (37%)	13/44 (29%)	0/6
Infection	37/141 (26%)	17/44 (39%)	0/6
Fall complication	10/141 (7%)	3/44 (7%)	3/6
Other	42/141 (30%)	11/44 (25%)	3/6

* All had underlying chronic obstructive pulmonary disease.

Table 3.2
Causes of death in the 490 necropsy patients aged 80–103 years

more frequent and heavier in the nonagenarians than in the octogenarians.

Numbers of patients with narrowing of one or more major epicardial coronary arteries

Among the 490 patients, 194 (40%) had none of the three major (right, left anterior descending and left circumflex) epicardial coronary arteries narrowed by plaque more than 75% in cross-sectional area; 89 (18%) had one artery so narrowed; 105 (21%) had two arteries so narrowed, and 94 (19%) had all three arteries so narrowed. The percentage of patients in each of the three groups with no arteries and one, two, and three arteries narrowed more than 75% was similar.

Numbers of major coronary arteries (three/patient) narrowed more than 75% in cross-sectional area by plaque

Among the 490 patients, a total of 1470 major epicardial coronary arteries were examined: 865 (59%) arteries had insignificant (<75% in cross-sectional area) narrowing and 605 (41%) had narrowing by plaque more than 75% in cross-sectional area. The percentage of arteries significantly narrowed was similar in each of the three groups (42% versus 39% versus 33%).

Acute and healed myocardial infarcts

Grossly visible foci of left ventricular wall (includes ventricular septum) necrosis (acute infarcts) without associated left ventricular scars (healed infarcts) were found in 64 (13%) patients; foci of left ventricular fibrosis without associated necrosis were observed in 123 patients (25%), and foci of both necrosis and fibrosis were found in 42 patients (9%). Thus,

a total of 229 (47%) of the 490 patients had grossly visible evidence of acute or healed myocardial infarcts or both. The percentages of patients with myocardial lesions of ischemia were similar among the octogenarians and nonagenarians.

Ventricular cavity dilatation

One or both ventricular cavities were dilated (by gross inspection) in 218 (44%) of the 490 patients and no significant differences were observed in the three groups.

Cardiac amyloidosis

Grossly visible amyloid (confirmed histologically) in ventricular and atrial myocardium as well as in atrial mural endocardium was present in 22 patients (4%). In these 22 patients the amyloidosis was symptomatic and fatal. A number of other patients who had no gross evidence of cardiac amyloidosis had small foci in the heart on histological study. These minute deposits did not cause symptoms of cardiac dysfunction. In the 22 patients with fatal cardiac amyloidosis, deposits of amyloid also were present in several other body organs at necropsy.

Electrocardiographic findings

Information on electrocardiograms was available on 30 of the 99 patients aged at least 90 years. Of the 30 patients, three had electrocardiograms recorded during acute myocardial infarction. The electrocardiograms in all three, however, disclosed only atrial fibrillation and complete left bundle branch block, and these findings in these patients were known to be present before the fatal acute myocardial infarction. The electrocardiograms in the other 27 patients were not recorded during periods of acute myocardial infarction. Of the 30 patients on whom electrocardiographic information was available, eight had clinical evidence of heart disease and 22 did not; the findings are summarized in Table 3.3. The total 12-lead QRS voltage ranged from 82 to 251 mm (mean 151; 10 mm = 1 mV). In the 19 women, the total voltage ranged from 82 to 251 mm (mean 158) and, in the five men, from 105 to 154 mm (mean 101; $P < 0.05$). The total 12-lead QRS voltage did not correlate with either heart ($r = -0.01$) or body weight ($r = -0.02$). The 24 patients in whom the total 12-lead QRS voltage was measured were separated into two groups: eight patients in whom clinical evidence of cardiac dysfunction was present (coronary heart disease in five, massive cardiac amyloid in two, and aortic valve stenosis in one) and 16 patients without such evidence (Table 3.3). Comparison of the total QRS voltage in the eight patients with and in the 16 patients without clinical evidence of heart disease disclosed no significant difference (mean 147 mm versus 152 mm). Breakdown on the eight patients with cardiac dysfunction did show some differences: the total 12-lead QRS voltage in the five patients with angina pectoris or acute myocardial infarction ranged from 123 to 163 mm (mean 143); in the two patients with massive cardiac amyloidosis it was 102 and 117 mm (mean 109); and in the one patient with aortic valve stenosis it was 238 mm. Of 29 patients on whom information was available, 18 (62%) received digitalis and only two appeared to have evidence of digitalis toxicity.

Comments

This study describes findings in a large group ($N = 490$) of patients at least 80 years of age studied at necropsy, and it compares certain clinical and necropsy findings in the octogenarians, nonagenarians and centenarians. Despite study of nearly 500 patients, only 6 (1%) lived 100 years or longer, and only 93 (19%) lived into the tenth decade of life. Nevertheless, the ratio of one centenarian for every 65 octogenarians is much higher than might be expected. In general, it takes 10 000 persons to reach age 85 before one reaches age 100.[8]

Another finding was the high frequency of men: 248 men (51%) and 242 (49%) women. A higher than expected percentage of men may have resulted in part from receiving a number of these cases from a Veterans Administration Hospital and from a retirement home filled almost entirely by men.

The causes of death were divided into three major types: cardiac, 228/490 (47%); vascular but noncardiac, 71/490 (14%); and noncardiac and nonvascular, 191/490 (39%). The frequency of a cardiac condition causing death decreased with increasing age groups (51% versus 32% versus 0), and the frequency of a noncardiac and nonvascular condition causing death increased with increasing age groups (36% versus 47% versus 100%). Among the cardiac conditions, coronary artery disease was the problem in 62% (141/228), and the other cardiac conditions, mainly aortic valve stenosis (36/228 (16%)) and cardiac amyloidosis (22/228 (10%)), in the other 38%. Stroke, rupture of an abdominal aortic aneurysm and complications of peripheral arterial atherosclerosis were the major vascular (noncardiac) conditions causing death. Of the noncardiac and nonvascular causes of death, cancer and infection, mainly pneumonia, were the major conditions, 35% (65/185) and 29% (54/185), respectively, among the octogenarians and nonagenarians.

The cardiac necropsy findings focused primarily on calcific deposits in the coronary arteries, aortic valve cusps, and mitral valve annulus and their consequences, and, to a lesser extent, on heavy amyloid deposits in the heart. Calcific

Abnormality	Clinical heart disease		Total	
	Present* (N = 8)	Absent (N = 22)	N	%
Atrial fibrillation	5	7	12	40
Abnormal QRS axis			12	40
Left (−30 to −90°)	4	6		
Right (+111 to +210°)	1	1		
Complete (QRS ≥0.12 second) BBB			12	40
Left	6	1		
Right	1	4		
Ventricular premature complexes	4	6	10	33
Atrial premature complexes	1	2	3	10
Heart block			8	27
P-R interval >0.2 second	3	3		
Second degree	0	1		
Third degree (complete)	1†	0		
Q-wave abnormality without BBB			4	13
Q II, III, aV₁	0	1		
Q-S V$_1$–V$_3$	0	1		
Both	0	2		
Left ventricular hypertrophy without BBB (R in V$_5$ or V$_6$ + S in V$_1$ ≥35 mm)	1	0	1	3
Low voltage (QRS ≤ 15 mm in I + II + III)	0	1	1–	3

* Coronary heart disease = 3; cardiac amyloidosis = 4; aortic valve stenosis = 1.
† Pacemaker inserted 6 years before death.
BBB = bundle branch block.
From Waller and Roberts[1].

Table 3.3
Electrocardiographic observations in 30 patients aged 90–103 years

deposits were present in the atherosclerotic plaques of one or more epicardial coronary arteries in 81% (398/490) of the patients, on the aortic aspects of the aortic valve cusps in 47% (228/490), in the mitral annular region in 39% (190/490), and in one or both left ventricular papillary muscles in 25% (122/490). The calcific deposits tended to be less frequent in the octogenarians. The frequent presence of calcific deposits in the coronary arteries, aortic valve cusps, and mitral annular region in the same patient suggests that the cause of the calcific deposits in each of these three locations is the same. The calcific deposits in the coronary arteries indicate the presence of atherosclerosis because calcium occurs in the coronary arteries, with one exception,[9] only in the plaques and not in the media. It is reasonable to believe that the calcific deposits in and on the aortic cusps, at least when this valve is tricuspid, are another manifestation of 'atherosclerosis.' Because mitral annular calcium in this older population is nearly always associated with calcium in the coronary arteries, it is also reasonable to believe that mitral annular calcium in persons at least 80 years of age is also a manifestation of 'atherosclerosis.' Calcium in a papillary muscle appears to be a consequence of 'aging' and not a direct manifestation of atherosclerosis.

When the deposits of calcium on the aortic aspect of the aortic valve cusps are extensive, the cusps may become relatively or absolutely immobile resulting in aortic valve stenosis. These valves usually lack commissural fusion, that is adherence of two cusps together near the lateral attachments, and, therefore, aortic regurgitation is usually absent. Although it most often is associated with some degree of mitral regurgitation, mitral annular calcium, if 'massive' and if the left ventricular cavity is also small and the wall quite thickened, may result in mitral stenosis.[10]

Although the calcific deposits in the epicardial coronary arteries were located entirely in atherosclerotic plaques, which are located in the intima, the presence of calcific deposits in the coronary arteries in this older population did not necessarily indicate the presence of significant (>75% cross-sectional area) luminal narrowing. In contrast, the presence of calcific deposits in epicardial coronary arteries in persons aged under 65 years generally indicates the presence of significant luminal narrowing. The calcific deposits tended to occur in each of the four major (right, left main, left anterior descending and left circumflex) epicardial arteries and were always larger in the proximal than in the distal halves of the right, left anterior descending and left circumflex arteries or, if small, limited to their proximal halves. The plaques consisted mainly (87 ± 8%) of fibrous tissue with calcific deposits forming 7 ± 6% of the plaques.[3]

The percentage of patients with narrowing more than 75% in cross-sectional area by plaque of one or more major epicardial coronary arteries was similar in all three age groups, as was the percentage of major coronary arteries narrowed significantly.

In 36 patients (all ≥90 years of age), each of the four major coronary arteries were divided into 5-mm-long segments and the degree of cross-sectional area narrowing by atherosclerotic plaque was determined for each segment. Of the 1789 5-mm segments in the 36 patients, the average amount of cross-sectional area narrowing by atherosclerotic plaques per segment was 42% (range 19–69). Of the 467 5-mm segments in the 10 patients with clinical evidence of coronary artery disease, the average amount of cross-sectional area narrowing per segment was 55% (range 43–69) and, of 1322 5-mm segments in the 26 patients without clinical evidence of coronary artery disease, 38% (range 19–40; $P < 0.01$).

These detailed morphological studies of the coronary arteries in these very elderly persons suggest that the degree of severe coronary narrowing necessary to have a fatal or nearly fatal coronary event is considerably less than that necessary to have a coronary event in younger patients. Moreover, these studies indicate that these very elderly patients without symptoms of coronary artery disease have distinctly more coronary luminal narrowing by atherosclerotic plaques than control subjects who are younger (mean age 52 years).[11] The latter observation suggests that coronary artery disease may be underdiagnosed clinically in the very elderly.

Clinical diagnosis of cardiac and other conditions in patients aged 80 years and over, particularly those 90 years of age and over, appears more difficult than in younger persons. Historical information may be difficult to obtain because of impaired intellect on the part of the patient and an impaired diagnostic pursuit on the part of the physician. Physicians caring for these very elderly persons may focus primarily on the prevention of suffering and only secondarily on accurate diagnosis or longer-term therapy. Patients aged 90 years and over generally have outlived their spouses and private physicians and are often 'inherited' by nursing home physicians, who may have limited access to earlier medical records.

Angina pectoris appears particularly difficult to diagnose in the very elderly because they may not be able to describe this symptom. Acute myocardial infarction is also difficult to diagnose clinically, but it is often fatal in the very elderly. Furthermore, the electrocardiogram is not as useful in diagnosis of acute myocardial infarction in the very elderly because left bundle branch block is frequent and, of course, it prevents the appearance of typical changes. Serial recordings of electrocardiograms also appear to be quite infrequent in the very elderly.

Physical examination in the very elderly may be both difficult and misleading. The lack of mobility may prevent proper positioning of the elderly patient for proper examining. Precordial murmurs, although common, infrequently indicate significant functional abnormality. Although calcific deposits in the aortic valve are common, actual aortic valve stenosis is not nearly as frequent. Likewise, although mitral annular calcific deposits are common, these calcific deposits rarely narrow the mitral orifice or produce significant mitral regurgitation.

Electrocardiographic abnormalities are common in elderly persons. Of the patients for whom electrocardiograms were available, all had one or more abnormalities recorded, the most frequent being abnormal axis, atrial fibrillation and complete left bundle branch block. Although 15 of the 30 patients had cardiomegaly (>350 g in women; >400 g in men) at necropsy, only one patient had voltage criteria for left ventricular hypertrophy. Likewise, only one patient had low voltage. Measurement of the QRS amplitude in each of the 12 leads was performed in 24 patients. The total QRS voltage was similar in the eight patients with and in the 16 patients without clinical evidence of cardiac disease (mean 147 versus 152 mm; 10 mm = 1 mV).

Summary

Certain clinical and necropsy cardiac findings are described and compared in 391 octogenarians (80%), 93 nonagenarians (19%) and in six centenarians (1%). The numbers of men and women were similar (248 (51%) and 242 (49%)). The cause of death was cardiac in 228 patients (47%), vascular but noncardiac in 71 (14%), and noncardiac and nonvascular in 191 (39%). The frequency of a cardiac condition causing death decreased with increasing age groups (51% versus 32% versus 0), and the frequency of a noncardiac nonvascular condition causing death increased with increasing age groups (36% versus 47% versus 100%). Among the cardiac conditions causing death, coronary artery disease was the problem in 61% (141/228) followed by aortic valve stenosis in 16% (36/228) and cardiac amyloidosis in 10% (22/228). Calcific deposits were found at necropsy in the coronary arteries in 81% (398/490) of the patients, in the aortic valve in 47% (228/490), in the mitral annular area in 39% (190/490), and in one or both left ventricular papillary muscles in 25% (122/490). The calcific deposits tended to be less frequent in the octogenarians. Three hundred (61%) of the 490 patients had one or more major coronary arteries narrowed more than 75% in cross-sectional area by plaque and the percentage of patients in each of the three age groups and the percentage of coronary arteries significantly narrowed in each of the three age groups were similar.

References

1. Waller BF, Roberts WC. Cardiovascular disease in the very elderly. Analysis of 40 necropsy patients aged 90 years or over. *Am J Cardiol* (1983) **51**:403–21.

2. Lie JT, Hammond PI. Pathology of the senescent heart: anatomic observations on 237 autopsy studies of patients 90 to 105 years old. *Mayo Clinic Proc* (1988) **63**:552–64.

3. Gertz SD, Malekzadeh S, Dollar AL et al. Composition of atherosclerotic plaques in the four major epicardial coronary arteries in patients ≥90 years of age. *Am J Cardiol* (1991) **67**:1228–33.

4. Roberts WC. Ninety-three hearts ≥90 years of age. *Am J Cardiol* (1993) **71**:599–602.

5. Shirani J, Yousefi J, Roberts WC. Major cardiac findings at necropsy in 366 American octogenarians. *Am J Cardiol* (1995) **75**:151–6.

6. Roberts WC. The heart at necropsy in centenarians. *Am J Cardiol* (1998) **81**:1224–5.

7. Roberts WC, Shirani J. Comparison of cardiac findings at necropsy in octogenarians, nonagenarians, and centenarians. *Am J Cardiol* (1998) in press.

8. Fries JF. Aging, natural death, and the compression of morbidity. *N Engl J Med* (1980) **303**:130–5.

9. Lachman AS, Spray TL, Kerwin DM et al. Medial calcinosis of Monckeberg. A review of the problem and a description of a patient with involvement of peripheral, visceral, and coronary arteries. *Am J Cardiol* (1977) **63**:615–22.

10. Hammer WJ, Roberts WC, deLeon AC Jr. 'Mitral stenosis' secondary to combined 'massive' mitral annular calcific deposits and small, hypertrophied left ventricles. *Am J Med* (1978) **64**:371–6.

11. Roberts WC. Qualitative and quantitative comparison of amounts of narrowing by atherosclerotic plaques in the major epicardial coronary arteries at necropsy in sudden coronary death, transmural acute myocardial infarction, transmural healed myocardial infarction and unstable angina pectoris. *Am J Cardiol* (1989) **4**:324–8.

4

Normal cardiovascular function in the octogenarian: rest and exercise

Susan J Zieman and Gary Gerstenblith

Introduction

One of the most consistent aspects of aging is the heterogeneity with which the process occurs. Whether this variability is due to intrinsic factors such as inherited genetic differences, personality and programmed cell death or to such extrinsic influences as disease, diet, exercise, lifestyle and toxin exposure or to a combination of these factors is unknown. The inability to distinguish the impact of these variables creates difficulty in defining which changes in the cardiovascular system are due to 'normal aging' and which are the result of, or can be modulated by, these influential factors. Interpretation of studies of normal cardiovascular physiology is further obscured in the octogenarian because of the high incidence of occult coronary disease.[1] One necropsy series of 366 octogenarians found greater than 75% occlusion in at least one major epicardial artery in 60% of the subjects although only approximately 30% had a history of angina pectoris, congestive heart failure or myocardial infarction.[2]

Our current understanding of age-related cardiovascular changes is mainly derived from cross-sectional studies, in which an attempt was made to exclude subjects with known coronary disease and to control for other significant variables. Although these cross-sectional studies form the foundation of our knowledge of age-related cardiovascular changes, the results must be interpreted with caution. Shortcomings of these studies include biases introduced by selective attrition and cohort effect and the inability to demonstrate trends over time and identify variables associated with these trends. Longitudinal studies, which examine the same population over an extended time period, are the best method to investigate age-related structural and functional changes.[3] The results of one such ongoing longitudinal study, the Baltimore Longitudinal Study on Aging (BLSA), provide significant insight into a multitude of cardiovascular issues in an aging population; some of the data presented in the text are drawn from this population.

Much of our current understanding of normal cardiovascular function in 80 year olds is based on the extrapolation of data from aging studies of the 'younger old'. The information presented in this chapter focuses on octogenarian studies, but also includes physiological studies of sexagenarians and septuagenarians when data on the very elderly are not available.

Rest physiology

Contrary to the widely accepted belief that aging leads to a decline in the function of various organs, the cardiovascular system in the octogenarian and beyond is remarkably resilient. Many adaptive physiological changes occur with age that preserve resting cardio-vascular function in the healthy older individual (see Lakatta[4] for a review). Cross-sectional data of cardiac volumes obtained using gated blood pool scans on healthy BLSA subjects, screened to exclude those with overt and occult cardiac disease, show no significant change in resting, seated ejection fraction in men and women with age[5] (Figure 4.1).

Although cardiac performance is often characterized by examining preload, afterload, myocardial contractility and heart rate, overall cardiovascular function represents the inter-action of all of these variables. For simplicity, these aspects of function will be discussed sep-arately with the recognition that, in vivo, they are inseparable. In addition to these factors, cardiovascular function is under constant reg-ulation by the autonomic nervous system.

Cardiac filling or preload

Cardiac filling or 'preload' refers to the ventricular volume that determines myocardial stretch prior to ventricular contraction. Although no significant change occurs in resting left ventricular end-diastolic volume (LVEDV) with age, echocardiographic[6] and gated-blood-pool studies[7] suggest that the diastolic filling pattern is altered (Figure 4.2). Early diastolic filling rate decreases by as much as 50% with advanced age, but EDV is maintained, in part because of enhanced atrial contribution late in diastole.[8,9] Higher left atrial pressure at this time may be responsible for the age-related increase in atrial size.[1] The etiology of slowed early diastolic filling is multi-factorial. One contributor is increased passive ventricular stiffness resulting in slower relax-ation and uncoiling after contraction. The increase may be caused by left ventricular hypertrophy, fibrosis and/or infiltrates such as amyloid. The incidence of cardiac amyloid infiltrates in one necropsy series was 10% in 80 year olds and increased to 50% in 90 year olds.[10] A cross-sectional study of diastolic fill-ing measured as E/A ratio on echocardiogra-phy in healthy subjects (age 67 ± 5.4 years) found that delayed early diastolic filling was independently predicted by left ventricular mass, but not by arterial compliance.[11] Alter-ation of active state properties that prolong ventricular contraction and delay early dia-stolic relaxation is another etiology for delayed early diastolic left ventricular filling.

Afterload

Components that contribute to the force against which the left ventricle ejects its blood, or 'afterload', include central arterial stiffness, peripheral vascular resistance, inertance, and ventricular wall stress. Histological examina-tion of the central arterial structure demon-strates an increase in disarrayed collagen and a decrease in elastin content with age. The increased central vascular stiffness leads to less elastic movement in systole during left ventric-ular ejection and less recoil during diastole.[12] These alterations in the pressure-strain and stress-strain moduli increase the propagation velocity of the pulse wave from the aortic valve to the aortoiliac bifurcation and the velocity of the reflected waves, which result from the reverberation of aortic pulse waves from the iliac bifurcation. In younger individu-als, with slower pulse-wave velocity, the reflected waves augment diastolic pressure and thus increase coronary perfusion.[13] In older individuals, however, the reflected waves return earlier, in late systole, and increase the pressure that must be developed by the left ventricle as it continues to eject blood at this time.[14–17] These arterial structural and physio-logical changes contribute to the widened pulse pressure and isolated systolic hyperten-

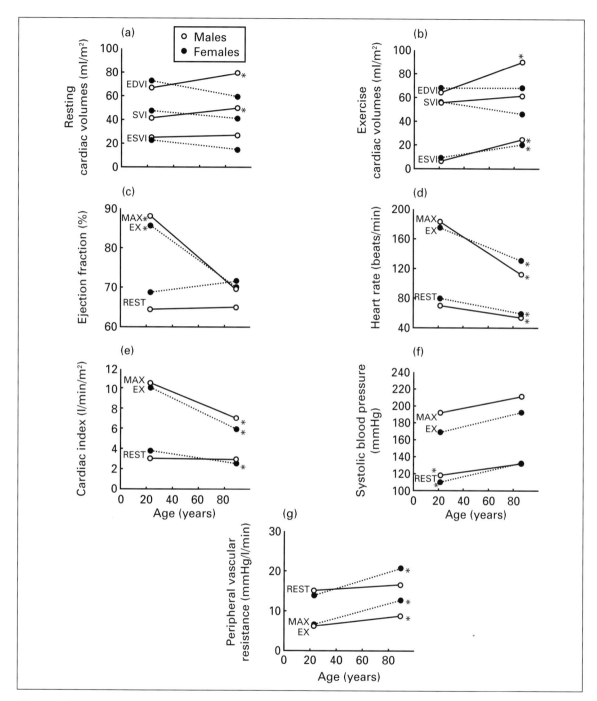

Figure 4.1
Linear regression of age on cardiac volume indices, heart rate, systolic pressure and peripheral vascular resistance in healthy men and women BLSA participants during rest and exercise.[5]
*Statistical significance of linear regression on age within sex.

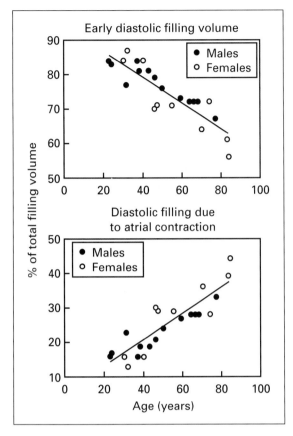

Figure 4.2
Linear regression of age on early diastolic filling and on atrial contribution to diastolic filling by echo-Doppler in healthy BLSA participants (EP Shapiro, personal communication).

sion common in the elderly.[18,19] The ascending aortic diameter also increases with age creating further impedance by inertial forces related to the enhanced cross-sectional blood volume which must be accelerated by the left ventricle at the onset of ejection. The cardiac component of afterload is wall stress, which, by LaPlace's law, depends on left ventricular radius, intracavitary pressure and wall thickness. At rest, there is no age-related change in

LVEDV, suggesting no change in radius. Wall thickness, however, increases. Therefore, at rest, an age-related increase in afterload is caused by an increase in arterial stiffness, which increases both the initial and late systolic load against which the left ventricle ejects its blood, and by a larger aortic diameter, which increases inertial resistance to left ventricular ejection. In response to the increased afterload, left ventricular myocytes hypertrophy[3] increasing wall thickness[6] so as to decrease left ventricular wall stress. It should be noted, however, that the age-related increase in arterial stiffness differs among cultural groups, possibly due to differences in dietary salt consumption.[20-22]

Myocardial contractility

Investigation of myocardial contractility is complicated by the inseparable influences of autonomic regulation, preload, afterload and heart rate. Studies of isolated older rat myocytes and trabeculae carneae suggest a prolongation of myocardial contraction and delayed relaxation. The duration and strength of each contraction is principally governed by the amount and persistence of Ca^{2+} on the troponin site. One of the major determinants of the former is the cytosolic calcium transient, which is largely regulated by calcium influx and efflux across the myocyte membrane and sarcoplasmic reticulum. Although there is no change in the myocyte resting membrane potential or the amplitude following a triggered action potential, repolarization duration is substantially increased in hearts from aged, as compared with young, animals.[23] The persistence of the Ca^{2+}–troponin interaction is determined by the rate of myofibril Ca^{2+} activated ATPase activity. In older rats, myosin isozyme predominance switches from a faster to a slower form, which may lead to a lengthier Ca^{2+}–troponin interaction and a longer contraction duration. Prolonged myocardial contraction is present in pathological conditions associated with increased ventricular afterload and left ventricular hypertrophy and may be an adaptive measure that increases the ability of the left ventricle to eject its stroke volume when confronted with increased impedance.

Heart rate

An age-related change in heart rate is not seen in the supine position; however, a slight decrease is noted in the resting heart rate of older men and women in the seated position.[5] Twenty-four hour ambulatory ECG monitoring of 101 healthy volunteers (age 16–68 years) shows a blunting of the respiratory and spontaneous heart-rate variation with age.[24,25] The blunted heart-rate response with age is consistent with another ambulatory ECG study of healthy individuals (age 40–102 years), although no significant age-related changes were found in the short-term modulation of heart-rate variability in this study.[26] This suggests that vagal modulation of heart rate in the elderly remains intact, but that the response to sympathetic stimulation is decreased.[27]

Neurohumoral control

Important aspects of cardiovascular function including heart rate, myocardial contractility, vascular tone and the response to stressors are modulated by constant input from the sympathetic and parasympathetic nervous systems. Basal plasma levels of epinephrine and norepinephrine are elevated or unchanged in older, healthy individuals compared with younger ones.[28] Any increase is thought to be secondary to diminished renal clearance and decreased postsynaptic uptake, rather than to increased production. Despite elevated levels, there is a blunted end-organ response to beta-adrenergic stimulation that is thought to be postsynaptic in nature.[28] This reduction in cardiovascular sympathetic responsiveness becomes more apparent during exercise and is described below.

Exercise physiology

The cardiovascular system of healthy older individuals adapts well to the physiological stress of exercise. Overall cardiovascular fitness is often evaluated by the determination of oxygen consumption at peak exercise. Maximum oxygen consumption is diminished in older, healthy, sedentary subjects free of overt evidence of coronary disease.[29,30] VO_2max is determined by cardiac output and the extraction of oxygen by peripheral tissues. A significant reduction of skeletal muscle mass occurs in older sedentary individuals and when oxygen consumption is corrected for creatinine clearance, there is no longer a significant age relationship.[31]

Autonomic influences during exercise

Exercise physiology of the older heart is sometimes likened to that of a younger heart exercising under the influence of beta-adrenergic blockade.[32] Although a slight increase in basal norepinephrine and epinephrine levels is described, there is a steeper age related augmentation of catecholamines during aerobic exercise stress.[28] Despite high circulating catecholamine levels, the cardiovascular responses to adrenergic stimulation, including the increase in heart rate, peripheral vasodilation and myocardial contractility, are all decreased.[33,34] The fact that the age change is clearly related to a decreased response to catecholamines, is demonstrated in studies showing age-related decreases in peak exercise heart rate, cardiac output and ejection fraction responses to a graded infusion of the beta-adrenergic agonist isoproterenol.[35] When younger and older healthy subjects are exercised while receiving beta-blocking drugs, their cardiovascular response parameters do not differ significantly from each other or from the exercise response of healthy, non-beta-blocked older subjects.[36]

Cardiac function in response to exercise

Multiple regression analysis of the effect of age, independent of gender and exercise capacity, on gated blood pool scan-derived cardiac volumes at peak cycle exercise in 200 healthy men and women BLSA participants was recently reported by Fleg et al.[5] Despite a significant reduction in heart rate at maximum exercise in older individuals, cardiac index is preserved by a compensatory augmentation in stroke volume index (SVI). Left ventricular end-diastolic and systolic volume indices are increased and ejection fraction and the systolic blood pressure/end-systolic volume index, an index of contractility, are significantly decreased with age at peak exercise. The reduction in early left ventricular filling, which is seen at rest, is unchanged at peak exercise, but does not compromise end-diastolic volume.[7] The increase in left ventricular end-systolic volume index (LVESVI) and the decline in left ventricular ejection fraction with age contribute to the 35% increase in preload (LVEDVI).[5] The increase in stroke volume of the exercising heart with advanced age is achieved through enhanced preload and a greater reliance on the Frank–Starling mechanism.[37] Peak systolic and diastolic blood pressures are also higher in older than in younger subjects during exercise.[38]

Physical conditioning status

The effects of physical conditioning on the heart of an octogenarian have also been studied. Although the overall age-related decline in physical fitness, as measured by VO$_2$max, is affected by skeletal muscle loss, the effects of diminished physical conditioning associated with age-related lifestyle changes may be underestimated. To determine the cardiovascular effects of physical conditioning status, several studies report the hemodynamic influences of routine exercise training programs in older persons. The effects of chronic endurance training in elderly people will also be addressed.

Influences of training

Routine exercise training affects the overall fitness level of older individuals and significantly influences hemodynamic parameters.[39,40] After 6 months of low intensity aerobic training for 90 minutes three times a week, followed by 6 months of the same amount of high intensity aerobic training, sedentary older subjects increased their VO$_2$max by 30%.[41] No change was seen in peak exercise cardiac output after training, suggesting an increase in peripheral oxygen extraction with exercise. When 13 sedentary healthy subjects (age 60–82 years) exercised regularly for 6 months, resting heart rate decreased by 12%, resting LVEDV increased by 13% and resting SVI increased by 18%.[42] Compared with 11 younger individuals (age 24–32) who underwent the same exercise program, peak exercise SVI in the older subjects was not significantly different, although the increase was achieved via a different mechanism. The older individuals relied on a higher preload (8% increase in LVEDV) and no change in LVESV, whereas the younger subjects decreased LVEDV by 10% and LVESV by 32% to achieve a 40% higher cardiac index. Peak heart rate in older trained subjects increased 105% from rest compared with 166% in younger subjects. A routine exercise program may diminish some of the age-related increase in central arterial stiffness, as was shown by a decrease in aortic pulse wave velocity with training.[15] Improved left ventricular performance was also demonstrated following a 4-days-a-week for 12-months exercise program in healthy, sedentary individuals (mean age 62 ± 3 years). After training sufficient to increase VO_2max from 29 to 37 ml/kg/min, resting to peak exercise ejection fraction increased from 66–70% (pre-training) to 67–77% (post-training).[43] An increase in echocardiographic LVEDV and posterior wall thickness occurred without a change in the wall thickness/radius ratio, indicating a hypertrophied, volume-overloaded left ventricular response to the training program. Training was also associated with an increase in the stroke volume/LVEDV relationship. Some age-associated cardiovascular parameters do not significantly change with routine exercise. After 6 months of intensive training of the older (60–82 years) subjects sufficient to achieve a 21% increase in maximum oxygen consumption, there was no significant change in the cardiovascular response to isoproterenol, suggesting a true age-related diminished response to catecholamines that appears to be postsynaptic.[35] Although regular exercise increases peak diastolic filling rate in both young and old healthy subjects, the significant age-associated slowing in early diastolic filling remains.[44]

Senior master athletes

The beneficial effects of chronic endurance training in the older population are evident in studies of resting and exercise cardiovascular hemodynamics of senior master athletes. These individuals engage in vigorous aerobic and anaerobic exercise such as running (i.e. 43 ± 6 miles/week), swimming and cycling. Resting. hemodynamic parameters of endurance-trained older individuals do not vary from their age-matched sedentary cohort. Specifically, one study found no significant change in resting heart rate, stroke volume, blood pressure or left ventricular end-diastolic or systolic volumes in those who engaged in routine, rigorous aerobic exercise compared with sedentary controls,[39] whereas another study found a slight decrease in resting heart rate and a slight increase in resting cardiac output in master athletes.[45] As with routine short-term training programs described above, master athletes may continue to demonstrate early diastolic filling impairment compared with younger individuals.[7,46] Endurance-trained athletes exhibit a remarkably higher cardiac reserve during exercise when compared with sedentary individuals. A significant increase in VO_2max is seen in master athletes[21,47] which declines with deconditioning.[39] Both augmented cardiac output and higher peripheral oxygen extraction contribute to this increase in overall cardiovascular fitness.[31,39,48] These changes are accompanied by a significant increase in cardiac index, stroke volume index, ejection fraction and contractile indices and a significant decrease in left ventricular end-systolic volume, diastolic blood pressure and total systemic vascular resistance at peak exercise compared with sedentary individuals.[39,45] There is no conditioning influence on maximum heart rate or left ventricular end-diastolic volume at peak exercise, suggesting that the age-associated decrease in catecholamine responsiveness is not influenced by physical conditioning status.[39,45,48] The ability of an older athlete to attain a higher exercise stroke volume and cardiac output than a sedentary older individual is based on a significant reduction in left ventricular end-systolic volume with a relatively unchanged end-diastolic volume at peak exercise.[45] The rise in blood pressure at peak exercise is unaffected by endurance training, but training does lower central arterial stiffness as measured by augmentation index and pulse wave velocity.[15] The relative contributions of enhanced contractility and decreased aortic impedance are unclear. In summary, endurance training in the older individual can create a consequential increase in overall cardiovascular fitness, increased muscle mass, a hypertrophied volume-overload left ventricle that has improved contractile abilities, better cardiovascular reserve and decreased arterial stiffness.[15,39,44,45]

Gender differences in cardiovascular function with age

Subtle gender differences are present in cardiovascular structure and function that may have important clinical implications.[5] At rest, the left ventricular cavity size and volume of a female is smaller than that of a male, yet the mass of a woman's heart increases at a greater rate over the years. From the third to the ninth decade of life, the resting LVEDVI, LVESVI and SVI increase by 20% in males in contrast to no significant age-related change in these parameters in women. Despite the smaller cavity and higher total systemic vascular resistance, the ejection fraction of a woman's heart at rest is greater than that of a male. Men demonstrate higher peak work rates than females at any given age. At peak exercise, there is no significant gender difference in SVI, yet the contributors of SVI vary between men and women. Men have a greater reliance on the Frank–Starling mechanism to achieve an increase in SVI and a lower peak exercise heart rate than do women. During exercise in men, LVEDVI increased by 35% and LVESVI increased three-fold, whereas in exercising women, there is no significant increase in LVEDVI and a two-fold increase in LVESVI. Despite the smaller cardiac volumes, the same cardiac index is attained by a higher peak exercise heart rate. The resting ejection fraction of a female left ventricle is higher than that of a male, but augments less with exercise.[5] VO_2max is 22–35% greater in men than women and remains 15% higher when normalized for lean body mass.[29]

Summary

Studies of normal and exercise cardiovascular physiology in the octogenarian are sparse. Cross-sectional studies and the extrapolation of data from the 'younger old', however, suggest a general preservation of cardiovascular function in this age group. Age-related cardiovascular changes that are reliably seen include increased central arterial stiffness, delayed early left ventricular diastolic filling and a diminished response to beta-adrenergic stimulation. During exercise, the older heart increases and maintains cardiac output in the setting of a decreased peak heart rate by augmenting stroke volume. This rise in stroke volume is due to an increase in preload (LVEDV) and an increased reliance on the Frank–Starling mechanism. Physical conditioning in the octogenarian can have significant hemodynamic consequences consistent with overall improvement in left ventricular function.

Acknowledgements

This work was supported in part by a contract from the National Institute on Aging (N01-AG-9-2116).

References

1. Waller BF, Roberts WC. Cardiovascular disease in the very elderly: analysis of 40 necropsy patients aged 90 years or older. *Am J Cardiol* (1983) **51**:403–21.

2. Shirani J, Yousefi J, Roberts WC. Major cardiac findings at necropsy in 366 American octogenarians. *Am J Cardiol* (1995) **75**:151–6.

3. Brandt LJ, Pearson JD, Morrell CH et al. Autonomy and well being in the aging population. In Deeg DJH, Knipscheer CPM, van Rilburg W, eds, *Longitudinal Methods of Assessing Vulnerability: Concepts and Design of the Longitudinal Aging Study. Amsterdam.* (NIG Trend Studies: Nijmegen, Netherlands, 1993) 185–97.

4. Lakatta EG. Cardiovascular regulatory mechanisms in advanced age. *Physiol Rev* (1993) **73**:413–67.

5. Fleg JL, O'Connor F, Gerstenblith G et al. Impact of age on the cardiovascular response to dynamic upright exercise in healthy men and women. *J Appl Physiol* (1995) **78**: 890–900.

6. Gerstenblith G, Fredericksen J, Yin FCP et al. Echocardiographic assessment of a normal aging population. *Circulation* (1977) **56**: 273–8.

7. Schulman SP, Lakatta EG, Fleg JL et al. Age-related decline in left ventricular filling at rest and exercise. *Am J Physiol* (1992) **263**: H1932–8.

8. Swinne CJ, Shapiro EP, Lima SD, Fleg JL. Age-associated changes in left ventricular diastolic performance during isometric exercise in normal subjects. *Am J Cardiol* (1992) **69**:823–6.

9. Miller TR, Grossman SJ, Schectman KB et al. Left ventricular diastolic filling in the healthy elderly. *Am J Cardiol* (1986) **58**:531–5.

10. Pomerance A. Senile cardiac amyloidosis. *Br Heart J* (1965) **27**:711–18.

11. Rajkumar C, Cameron JD, Christophidis N et al. Reduced systemic arterial compliance is associated with left ventricular hypertrophy and diastolic dysfunction in older people. *J Am Geriatr Soc* (1997) **45**:803–8.

12. Hass GM. Elastic tissue. III. Relations between the structure of the aging aorta and the properties of the isolated aortic elastic tissue. *Arch Pathol* (1943) **35**:29–45.

13. Saeki A, Recchia F, Kass DA. Systolic flow augmentation in hearts ejecting into a model of stiff aging vasculature: influence on myocardial perfusion–demand balance. *Circ Res* (1995) **76**:132–41.

14. Nichols WW, O'Rourke MF, Avolio AP et al. Effects of age on ventricular–vascular coupling. *Am J Cardiol* (1985) **55**:1179–84

15. Vaitkevicius PV, Fleg JL, Engel JH et al. Effects of age and aerobic capacity on arterial stiffness in healthy adults. *Circulation* (1993) **88**(Pt l): 1456–62.

16. Sharir T, Marmor A, Ting CT et al. Validation of a method for noninvasive measurement of central arterial pressure. *Hypertension* (1993) **21**:74–82.

17. O'Rourke MF, Kelly RP. Wave reflection in the systemic circulation and its implications in ventricular function. *J Hypertens* (1993) **11**: 327–37.

18. Pearson JD, Morrell CH, Brant LJ et al. Age-related changes in blood pressure in a longitudinal study of healthy men and women. *J Gerontol* (1997) **52A**:M177–83.

19. Jenson E, Hagberg B, Samuelsson G et al. Blood pressure in relation to medical, psychological and social variables in a population of 80-year-olds. Survival during 6 years. *J Int Med* (1997) **241**:205–12.

20. Weinberger MH, Fineberg NS. Sodium and volume sensitivity of blood pressure: age and pressure change over time. *Hypertension* (1991) **18**:67–71.

21. MacGregor GA. Sodium is more important than calcium in essential hypertension. *Hypertension* (1985) **7**:628–37.

22. Avolio AP, Chen SG, Wang RP et al. Effects of aging on changing arterial compliance and left ventricular load in a northern Chinese urban community. *Circulation* (1983) **68**: 50–8.

23. Wei JY, Spurgeon HA, Lakatta EG. Excitation-coupling in rat myocardium: alterations with adult aging. *Am J Physiol* (1984) **246:** H784–91.

24. Davies HEF. Respiratory change in heart rate, sinus arrhythmia in the elderly. *Gerontol Clin* (1975) **17:**96–100.

25. Kostis JB, Moreyra AE, Amendo MT et al. The effect of age on heart rate in subjects free of heart disease. Studies by ambulatory electrocardiography and maximal exercise stress test. *Circulation* (1982) **65:**141–5.

26. Reardon M, Malik M. Changes in heart rate variability with age. *Pacing and Clin Electrophys* (1996) **19:**1863–6.

27. De Meersman RE. Aging as a modulator of respiratory sinus arrhythymia. *J Gerontol* (1993) **48:**B74–8.

28. Fleg JL, Tzankoff SP, Lakatta EG. Age-related augmentation of plasma catecholamines during dynamic exercise in healthy older men. *J Appl Physiol* (1985) **59:**1033–9.

29. Ogawa T, Spina RJ, Martin WH et al. Effects of aging, sex, and physical training on cardiovascular response to exercise. *Circulation* (1992) **86:**494–503.

30. Julius S, Amery A, Whitlock L, Conway J. Influence of age on the hemodynamic response to exercise. *Circulation* (1967) **26:**222–30.

31. Fleg JL, Lakatta EG. Role of muscle loss in the age-associated reduction in VO$_2$max. *J Appl Physiol* (1988) **65:**1147–51.

32. Fleg JL. The effect of normative aging on the cardiovascular system. *Am J Geriatr Cardiol* (1994) **3:**25–31.

33. Davies CH, Ferrara N, Harding SE. β-Adrenoceptor function changes with age of subject in myocytes from non-failing human ventricle. *Cardiovasc Res* (1996) **31:**152–6.

34. Pan HYM, Hoffman BB, Pershe RA, Blaschke TF. Decline in beta adrenergic receptor-medicated vascular relaxation with aging in man. *J Pharmacol Exp Ther* (1986) **239:** 802–7.

35. Stratton JR, Cerqueira MD, Schwartz RS et al. Differences in cardiovascular responses to isoproterenol in relation to age and exercise training in healthy men. *Circulation* (1992) **86:** 504–12.

36. Fleg JL, Schulman SP, O'Connor F et al. Effects of acute β-adrenergic receptor blockade on age-associated changes in cardiovascular performance during dynamic exercise. *Circulation* (1994) **90:**2333–41.

37. Plotnick GD, Becker LC, Fisher ML et al. Use of the Frank–Starling mechanism during submaximal versus maximal upright exercise. *J Appl Physiol* (1986) **251:**H1101–5.

38. Daida H, Allison TG, Squires RW et al. Peak exercise blood pressure stratified by age and gender in apparently healthy subjects. *Mayo Clin Proc* (1996) **71:**445–52.

39. Schulman SP, Fleg JL, Goldberg AP et al. Continuum of cardiovascular performance across a broad range of fitness levels in healthy older men. *Circulation* (1996) **94:**359–67.

40. Morey MC, Pieper CF, Sullivan RJ et al. Five-year performance trends for older exercisers: a hierarchical model of endurance, strength and flexibility. *J Am Geriatr Soc* (1996) **44:** 1226–31.

41. Seals DR, Hagberg JM, Hurley BF et al. Endurance training in older men and women: I. Cardiovascular response to exercise. *J Appl Physiol* (1984) **57:**1024–9.

42. Stratton JR, Levy WC, Cerqueira MD et al. Cardiovascular response to exercise: effect of aging and exercise training in healthy men. *Circulation* (1994) **89:**1648–55.

43. Ehsani AA, Ogawa T, Miller TR et al. Exercise training improves left ventricular systolic function in older men. *Circulation* (1991) **83:** 96–103.

44. Levy WC, Cerqueira MD, Abrass IB et al. Endurance exercise training augments diastolic filling at rest and during exercise in healthy young and older men. *Circulation* (1993) **88:**116–26.

45. Seals DR, Hagberg JM, Spina RJ et al. Myocardial function/valvular heart disease/hypertensive heart disease: enhanced left ventricular performance in endurance trained older men. *Circulation* (1994) **89:**198–205.

46. Fleg JL, Shapiro EP, O'Connor FC et al. Left ventricular diastolic filling performance in older male athletes. *JAMA* (1995) **273:** 1371–5.

47. Heath GW, Hagberg JM, Ehsani AA, Holloszy JO. A physiological comparison of young and older endurance athletes. *J Appl Physiol* (1981) **51:**634–40.

48. Fleg JL, Schulman SP, O'Connor FC et al. Cardiovascular responses to exhaustive upright cycle exercise in highly trained older men. *J Appl Physiol* (1994) **77**:1500–6.

5

The importance of preclinical disease: lessons from the Cardiovascular Health Study

Lewis H Kuller, Linda P Fried and Richard A Kronmal

Introduction

The traditional approaches for studying cardiovascular risk factors and disease among older individuals have important limitations. First, many older individuals have subclinical cardiovascular disease such as extensive atherosclerosis.[1] Thus, the amount of disease in the 'incident' cases may be very similar to that in the comparison group (or controls) without clinical disease. Risk factors such as low density lipoprotein (LDL) cholesterol, that primarily relate to the risk or extent of atherosclerosis may be less powerful predictors of disease (that is, have lower relative risk among the older individuals) because there is not a clear separation of cases and noncases with regard to the extent of atherosclerosis.

Second, the levels of the risk factors may change with increasing age and associated comorbidity. Thus, weight loss or declines in total cholesterol and LDL cholesterol and blood pressure (especially diastolic blood pressure) with increasing age may be markers of disease.[2] The measurement of the risk factors at older age may be difficult to interpret or even be falsely interpreted, because of the lack of knowledge of the prior level or changes of the risk factors of interest at younger ages over time.

Third, the association of the level of risk factor and disease may be time dependent. The development of atherosclerosis and coronary artery disease at older ages is probably a function of both the level of the risk factor (such as LDL cholesterol or blood pressure) and the duration of exposure. At older ages, individuals with lower levels of risk factors but for longer duration, may be at risk while individuals with higher risk factor levels may either have already developed clinical disease or are no longer at risk of incident disease, or may be less susceptible (i.e. host susceptibility) as measured by genetic factors to these higher levels of risk factors since they have survived without clinical disease to older ages.

Fourth, the development of subclinical vascular disease with increasing age may be the primary determinant of the level of some risk factors. For example, increased carotid artery wall thickness and stiffness of large arteries may be important determinants of higher systolic blood pressures and lower diastolic blood pressures, especially if there is little change in overall vascular resistance.[3]

Fifth, the primary determinants of clinical cardiovascular disease may be other risk factors that modulate the determinants of transition from subclinical vascular disease to clinical disease. These may reflect changes in the vascular wall, thrombosis, fibrinolysis and various adhesion molecules. Measurement of these risk factors related to vascular wall changes, thrombosis and fibrinolysis may have to be done in close proximity to the incident event and, probably also, in association with the extent of the underlying vascular disease.[4]

Many of these important issues led to the development of the Cardiovascular Health Study (CHS). The major goal of the CHS was to utilize new or clinical technology, or technology that had primarily been limited to clinical studies, in population studies in order to evaluate the prevalence of subclinical cardiovascular disease among older individuals age 65 and over, determine risk factors for subclinical disease, and the relationship of subclinical disease to clinical disease and functional status. The study included the measurement of the incidence of cardiovascular disease, including myocardial infarction (MI), angina, congestive heart failure (CHF), peripheral vascular disease and stroke. The study also included measures of thrombosis, fibrinolysis and inflammation, and the subsequent relationship of these measures to risk factors, subclinical disease and clinical disease.[5]

Methods

The original sample of the Cardiovascular Health Study was recruited from Medicare Part A listings in four communities in the United States (Forsyth County, NC; Sacramento County, CA; Washington County, MD; and Allegheny County, PA). Letters were initially mailed to 11 955 sampled individuals. Persons who were then recruited were required to complete an extensive home interview and a 4-hour in-clinic examination. From the baseline sample, 3654 participants were recruited from those randomly selected from the Medicare sampling frame, and an additional 1547 were other age-eligible individuals living in the household with the sampled individuals, giving an initial sample of 5201 participants.[5]

In 1992–93 (year 5 of the study) a new cohort of 249 black men and 424 women and 14 other races were added to the study. The recruitment of the new black participants was similar to that of the original cohort of black and white participants. There were 244 blacks in the original cohort, 91 men and 153 women. Thus, the final sample consisted of 2791 white women (48%) and 2135 white men (36%), 577 black women (10%) and 340 black men (6%) and 45 other races.

The baseline examinations included both a home interview and physical examination in the clinic. The prevalence of clinical and subclinical disease in this cohort was based on measurements of the resting electrocardiogram, echocardiogram, carotid artery sonography, ankle–brachial blood pressure measurements, history of vascular disease, cardiovascular surgery and selective symptomatology (Rose angina and claudication).[5]

Cognitive testing

At the baseline examination for the original cohort (year 2), participants completed the Mental State Exam (MMSE). In the first follow-up examination (year 3 of the study) the Modified Mini-Mental State Exam (3MSE) replaced the MMSE and was then administered annually at all clinic visits and at-home visits when appropriate. The 3MSE sampled a wider range of cognitive abilities, including a short-term and delayed recall and a temporal and spatial orientation. Scores on the 3MSE range from 0–100. A cut-off point of below 80 has been used to classify individuals as at high-risk of dementia. The Digit Symbol Substitution Test (DSST) and the Benton Visual Retention Test were also administered to the participants.[6]

MRI examinations

The MRI exams were completed on 3660 (62%) of the 5888 participants in the CHS in year 5 of the study. Detailed descriptions of the CHS MRI methods of analysis have previously been published.[7]

Results

Clinical disease

For the baseline cohort of women (1989–90), the prevalence of myocardial infarction increased from 9.7% at age 65–69, 10.2% at age 70–74, 16.1% at age 75–79, 9.5% at age 80–84 and 17.9% at age greater than 85. Similarly, the prevalence of stroke increased from 2.2% at age 65–69 to 7.8% at age 85 and over, and for congestive heart failure from 1.8% at age 65–69 to 3.3% at age 85 and over. In men, the prevalence was much higher than in women—18% of men had MIs among those at age 65–69 increasing to 29.6% at age 80–84, and stroke varied from 5.3% at age 65–69 to 9.8% at age 80–84. The prevalence of congestive heart failure in men varied from 2.0% at age 65–74 to 2.9% at age 85 and over.[8]

Subclinical disease

Ankle–brachial blood pressure

The ankle–arm index was measured in 5084 participants at the baseline examination in the CHS. An ankle–arm index below 0.9 was considered to be abnormal. The prevalence of low ankle–arm blood pressures below 0.9 was substantially higher in individuals with prevalent cardiovascular disease at baseline and increased dramatically with age. Approximately 20% of men and women age 80–84 and 30–35% age 85+ had a decreased ankle–brachial blood pressure. The frequency of a decreased ankle–brachial blood pressure

was strongly associated with the prevalence of myocardial infarction, angina, CHF, stroke and transient ischemic attack (TIA) at the baseline examination (Figure 5.1).[9]

Carotid artery intimal medial thickness and stenosis

The maximal carotid intimal medial thickness increased with age and was greater at all ages in men than in women. Mean internal carotid artery wall thickness (mm) in men was 1.50 at ages 65–74, 1.66 for ages 75–84, and 1.84 in ages over 85 for participants without clinical cardiovascular disease, and 1.79 for ages 65–74, 1.92 in ages 65–74, and 2.04 in ages over 85 for those with cardiovascular disease. The results for women were similar.[10,11]

The prevalence of maximal carotid artery stenosis greater than 50% in the CHS increased from 4.3% at age 65–69, to 14.3% at age 85 or over for men and from 4.3% at age 65–69, to 11.4% at age 85 or over for women without a history of cardiovascular disease. Stenosis was significantly related to history of hypertension, cigarette smoking, diabetes, left ventricular hypertrophy, major electrocardiographic abnormalities, carotid artery bruit, history of heart disease and stroke (Figure 5.2).[11]

ECG abnormalities

Major electrocardiographic abnormalities increased substantially with age and with the prevalence of either coronary heart disease or hypertension. Among women without a history of coronary heart disease or hypertension, the prevalence increased from 10.5% at age 65–69 to 31.6% at age 85 and over and, in men from 16% at age 65–69 to 45.9% at age 85 and over. For women who had either a history of hypertension or coronary artery disease at entry, the prevalence of major ECG abnormalities increased from 25.8% at age

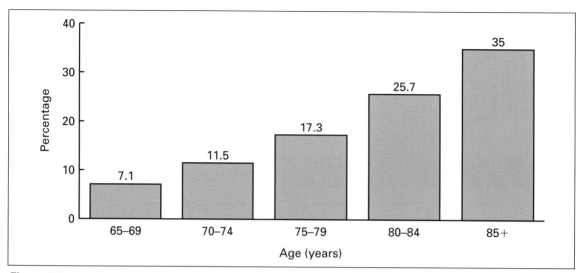

Figure 5.1
Distribution of CHS participants by ankle–arm index less than 0.9 by age.

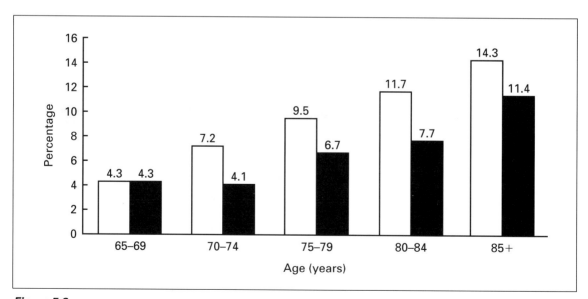

Figure 5.2
Distribution of carotid artery maximal stenosis at least 50% by age and sex (either artery). (■, Women; □, men.) From O'Leary et al[11] with permission.

65–69 to 38.8% at age 85 and over and, for men from 37.9% at age 65–69 to 61.1% at age 85 and over.[12]

Echocardiography

Left ventricular mass, as estimated by an M-mode echocardiogram, has previously been shown to be an independent predictor of incident cardiovascular disease, morbidity and mortality. The relationship of left ventricular mass to cardiovascular disease and covariates was evaluated in the Cardiovascular Health Study among 5201 men and women at baseline. Left ventricular mass was substantially increased in participants with a history of hypertension or on antihypertensive medication, among diabetics, among those with a history of MI, history of congestive heart failure,

history of coronary heart disease, and major ECG abnormalities. Left ventricular mass was greater in men than in women, but there was no consistent relationship with age.[13]

Abdominal aortic aneurysm

Risk factors for abdominal aortic aneurysm in the Cardiovascular Health Study were evaluated. Ultrasound techniques provided a non-invasive method of detecting aortic aneurysms. Images of the abdominal aorta were obtained in both transverse and longitudinal projections. Abdominal aortic aneurysms were defined as: (1) an infrarenal aortic diameter at least 3 cm; (2) an infrarenal to suprarenal ratio at least 1.2; or (3) a history of aortic aneurysm repair. The studies were done in years 5,6 (1992–93) of the CHS (Figure 5.3).[14]

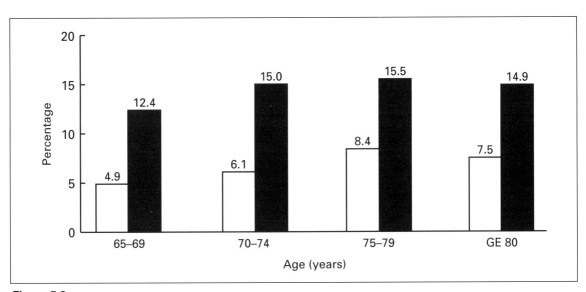

Figure 5.3
Distribution of prevalent abdominal aortic aneurysms by age and sex (■, women; □, men) in the CHS. From Alcorn et al[14] with permission.

The prevalence of aortic aneurysm increased slightly with age—7.7% at age 65–69, 10% at age 70–74, 11.3% at age 75–79 and 11% at age 80 and over, with an overall prevalence of 9.5%. Aneurysms occurred much more frequently in men (14.2%) than in women (6.2%). There was little difference in aneurysms in blacks and whites. Aneurysms were much more frequent among current smokers and among individuals who were taller and weighed more. Prevalence of aortic aneurysms was higher among participants who had a history of coronary heart disease, including both angina pectoris and myocardial infarction, and a history of stroke. Aneurysm prevalence was higher for participants with other measures of subclinical disease including ankle–arm index, maximum carotid artery stenosis, and maximum internal and maximum intimal medial thickness in the internal carotid artery. There was also a positive association between the prevalence of aneurysms and LDL cholesterol, inversely with high density lipoprotein (HDL) cholesterol, and a direct relationship to creatinine level. There was no relationship in this study between aneurysms and blood pressure levels.

Composite index of subclinical disease

A composite subclinical disease index was defined as major electrographic abnormalities, echocardiograms with wall motion abnormalities or low ejection fractions, increased carotid or internal carotid artery wall thickness greater than the 80th percentile or stenosis greater than the 25th percentile, a decreased ankle–brachial blood pressure below 0.9, and a positive response to the Rose Questionnaire for angina and intermittent claudication. Based on these criteria, the initial prevalence of subclinical disease increased from 21.7% at

age 65–69 in women to 43.3% at age 85 and over, and for men from 32.9% at age 65–69 to 44.7% at age 85 and over. Among the older age groups, approximately 80% of women age 80–84 and close to 90% at age 85 and over had either manifestation of subclinical or clinical disease, while for men approximately 90% at age 80–84 had either clinical or subclinical disease, as well as at age 85 and over.

The risk factors for the composite index of subclinical disease included higher LDL cholesterol, triglycerides, fasting glucose and insulin, body mass index and waist circumference, cigarette smoking, hypertension, diabetes and family history of heart disease in first-degree relatives. There were only small differences in the association of risk factors by race and sex. In multivariate analysis, the association with lipids was stronger in women than men (Table 5.1).[15]

Incident events: longitudinal analysis

Myocardial infarction

At baseline, 1967 men and 2979 women had no history of myocardial infarction. After a follow-up of an average of 4.8 years, the 302 cardiac events included 263 patients with a myocardial infarction and 39 with definite fatal coronary artery disease; the incidence was higher in men (20.7/1000) than in women (7.9/1000). The incidence also increased strongly with age, from 7.8/1000 in participants at age 65–69 to 25.6/1000 in subjects age 85 and older (Figure 5.4). Diabetes, fasting blood glucose at least 127 mg%, and systolic blood pressure were associated with an increased incidence of myocardial infarction in this older age group. Subclinical measures related to myocardial infarction included abnormal ejection fraction on echocardiogram, higher levels of intimal medial thickness

Variable	White		Black	
	Odds ratio	95% CI	Odds ratio	95% CI
Women (N = 1810 white, 299 black)				
Age	1.064*	1.041–1.087	1.043	0.994–1.0095
Average systolic BP	1.016*	1.009–1.022	1.024†	1.009–1.040
Average diastolic BP	0.969*	0.958–0.980	0.983	0.955–1.013
LDL cholesterol	1.007*	1.004–1.009	1.011†	1.004–1.018
Glucose	1.006†	1.002–1.011	1.004	0.999–1.010
White blood cells	1.088†	1.024–1.155	1.039	0.905–1.193
Present smoker	2.104*	1.518–2.915	3.162†	1.435–6.966
History of hypertension	1.514*	1.220–1.880	0.815	0.474–1.401
Family history of MI	1.258‡	1.017–1.555	1.686	0.922–3.082
Men (N = 1197 white, 188 black)				
Age	1.080*	1.050–1.110	1.194*	1.083–1.317
Average systolic BP	1.028*	1.019–1.036	1.010	0.986–1.035
Average diastolic BP	0.966*	0.951–0.981	0.972	0.930–1.016
Triglycerides	1.001	0.999–1.003	1.010‡	1.002–1.019
Body mass index	1.067*	1.028–1.108	0.931	0.840–1.032
Present smoker	2.165*	1.368–3.427	2.555	0.964–6.766
Family history of MI	1.086	0.816–1.446	0.316‡	0.132–0.760
Anti-hypertensive meds	1.462‡	1.087–1.967	5.083*	2.176–11.877

Notes. Variables were selected in a forward stepwise fashion. The resulting model was then refit using a common set of variables across races within a gender (the union of the variables selected in the stepwise procedure). * $P < 0.001$, † $P < 0.01$, ‡ $P < 0.05$
From Kuller et al[15] with permission

Table 5.1
Logistic regression analysis of the risk of subclinical disease excluding individuals with clinical disease by sex and race: common set of variables across races within a gender

of the internal carotid artery, and lower ankle–brachial blood pressure. Neither LDL nor HDL cholesterol levels were related to the incidence risk of myocardial infarction.[16]

Congestive heart failure

At a mean follow-up of 3.3 years, 92 participants (3.4%) of the 2762 with technically adequate echocardiograms in the CHS developed congestive heart failure. Approximately 90% (83) had greater than 25% left ventricular shortening at baseline. Echocardiographic variables associated with incident congestive heart failure included increased left ventricular mass and relative wall thickness, left atrial size, left ventricular fractional shortening and peak velocity of late, but not early, diastolic filling. Participants who developed congestive

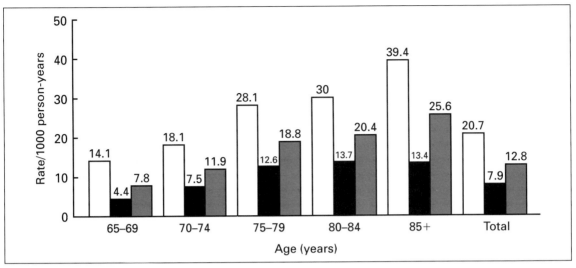

Figure 5.4
Incidence of myocardial infarction by age and sex (■, women; □, men; ■, total) per 1000 person-years in the CHS. Rates were significantly higher in men than in women and strongly associated with age in both men and women (P < 0.01).

heart failure were older, had higher systolic blood pressure, low ankle–arm index, greater carotid artery wall thickness, diabetes, history of hypertension and consumed more alcohol.[17]

Stroke

During approximately 3.3 years of follow-up in the Cardiovascular Health Study there were 188 incident strokes. The incidence of stroke was similar in men and women. The incidence of stroke per thousand person years in women varied from 4.4/1000 person years at age 65–69 to 22.3/1000 person years at age 80 and over, and in men from 7.9/1000 person years at age 65–69 to 22.4 at age 80 and over (Figure 5.5). Factors associated with increased stroke risk in multivariate analysis included increasing age, aspirin use, diabetes, impaired glucose tolerance, higher systolic blood pressure and increased time to walk 15 feet. Other risk factors related to increased risk of stroke included elevated creatinine levels, abnormal left ventricular wall motion, increased left ventricular mass on echocardiography, ultrasound-defined carotid stenosis and atrial fibrillation.

Increased left ventricular mass and carotid stenosis were associated with a two- to three-fold increase in the incidence of stroke. Aspirin users without a prior history of coronary heart disease, atrial fibrillation, claudication or transient ischemic attack had an 84% higher risk (relative risk 1.84, confidence limits 1.2–2.8) of stroke. Seventy-nine incident

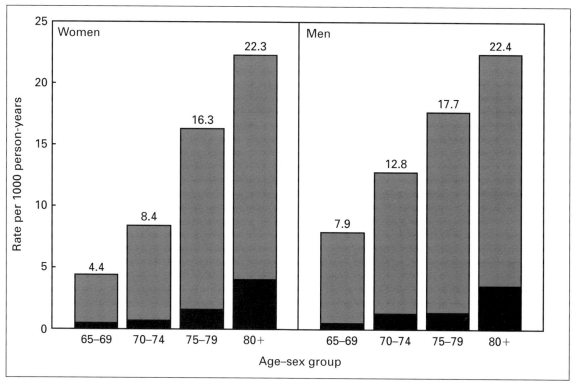

Figure 5.5
Incident stroke by age and sex (■, fatal stroke; ■, nonfatal stroke). From Manolio et al[18] with permission.

strokes occurred among the 2799 subjects who were not on antihypertensive therapy and there were 109 (58%) of 188 strokes among the 2163 users on antihypertensive therapy. Of the 188 strokes, 111 (59%) occurred among individuals who had systolic blood pressures over 140 at baseline.[18]

Composite index of subclinical disease
For participants without evidence of clinical cardiovascular disease at baseline, the prevalence of subclinical disease compared with no subclinical disease was associated with signifi-

cantly increased risk of incident total coronary heart disease, including CHD death and nonfatal MI and angina, for both men and women. For individuals with subclinical disease, the increased risk of total coronary heart disease was two-fold for men and 2.5-fold for women. The increased risk for total mortality was 2.9-fold for men and 1.7-fold for women. This increase in risk changed little after adjustment for other risk factors, including the lipoproteins, blood pressure, smoking and diabetes (Figure 5.6).

Incidence of fatal CHD over 2.4 years was

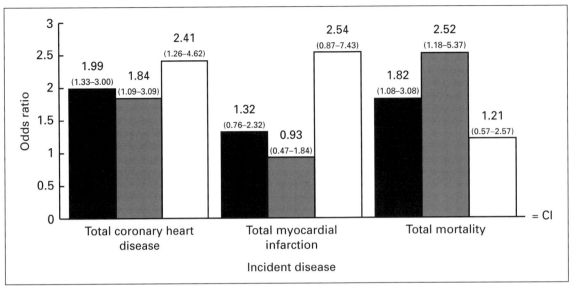

Figure 5.6
Multivariate assessment of group differences in incident clinical cardiovascular diseases: subclinical disease compared with no subclinical disease group. (■, Men and women combined; ■, men only; □, women only.) Confidence intervals are given beneath the odds ratios which appear above the columns. Included in the model are age, systolic blood pressure, LDL cholesterol level, HDL cholesterol level, triglyceride level, diabetes, hypertension, weight and current smoking status. From Kuller et al[19] with permission.

4.2% in men with a history of clinical disease, 1.0% for those with subclinical disease, and 0.4% for those with no subclinical disease. In women, the incidence of definite fatal CHD was 2.9% for those with clinical cardiovascular disease at entry, 0.1% for those with subclinical and none over 3 years for those who had neither subclinical nor clinical disease. For total CHD (fatal and nonfatal) incidence, the rates were 8.2% for men with subclinical disease versus 4.3% for men without subclinical disease and, for women, 3.8% for those with subclinical disease and only 1.5% for those with no subclinical disease.[19]

Measures of subclinical disease were also independently predictive of all-cause mortality. In 5-year follow-up of the original CHS cohort ($N = 5201$), the following measures were predictive of total mortality over the subsequent 5 years, adjusting for clinical history of disease, socio-economic status, health habits and functioning: brachial artery (>169 mmHg) and tibial artery (≤127 mmHg) systolic blood pressure, aortic stenosis (moderate or severe) and abnormal left ventricular ejection fraction (by echocardiography), major ECG abnormality, and stenosis of the internal carotid artery (by ultrasound) (Figure 5.7).[20]

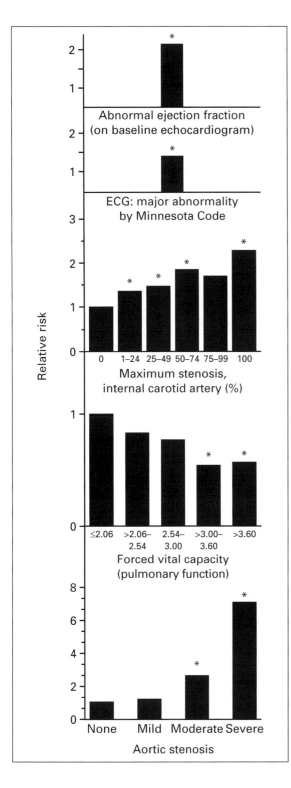

Cranial MRI examination

Ventricular size, sulci, ventricular and white matter changes and MRI

Sulci size, ventricular size and white matter signal intensity changes were graded on the cranial MRI of 3660 participants in the CHS. Sulci grade, ventricular size and white matter signal intensity changes all increased with age. Sulci grade was also greater in men and in whites compared with blacks, and was positively associated with ventricular size, but not with white matter grade. Ventricular grade was also significantly associated with age and was also substantially greater in men than women. Ventricular grade was significantly higher in whites than in blacks. Ventricular grade was independently associated with sulci grade and with white matter grade. Planimetric frontal horn ratio, the ratio of frontal horn with inner table distance, also increased with age and was greater in men but was not different between blacks and whites.[21,22]

One or more MRI infarcts, lesions greater than 3 mm, were detected in 1131 of the 3647 participants (31%). MRI infarcts were detected in 68% of 250 participants with prior clinically recognized stroke and in 28% (961) of the 3397 without a prior history of stroke. Prevalence of MRI infarcts increased with age. There was no difference in prevalence of MRI infarcts between black and white participants. MRI infarcts were also associated with systolic blood pressure, cigarette smoking and diabetes (Figure 5.8).[23]

Figure 5.7
Associations with 5-year mortality from the Cardiovascular Health Study: relative risks of total mortality. *P < 0.005.

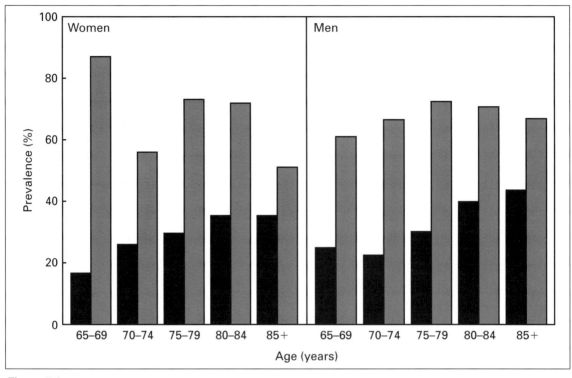

Figure 5.8
Prevalence of MRI infarct by sex, age and prior stroke (■, no prior stroke; ■, prior stroke). From Price et al[29] with permission.

Higher white matter grade, greater ventricular scores and number of infarcts on MRI were related to low scores on cognitive function tests and decline in scores between years 5–7. Prevalent stroke was associated with lower cognitive scores, and incident stroke after MRI year 5–7 was associated with a substantial decline in cognitive scores (Figure 5.9).[6]

In preliminary analysis, MRI infarct-like lesions were associated with an increased risk of clinical stroke.

Discussion

The initial findings from the Cardiovascular Health Study have provided a better interpretation of the determinants of cardiovascular and cerebrovascular disease in the elderly.

The implications of these results from the CHS are many and important. There are potential pharmacological and surgical therapies that can reduce the risk of clinical vascular disease and disability. The most effective use of these therapies requires the identification of high-risk individuals (i.e. older age is probably the most important risk factor for

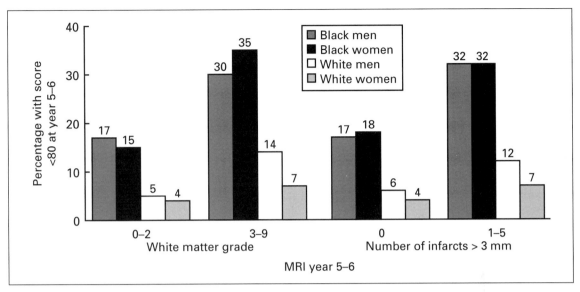

Figure 5.9
*Relationship between MRI variables and 3MSE at years 5–6 by race and with no prior history of stroke.
(■, Black men; ■, black women; □, white men; ▨, white women.)*

vascular disease). However, even in older individuals, the risk of MI or stroke per year is probably still too low to recommend universal drug therapy (such as lipid-lowering drugs or antiplatelet aggregating agents) for all older individuals. In the CHS, for example, there was some suggestion that use of aspirin therapy in individuals without cardiovascular disease or at high-risk might be deleterious.[18] The addition of measures of subclinical disease that may double or triple the risk will identify very high-risk populations of both men and women who might well be candidates for more aggressive (especially pharmacological) therapies.

Performance-based measures of physical functioning, such as 6-minute timed walk,

may provide a further potential measure of cardiovascular status and risk of disease. Performance-based measures, as well as certain subclinical measures (such as ankle–brachial blood pressure and electrocardiography) can be completed in a doctor's office, at low cost, and are powerful predictors of clinical vascular disease. Some of the other subclinical measurements are primarily technician-driven and can be done fairly quickly, noninvasively, and at relatively reasonable cost with high levels of reproducibility. It is likely, in the elderly, that the prevalence of subclinical disease is a marker of the long-term effects of risk factors (such as LDL cholesterol, systolic blood pressure, etc.) and it is an important determinant of vascular disease. Thus, intervening on subclinical disease may be more powerful than attempting to base interventions strictly on levels of traditional risk factors. Therefore, even though LDL cholesterol may not be a major risk factor for cardiovascular disease in the elderly, reduction of LDL cholesterol by stabilizing plaques, especially among individuals with subclinical disease, can reduce the incidence of cardiovascular disease.[24] Thus, the selection of older individuals for lipid lowering may be better if based on measures of subclinical and clinical vascular disease rather than on LDL cholesterol levels only. Further evaluation of this important question is clearly indicated.

Similarly, individuals with elevated systolic blood pressure benefit from decrease in the blood pressure.[25] However, individuals with elevated systolic blood pressure and subclinical disease may be at very high risk and the potential benefits of more aggressive lowering of systolic blood pressure, both the level at which therapy is introduced and the reduction to lower levels by treatment, may be of considerable value. Again, this issue needs further evaluation.

The association of measures of inflammation, thrombosis and fibrinolysis with increased risk, especially in the short-term, may offer a new approach to identify very high risk older individuals or candidates for therapies. With the development of new therapies to prevent thrombosis and increase fibrinolysis,[26] there is an opportunity to use some of these new tests to identify individuals at very high risk and test the efficacy of some of these new therapies in individuals without clinical cardiovascular disease but with subclinical disease.

The association of subclinical brain changes on the MRI with possible dementia may offer an approach to prevent, or at least delay, the onset of some dementia in the population and, in fact, aggressive therapy to prevent vascular disease may be the best approach we currently have to reduce dementia in the community.[27-29]

The risk factors for MRI infarction and white matter grade abnormalities are similar to other risk factors for both stroke and cardiovascular disease. Thus, it is important to determine whether aggressive therapy to modify risk factors related to vascular disease, possibly in combination with anti-inflammatory agents and, perhaps, antiplatelet aggregating agents or anticoagulants, could prevent or slow the progression of dementia in these high-risk individuals.

Finally, and worrisome, the majority of strokes still occur among individuals with systolic blood pressures of 140 mmHg and over and the highest attributable risk of stroke and MI is still due to systolic hypertension. Diabetes is the second most important attributable risk, especially for myocardial infarction. Effective hypertensive therapy is, therefore, still not reaching the at-risk population, at least in terms of lowering systolic blood pressures below 140 mmHg. Diabetes mellitus is also a major determinant of MI and stroke in the CHS. There remains an important need to determine the efficacy of blood glucose lowering in clinical trials, as well as modification of other risk factors to reduce the prevalence of macrovascular disease, including MI and stroke, among non-insulin-dependent older diabetics. The results of the Cardiovascular Health Study provide an important document for more effective therapies in older individuals.

Acknowledgements

This study was supported by contracts NO1-HC-85079, NO1-HC-85080, NO1-HC-85082, NO1-HC-85083, NO1-HC-85084, NO1-HC-85085, NO1-HC-85086, and NO1 to 9 from the National Heart, Lung, and Blood Institute.

References

1. Kuller L, Borhani N, Furberg C et al. Prevalence of subclinical atherosclerosis and cardiovascular disease and association with risk factors in the Cardiovascular Health Study. *Am J Epidemiol* (1994) **139**:1164–79.

2. Manolio TA, Ettinger WH, Tracy RP et al, for the CHS Collaborative Research Group. Epidemiology of low cholesterol levels in older adults. *Circulation* (1993) **87**:728–37.

3. Franklin SS, Sutton-Tyrrell K, Belle SH et al. The importance of pulsatile components of hypertension in predicting carotid stenosis in older adults. *J Hypertens* (1997) **15**:1143–50.

4. Tracy RP, Lemaitre RN, Psaty BM et al. Relationship of C-reactive protein to risk of cardiovascular disease in the elderly. Results from the Cardiovascular Health Study and the Rural Health Promotion Project. *Arterioscler Thromb Vasc Biol* (1997) **17**:1121–7.

5. Fried LP, Borhani NO, Enright P et al. The Cardiovascular Health Study: design and rationale. *Ann Epidemiol* (1991) **1**:263–76.

6. Kuller LH, Shemanski L, Manolio T et al. Relationship between Apo E, MRI findings, and cognitive function in the Cardiovascular Health Study. *Stroke* (1998) **29**:388–98.

7. Manolio TA, Kronmal RA, Burke GL et al. Magnetic resonance abnormalities and cardiovascular disease in older adults. The Cardiovascular Health Study. *Stroke* (1994) **25**:318–27.

8. Bild DE, Fitzpatrick A, Fried LP et al. Age-related trends in cardiovascular morbidity and physical functioning in the elderly: the Cardiovascular Health Study. *J Am Geriatr Soc* (1993) **41**:1047–56.

9. Newman AB, Siscovick DS, Manolio TA et al. Ankle–arm index as a marker of atherosclerosis in the Cardiovascular Health Study. *Circulation* (1992) **70**:1147–51.

10. O'Leary DH, Polak JF, Kronmal RA et al. Thickening of the carotid wall. A marker for athenosclerosis in the elderly? *Stroke* (1996) **27**:224–31.

11. O'Leary DH, Polak JF, Kronmal RA et al, on behalf of the CHS Collaborative Research Group. Distribution and correlates of sonographically detected carotid artery disease in the Cardiovascular Health Study. *Stroke* (1992) **23**:1752–60.

12. Furberg CD, Manolio TA, Psaty BM et al. Major electrocardiographic abnormalities in persons aged 65 years and older (the Cardiovascular Health Study). *Am J Cardiol* (1992) **69**:1329–35.

13. Gardin JM, Siscovick D, Anton-Culver H et al. Sex, age, and disease affect echocardiographic left ventricular mass and systolic function in the free-living elderly. The Cardiovascular Health Study. *Circulation* (1995) **91**:1739–48.

14. Alcorn HG, Wolfson SK Jr, Sutton-Tyrrell K et al. Risk factors for abdominal aortic aneurysms in older adults enrolled in the Cardiovascular Health Study. *Arterioscler Thromb Vasc Biol* (1996) **16**:963–70.

15. Kuller L, Fisher L, McClelland R et al. Differences in prevalence and risk factors for subclinical vascular disease among black and white participants in the Cardiovascular Health Study. *Arterioscler Thromb Vasc Biol* (1998) **18**:283–93.

16. Psaty BM, Furberg CD, Bild D et al. Traditional risk factors and sub-clinical-disease measures as predictors of myocardial infarction (MI) in older adults: the Cardiovascular Health Study (CHS). *Can J Cardiol* (1997) **13**(Supplement B):271B (abst).

17. Gottdiener JS, Shemanski L, Gardin JM et al. Echocardiographic predictors of incident congestive heart failure in elderly without prevalent cardiovascular disease: the Cardiovascular Health Study. *Circulation* (1996) **94**(Supplement 1):I-691 (abst).

18. Manolio TA, Kronmal RA, Burke GL et al. Short-term predictors of incident stroke in older adults. *Stroke* (1996) **27**:1479–86.

19. Kuller LH, Shemanski L, Psaty BM et al. Subclinical disease as an independent risk factor

for cardiovascular disease. *Circulation* (1996) **92**:720–6.

20. Fried LP, Kronmal RA, Newman AB et al. Risk factors for 5-year mortality in older adults: the Cardiovascular Health Study. *JAMA* (1998) **279**:585–92.

21. Yue NC, Arnold AM, Longstreth WT et al. Sulcal, ventricular, and white matter changes at MR imaging in the aging brain: data from the Cardiovascular Health Study. *Radiology* (1997) **202**:33–9.

22. Longstreth WT, Manolio TA, Arnold A et al. Clinical correlates of white matter findings on cranial magnetic resonance imaging of 3301 elderly people. The Cardiovascular Health Study. *Stroke* (1996) **27**:1274–82.

23. Bryan RN, Wells SW, Miller TJ et al. Infarct-like lesions in the brain: prevalence and anatomic characteristics at MR imaging of the elderly: data from the Cardiovascular Health Study. *Radiology* (1997) **202**:47–54.

24. Shepherd J, Cobbe SM, Ford I et al, for the West of Scotland Coronary Prevention Study Group. Prevention of coronary heart disease with pravastatin in men with hypercholesterolemia. *N Engl J Med* (1995) **333**:1301–7.

25. SHEP Cooperative Research Group. Prevention of stroke by antihypertensive drug treatment in older persons with isolated systolic hypertension: final results of the Systolic Hypertension in the Elderly Program (SHEP). *JAMA* (1991) **265**:3255–64.

26. Cannon CP, McCabe CH, Borzak S et al. A randomized trial of an oral platelet glycoprotein IIb/IIIa antagonist, sibrafiban, in patients after an acute coronary syndrome: results of the TIMI 12 trial. *Circulation* (1998) **97**:340–9.

27. Tatemichi TK, Foulkes MA, Mohr JP et al. Dementia in stroke survivors in the stroke data bank cohort. Prevalence, incidence, risk factors, and computer tomographic findings. *Stroke* (1990) **21**:858–66.

28. Hachinski V. Preventable senility: a call for action against the vascular dementias. *Lancet* (1992) **340**:645–8.

29 Price TR, Manolio TA, Kronmal RA et al. Silent brain infarction on magnetic resonance imaging and neurological abnormalities in community-dwelling older individuals. The Cardiovascular Health Study. *Stroke* (1997) **28**:1158–64.

6

Geriatric medicine and cardiology: where the disciplines intersect

Focus on geriatric assessment

Paul E McGann and William R Hazzard

Case history: 72 year old man

A 72 year old man was brought to the hospital emergency room because of 'funny spells'. He had a strongly positive history for coronary artery disease with a totally occluded right coronary artery and a 70% circumflex lesion treated with percutaneous transluminal coronary angioplasty (PTCA) in 1992. Nonobstructive disease of the left anterior descending coronary artery was also visualized. The patient's ongoing exertional angina was treated with Toprol XL, 50 mg p.o. q.d.; he also received Pravachol, 20 mg p.o. q.d. for hypercholesterolemia, and ASA 325 mg p.o. q.d. History as obtained in the emergency department was somewhat ambiguous, but because of the question of intermittent chest pain and the possibility of a significant cardiac dysrhythmia, the patient was admitted to the cardiology service with ECG monitoring. Initial physical examination revealed a left carotid bruit and a harsh grade 3/6 systolic murmur heard over the entire precordium with radiation to the base, neck and apex. Neurological examination was normal. Initial twelve-lead ECGs revealed normal sinus rhythm; the patient was ruled out for an acute myocardial infarction. However, he manifested labile blood pressure, including both hyper- and hypotension, and had episodes of chest discomfort which were poorly described to floor nursing personnel.

Because of ongoing concern about the possibility of unstable coronary disease, the patient was taken to coronary angiography on the second hospital day. This revealed patent coronary artery grafts with no evidence of progression of his coronary artery disease in the last 3 years. The evening following his angiogram, the patient became acutely disoriented. He had paranoid ideation centered around the concept that the nurses were playing illegal card games at the desk. His interpretation of the events on the busy cardiology ward caused him to become fearful and agitated. When approached by a nurse who tried to reassure him and reorient him to his surroundings, he became so frightened that he lashed out at and pushed and shoved her in an effort to escape from the ward. News of these events greatly concerned his wife and daughter. The caregiver stress that resulted precipitated a request from the family for a flurry of consultative opinions. Requests for both neurology and geriatric medicine consultations were submitted on Friday afternoon prior to a long weekend.

The neurology consultant emphasized the cause of the acute cognitive decompensation following coronary angiography. No focal neurological deficits were demonstrated. It was suggested that the acute decompensation might be related to the medications administered during the arteriogram.

Cognitive and functional assessment by the geriatrician revealed serious cognitive deficits, including those antedating hospitalization. History taken from the family indicated a decline in memory and instrumental activities of daily living function over the preceding 6–12 months. Significant caregiver stress and a substantial amount of denial on the part of the wife was identified. Family members who requested the consultation resisted the notion that the patient suffered from a permanent and progressive brain disease. Only after an hour of counselling did the famile accede to the idea that the events observed in the hospital may have been linked to the abnormal behaviors observed over the preceding year at home, with the acute illness and hospitalization causing the behaviors so distressing to the staff, family, and, in all likelihood, the patient. A plan was established to complete the diagnostic work-up of the identified dementia as an outpatient. Concrete arrangements were made with the daughter to further investigate the patient in the ambulatory care clinic in the Center on Aging. After discussion with the attending cardiologist, it was decided that it was in the patient's best interest to be discharged from the hospital that same day. Arrangements were made to complete cardiological investigations for an underlying arrhythmia or autonomic nervous system disorder as an outpatient. No new medications were started. (To be continued.)

Introduction

The preceding case illustrates clinical challenges that are becoming more common in routine cardiology practice as our population ages. From the geriatrician's perspective, the patient described is actually a relatively young, robust man. Numerous other examples may be found on cardiology wards and in coronary care units of patients 20 or even 30 years his senior with substantially more complicated medical and cognitive histories. Medical students, postgraduate medical trainees and subspecialists often find themselves confronted with clinical challenges related to the multiple complex processes associated with aging for which their undergraduate and postgraduate training has ill-prepared them. Despite the limitations of our medical education system in this regard, the graying of America is a well-established, irreversible trend, and practising cardiologists today already face complicated, medical, cognitive and ethical dilemmas with respect to the management of their sick, frail, elderly patients. This chapter provides a brief overview of particular approaches to these complex problems that have evolved within the growing discipline of geriatric medicine in the USA over the last 20 years.

The concept of geriatric assessment: a keystone for successful management of the frail elderly patient

The discipline of geriatric medicine is difficult for most subspecialists and even for many generalists to understand. The training that qualifies the board-certified internist or family physician to take the American Board of Internal Medicine–American Board of Family Practice (ABIM–ABFP) examination in geriatric medicine is not formally described as subspecialty training, nor is the certificate awarded a subspecialty certificate; rather it is a 'certificate of added qualifications' (CAQ), reflecting the close and ongoing relationship between the bodies of knowledge and practice between the parent specialty and the domain of geriatric medicine. Currently over 7000 board-certified internists and family physicians hold this certificate, the vast majority by virtue of having passed the certifying examination jointly developed by both boards beginning in 1988 but without having had formal fellowship training in geriatrics (via 'grandfathering'). Since 1994, however, only those candidates who have satisfactorily completed at least a year of training in an accredited fellowship program have been eligible to take the examination. Despite the fact that other 'CAQs' are available (such as in critical care medicine), it is not commonly appreciated what added skills those physicians who have focused in geriatrics may have acquired during their training. These added skills are perhaps best illustrated by what many of its practitioners regard as the highest form of expression of the contribution of this discipline: comprehensive geriatric assessment.

Comprehensive geriatric assessment is a process and a philosophy more than it is a body of knowledge.[1] It is a way of approaching the complex interacting medical problems of frail older adults such that the difficulties that are troubling to them and their caregivers are adequately tabulated, appropriate patient and family education is delivered, and, most importantly, a plan is developed to enable the patient and caregivers to cope as best as possible with multiple chronic, often progressive and irreversible illnesses. Comprehensive geriatric assessment is successful when the patient and family are able to cope with these chronic disease states after the assessment in ways that are much more productive and adaptive and when the assessment is translated into an effective, coordinated plan of management through time.

Over the last 20–50 years it has become clear that physicians by themselves are rarely able or willing to complete such a comprehensive assessment, which by definition is multidisciplinary. Neither are there compensation structures available in the US in the fee-for-service arena to reimburse them and their team members adequately for these activities. Nevertheless, the first rule of geriatric assessment is that it can only be adequately developed with resources available to enable a multidisciplinary evaluation. Without recognition by health-care providers of its essential role in the management of frail elderly patients in the most cost-effective manner and their provision of cross-subsidies from better funded lines of clinical service, such an essential multidisciplinary assessment is not feasible. Thus, each health-care system that has developed comprehensive geriatric assessment has done so with a unique combination of multidisciplinary resources. Nor is a single model of such assessment appropriate to all patients and all circumstances. Indeed, it is difficult to specify a single or ideal composition for a multidisciplinary geriatric team. In the authors' experience, however, the essential members of such a team usually include a physician, nurse and social worker, each with special training in geriatrics. Other team members often added to this process include, but are not limited to, occupational therapists, physiotherapists, speech therapists, recreation therapists, pastoral care workers, pharmacists, dieticians, respiratory therapists, and nondiscipline-specific case managers. The mission of such a team is to identify the multiple problems of the frail older individual. Furthermore, while identification of such problems is necessary, without their synthesis and translation into a coordinated plan for action through time, identification is not sufficient for clinical success. The many problems must also be explained in a way that makes sense to the patient and/or caregivers. This is a familiar theme to physicians, who have been trained to recognize and identify diseases. However, the physician who ventures into the realm of geriatrics must be especially prepared to identify and manage problems that do not fit into traditional diagnostic categories. These problems often fall into other realms of human life experience, which can be grouped under functional, psychological and social categories. The problems in these other realms are often perceived by the patient and family as much more pressing and important than the medical issues.

Experience has shown that it is not just the identification, tabulation and explanation of problems that is essential to effective geriatric assessment, it is equally important to identify resources and strengths. Without their identification, the family and even the health-care team can frequently be overwhelmed by feelings of helplessness in dealing with what are often formidable collections of problems that are seemingly irreversible and threaten to exhaust their coping skills. Identification of resources and strengths ultimately enables the patient and family to cope with chronic disease states. This is one area where nonphysician team members often excel and teach their physician colleagues much that is of value in the healing process.

Armed with the information collected in the multidisciplinary format, the team then develops a coordinated care plan, using all the resources in the community and emphasizing continuity of care, which then, if successful, enables the patient to remain as independent and with as high a quality of life as possible for as long as possible.

The essential components of this geriatric assessment are shown in Table 6.1.

Nonphysician team members approach the process in somewhat different ways, but these four main activities are those with which physicians must be conversant in order to participate as valuable members of the geriatric team.

1. Problem identification (multisystem)
2. Functional assessment
3. Medication review (for appropriateness and potential elimination)
4. Coordinated, multidisciplinary care plan construction

Table 6.1
Comprehensive geriatric assessment: essence of the process

Relevance to cardiology

These basic principles are clearly of central, everyday importance for physicians who pursue careers in nursing homes and subacute care units, but subspecialists in internal medicine (as well as specialists in nonmedical disciplines) often have a difficult time linking the principles of geriatric assessment to their busy practice in patients with diseases of the organ system of their specialty. What makes these considerations relevant to cardiology?

This question has many answers, but the answers provided below focus on considerations of the epidemiology of illness in the late twentieth century.

The first fact, of course, is that heart disease is the number-one cause of mortality in the elderly, and the relationship between age and cardiovascular mortality rises exponentially with advancing age beginning in the 30s and 40s.[2] Everyone knows that the population is aging and that heart disease is by far the most common cause of serious, mortal events in old age. However, not only is heart disease important as the leading cause of death in old age, diseases of the cardiovascular system in general, notably stroke and heart failure, also comprise the number-one cause of long-term disability in the elderly.[3] Thus, even when patients are not dying of cardiovascular diseases, they often become very disabled, and it is this disability that often gives rise to difficulties in chronic disease management.

One particular aspect of vascular disease of the brain, which perhaps is more debilitating than any other, is its contribution to the syndrome of dementia, which permeates everything a practicing geriatrician does in his or her daily work. Unlike the degenerative dementias (principally Alzheimer's disease), for which significant preventive intervention is not yet available, these dementias with a vascular component have a substantial potential for prevention through control of disease processes such as hypertension and dysrhythmias. There is now overwhelming evidence, for example, that proper treatment of atrial fibrillation can significantly reduce the incidence of stroke, and, by inference, multi-infarct dementia.[4-10]

Congestive heart failure is also now recognized as an important contributor to both morbidity and mortality in the elderly.[11] It is the number-one Diagnosis Related Group (DRG) in the elderly for admission to acute-care hospitals. Its often multiple etiologies (e.g. systolic dysfunction secondary to ischemic heart disease and diastolic dysfunction secondary to aging and hypertension) frequently coincide with multiple comorbidities in noncardiovascular domains (including those reflecting iatrogenesis) and require the most detailed and sophisticated comprehensive geriatric assessment for optimal management.

Finally, the dementias in general, whether vascular or degenerative in origin, are of epidemic proportion among elderly people and will only grow in their burden as the number of people surviving into advanced old age grows dramatically over the next 50 years. It is estimated that up to 50% of community-dwelling people over the age of 85 suffer from significant cognitive impairment.[12] Thus, as people live into even more advanced ages this prevalence will increase even more. As cardiologists encounter ever greater numbers of people aged between 80 and 100 in their practices, they must have at least basic skills in identifying dementia and its differentiation from delirium, with which it often coexists.

How a complete geriatric assessment is done

When geriatricians, in conjunction with other members of the multidisciplinary team, undertake comprehensive geriatric assessment, they typically focus on four major domains of investigation. These domains are shown in Table 6.2.

Medical

The collection of medical data on the geriatric patient presenting to the physician for a disease of the cardiovascular system should properly focus on all aspects of examination in

1. Medical
2. Functional
3. Psychological
4. Social

Table 6.2
Four major domains of investigation during geriatric assessment

which the cardiologist acquired skills during the course of internal medicine and cardiology subspecialty training. There are four additional areas of expertise that have relevance to the complete understanding of vascular disease in the elderly patient. These are:

1. An analysis of gait and transfers
2. Examination of the neurological system
3. Examination of visual function
4. Examination of hearing function

The cardiologist of the twenty-first century should be familiar with basic methods to collect physical examination data in these areas, despite the fact that they do not necessarily directly impinge on disease of the cardiovascular system. The cardiologist's knowledge in this area should be that of a manager of complex medical illness rather than the knowledge of an organ-system subspecialist. The specific geriatric knowledge-base acquired during fellowship training (mandated by the 1998 revision of listed requirements by the Residency Review Committee—Internal Medicine (RRC–IM)) should include awareness of the major causes of disability in elderly people related to these four medical areas. More importantly, the cardiologist must also have knowledge of how other members of a multidisciplinary health-care team might be able to help in the detection and screening of disability in these areas, as well as the management of any disability that might be uncovered by such examinations. This is particularly evident when discussing common clinical methods for screening for visual and hearing impairment in elderly people. These screening techniques can be easily incorporated into an office practice by nonphysician health-care professionals.

Many physicians find the neurological examination difficult, and it is unlikely that sufficiently detailed and accurate neurological data will be collected by nonphysician health care professionals. Therefore, it behooves the cardiologist who looks after geriatric patients to become proficient during fellowship training in the rapid assessment of neurological function, especially gait and transfer ability, in the elderly. Analysis of difficulties in gait and transfer ability also relates to a good neurological examination, but physiotherapists can also help for the less medical aspects of the gait examination.

Functional

Functional assessment of all geriatric patients, no matter what the organ system of principal focus and attention, is a mandatory part of understanding the impact of the illness on the patient's quality of life. All practicing physicians, including cardiology subspecialists, should be quite familiar with the terminology and methods of assessing the categories of human functional performance as described by the acronyms: BADL, IADL and AADL. These categories are explained in Table 6.3. Again, it may not necessarily be the case that the physician him- or herself will collect the functional data from the patient or the family, but the health-care delivery system must be developed in such a way that these functional data are available in at least synopsis form to the physician as he or she incorporates the treatment plan into the lives of patients and their families. Nonphysician health-care professionals, or in this case even nonhealth-care professional secretarial or administrative staff, can be trained to collect simple functional data in a reliable fashion.

Psychological

In dealing with the geriatric patient with cardiovascular disease, psychological and often psychiatric assessment is of the utmost importance. Detailed multiaxial DSM IV diagnostic

Categories (abbreviation)	Examples	Consequences of serious deficits	Published methods of assessment
Basic activities of daily living (BADL)	Feeding Bathing Toileting/continence Dressing Transfers	Puts patient at risk for institutional placement	Katz ADL Scale[14] Barthel ADL Scale[15]
Instrumental activities of daily living (IADL)	Shopping Driving Telephoning Financial management Housework Taking medication	Patient requires weekly support to remain independent at home	Lawton IADL Scale[16] Fillenbaum IADL Scale[17]
Advanced activities of daily living (AADL)	Booking complex travel itinerary Executive-level work or consultation Lecturing Complex or intellectually demanding hobbies Participating in exercise program	Interferes with quality of life Problems are generally 'early warning indicators' for cognitive loss or depression	Guttman Scale for Elderly[18] Reuben AADL Scale[19]

Table 6.3
Categories of human functional performance of importance to geriatric medicine[13]

interviews by the cardiologist are neither practical nor desirable when dealing with the geriatric patient with cardiovascular disease unless specifically required for management; here geropsychiatric consultation may be indicated. Psychological aspects of the evaluation with which all cardiologists must be familiar and in which skills must be developed are detection of the major disorders of cognition and affect. The two principal cognitive disorders that cardiologists will encounter in their practice are delirium and dementia. The most significant disorder of affect, one which is very common in geriatric cardiology practice, is depression. Depression is a treatable disease with a known biological basis and is very common in medically ill elderly patients. The treatment of depression has been revolutionized recently with the introduction of new classes of therapeutic agents.[20-22] The practicing cardiologist must be familiar with the recognition and identification of depression in elderly patients as well as with the full repertoire of treatment modalities for this illness. The reason it is so important that the cardiologist understand depression in elderly patients is because the disease may be completely reversible, and proper treatment can have a dramatic and positive impact on the patient's quality of life. Also, all known treatment modalities for depression have direct impact on the health and function of the cardiovascular system, and the consulting psychiatrist will depend on the cardiologist for reliable advice when selecting the proper therapeutic modality and selection of alternate modalities when initial selections prove to be ineffective or not well tolerated by the patient. Any of the psychological disorders of old age: delirium, dementia or depression, when present in a patient with cardiovascular disease, can have dramatic impact on the compliance and response of a patient to standard cardiovascular therapy. The cardiologist must be aware of the potential for delirium, dementia and depression to cause treatment failure in his/her elderly patients so that proper corrective actions can be taken to ensure that patients receive the cardiovascular treatment that is being prescribed for them. In the absence of such an assessment even the most advanced cardiovascular knowledge base will not result in optimal clinical outcomes.

Social

Although the practicing cardiologist might not have sufficient time to collect all the primary social information on geriatric patients, these data are equally as important as the psychological data in terms of the ultimate disposition of the patient. Proper treatment cannot be delivered to frail elderly patients without extensive knowledge of living arrangements, financial security and the social support network. Office staff can be trained to collect this information for physicians so it is available at the time of development of a treatment plan. Moreover, such information tends to be relatively stable over time (the death of a spouse or a change in living circumstances are notable exceptions) and hence need not be elicited at frequent intervals other than for changes.

Two other social issues are of great importance to the care of the geriatric patient with cardiovascular disease. The first is the identification and treatment of caregiver stress and the second is the development of advance directives, hopefully before the onset of critical illness. Currently, cardiologists often encounter geriatric patients in whom advance directives have not been established prior to critical illness. In this situation cardiologists must develop expertise in skilfully eliciting advance directive information at the time of critical illness. This is considerably more challenging than obtaining this information in advance of the onset of the crisis.

Caregiver stress was well illustrated in the clinical vignette which began this chapter. Caregiver stress is important because it diminishes both patient and caregiver quality of life and it frequently also interferes with the ability to deliver appropriate medical treatment to the geriatric patient and his or her family. Caregiver stress also transmits conflict and disruption to the health-care team and causes anxiety and nonproductive, nonhealing interactions during the course of hospitalizations and other encounters with the health-care system. In its worst manifestations, severe caregiver stress can result in litigious behavior on the part of the family, the majority of which is preventable.

Advance directives is a complex topic, the complete discussion of which is beyond the scope of this chapter. There are many good guides available to the entire spectrum of decisions related to advance directives in the elderly to which the interested reader is referred.[23–29] A more complex area, which has a smaller body of literature, is the determination of advance directive information during the crisis situation of an acute hospital or intensive care unit admission.

How is this relevant to me?

What is a practicing cardiologist to do?

Geriatric medicine is a field riddled with complexity. It concerns every organ system of the body, it involves all health-care professionals, and it impinges on aspects of human behavior and chronic disease management and ethical issues of death and dying to an extent greater than that historically characteristic of other, more focused subspecialties. One of the aspects of geriatric medicine that organ-system or disease-based subspecialists have had difficulty appreciating is this very quality of not being focused in any one particular area. At a given time one might be talking about antibiotic selection for parapneumonic effusions and empyemas and 2 minutes later about how to do a home assessment by an occupational or physiotherapist to put in grab bars for a patient with atrial fibrillation, multi-infarct dementia and unclear advance directives. Out of this chaotic array of complex decision-making tasks in geriatrics, how is it possible to identify manageable sections of knowledge that will be useful to the cardiologist and upon which the cardiology fellow can focus during his/her highly technical and demanding period of training?

The answers to these questions are not simple, but experience has taught that the common principles and philosophies that cardiologists could incorporate into their regular practice without becoming geriatricians include the following 'pearls of wisdom':

1. Recognize dementia;
2. Recognize (better, anticipate) delirium;
3. Know when your patients suffer functional impairment;
4. Recognize and acknowledge caregiver stress;
5. Minimize medication;
6. Establish advance directives for health care;
7. When faced with a difficult intervention choice, focus primary decision-making on quality rather than quantity of life and resist the urge to collect yet more quantitative data unless they will materially assist in management with that focus;
8. Teach your team how to 'think geriatrics';
9. Learn, respect and use your local geriatric health-care delivery system;
10. Insist that your complex, frail geriatric patients have regular contact with a

primary-care physician with interest, training and experience in caring for this special population of patients.

Epilogue for the case

The attending cardiologist for the 72 year old man described in the introduction to this chapter was pleased to have advice on Friday afternoon from both his neurology and geriatric medicine colleagues. Particularly after the investment of counseling time by the geriatrician, but also because of the reassurance of the neurologist that the patient was not 'going crazy', the family was persuaded that the best course of action was, in fact, to discharge the patient from the hospital immediately. This avoided prescription of new, potentially 'deliriogenic' medication, and achieved high patient satisfaction by respecting the patient's most intense wish, which was to leave the threatening environment of the hospital ward. Both cardiologist and neurologist agreed that no immediately threatening disorder of either the heart or the brain would make his return home unsafe. However, without the functional and cognitive assessment of the geriatrician, the fears of the family would very likely have prevented discharge and resulted in prescriptions of additional 'anti-anxiety' or sedating medication which could have made the situation worse.

Discharge from the hospital was uneventful. The patient returned to his home approximately 1 hour from the University Medical Center, and resumed primary care with his local medical doctor.

Under nonemergency, nonthreatening conditions, he returned 1 week later to the Multidisciplinary Geriatric Assessment Clinic at the Center on Aging. Here, under controlled circumstances, a comprehensive geriatric assessment was completed. Significant cognitive impairment was identified, which, by history, clearly antedated the recent hospitalization. The patient was screened for the so-called 'reversible' causes of dementia, and none was found. A diagnosis of early Alzheimer's disease was made and the patient was started on a new central acetyl cholinesterase inhibitor now available for the treatment of this disease (donepezil, 5 mg *q.h.s.*). The issue of caregiver stress was addressed by counseling with the clinic social worker. She organized participation of the family in a local Alzheimer's disease support group. Advance directives for health care were established with the patient, with the family's active participation. The occupational therapy department performed an on-road driving assessment (which the patient failed) and the patient and family were counseled about the inadvisability of driving. Important implications of this disease on the couple's financial well-being were addressed by counselors in the legal clinic for the elderly at the Center on Aging. Options for intelligent asset management were discussed now, years before the necessity for long-term institutional care would arise, to enable advanced planning for these eventualities, which can literally drive even the most well-off couples into financial ruin. Genetic implications of the illness were discussed with the couple's children who expressed considerable anxiety arising from their reading about apo-lipoprotein E4 testing gleaned from Internet searches. Family questions about new and experimental treatment approaches to dementing illnesses were answered. Questions were specifically addressed about aspirin, hormones, Tacrine, NSAIDs, and antioxidants such as vitamins C and E.

As can be readily appreciated, all 10 principles described in the previous section are illustrated by this case. Interestingly, the cause for the initial symptoms ('pre-syncope') that led to the original hospitalization and cardiac catheterization was never identified. These symptoms never recurred. Although difficult to prove, the geriatric consultant entertained a hypothesis that anxiety over the patient's unrecognized cognitive disorder may actually have been partially responsible for his presentation to the emergency department on the day of admission to the cardiology service. It is very common for geriatric patients to 'somatize' cognitive deficits to problems in one or more organ system areas, especially when contact has previously been established with a subspecialty service in a large medical center. With symptoms as serious as chest pain and syncope it is always appropriate to investigate fully for organic illness, but in the absence of documentable objective evidence of disease causing ill-defined symptoms, comprehensive geriatric cognitive and functional assessment should be the next step in an elderly patient. Sometimes, as in this case, the comorbidity uncovered by this process can lead to therapeutic interventions that both reduce healthcare expenditures over the subsequent months and also improve patient and caregiver quality of life. The more practicing cardiologists can be aware of these relatively new geriatric resources, the more complete and successful care their complex elderly patients can receive, to the enhanced professional satisfaction of the cardiologist.

References

1. Solomon D et al. NIH consensus development conference statement: geriatric assessment methods for clinical decisionmaking. *J Am Geriatr Soc* (1988) **36**:342–7.

2. Siegel JS. Recent and prospective demographic trends for the elderly population and some implications for health care. In Haynes SG, Feinleib M, eds, *Second Conference on the Epidemiology of Aging.* NIH Publication No. 80-969 (Washington, DC, US Department of Health and Human Services: Bethesda, MD, 1980).

3. Roth EJ, Mueller K, Green D. Stroke rehabilitation outcome: impact of coronary artery disease. *Stroke* (1988) **19**:42–7.

4. Stroke Prevention in Atrial Fibrillation Investigators. Preliminary report of the Stroke Prevention in Atrial Fibrillation Study. *N Engl J Med* (1990) **322**:863–8.

5. Petersen P, Boysen G, Godtfredsen J et al. Placebo-controlled randomized trial of warfarin and aspirin for prevention of thromboembolic complications in chronic atrial fibrillation. The Copenhagen AFASAK Study. *Lancet* (1989) **i**:175–9.

6. The Boston Area Anticoagulation Trial for Atrial Fibrillation Investigators. *N Engl J Med* (1990) **323**:1505–11.

7. Connolly SJ, Laupacis A, Gent M et al. Canadian atrial fibrillation anticoagulation. *J Am Coll Cardiol* (1991) **18**:349–55.

8. Ezekowitz MD, Bridgers SL, James KE et al. Warfarin in the prevention of stroke associated with non-rheumatic atrial fibrillation. *N Engl J Med* (1992) **327**:1406–12.

9. EAFT (European Atrial Fibrillation Trial) Study Group. Secondary prevention in non-rheumatic atrial fibrillation transient ischaemic attack or minor stroke. *Lancet* (1993) **342**:1255–62.

10. Stroke Prevention in Atrial Fibrillation Investigators. Warfarin versus aspirin for prevention of thromboembolism in atrial fibrillation: Stroke Prevention in Atrial Fibrillation II Study. *Lancet* (1994) **343**:687–91.

11. Kannel WB. Epidemiological aspects of heart failure. *Cardiol Clin* (1989) **7**:1–9.

12. Beck JC, Benson DF, Schiebel AB et al. Dementia in the elderly: the silent epidemic. *Ann Intern Med* (1982) **97**:231–41.

13. Applegate WB, Blass JP, Williams TF. Instruments for the functional assessment of older patients. *N Engl J Med* (1990) **322**:1207–14.

14. Katz S. Progress in development of the index of ADL. *Gerontologist* (1970) **10**:20–30.

15. Maloney FI, Barthel DW. Functional evaluation: the Barthel index. *Md State Med J* (1965) 61–65.

16. Lawton MP, Brody EM. Assessment of older people: self-maintaining and instrumental activities of daily living. *Gerontologist* (1969) **9**:179–86.

17. Fillenbaum GG. Screening the elderly: a brief instrumental activities of daily living measure. *J Am Geriatr Soc* (1985) **33**:698–708.

18. Rosow I, Breslau N. A Guttman health scale for the aged. *J Gerontol* (1966) **21**:556–9.

19. Reuben DB et al. A hierarchical exercise scale to measure function at the advanced activities of daily living (AADL) level. *J Am Geriatr Soc* (1990) **38**:855–61.

20. Dunbar GC. Paroxetine in the elderly: a comparative metanalysis against standard antidepressant pharmacotherapy. *Pharmacology* (1995) **51**:137–44.

21. Preskorn SH. Recent pharmacologic advances in antidepressant therapy for the elderly. *Am J Med* (1993) **94**:2–11S.

22. Salzman C. Pharmacologic treatment of depression in the elderly. *J Clin Psychiatry* (1993) **54**:23–8.

23. Jonsen AR, Cassel C, Lo B, Perkins HS. The ethics of medicine: an annotated bibliography of recent literature. *Ann Intern Med* (1980) **92**:136.

24. Jonsen AR et al. *Clinical Ethics: A Practical Approach to Ethical Decisions in Clinical Medicine.* 3rd edn. (McGraw-Hill: New York, 1992).

25. Perkins HS. Ethics at the end of life: practical

principles for making resuscitation decisions. *J Gen Intern Med* (1986) **1:**170–6.

26. Mahowald MB. So many ways to think: an overview of approaches to ethical issues in geriatrics. *Clin Geriatr Med* (1994) **10:**403–18.

27. Deon M, Sachs GA. Advance directives and the patient self-determination act. *Clin Geriatr Med* (1994) **10:**431–44.

28. Annas GJ. The health care proxy and the living will. *N Engl J Med* (1991) **321:**1210–13.

29. Uhlman RF, Clark H, Pearlman RA et al. Medical management decisions in nursing home patients: principles and policy recommendations. *Ann Intern Med* (1987) **106:**879–85.

7

Heart failure: epidemiology, pathophysiology and management

Michael W Rich

Introduction

Heart failure is the prototypical disorder of cardiovascular aging in that it represents the confluence of age-related changes in cardiovascular structure and function in combination with an increasing prevalence of cardiovascular risk factors and diseases. Indeed, heart failure is the final common pathway arising from diverse pathophysiological influences, and it represents a distinct geriatric syndrome, in much the same way that dementia and incontinence are geriatric syndromes. Individuals over 80 years of age comprise the most rapidly growing segment of the population in many industrialized nations. Moreover, the prevalence of heart failure is highest in this age group. In this chapter, current knowledge about the epidemiology, pathophysiology, diagnosis and management of heart failure in the very elderly is reviewed.

Epidemiology

Heart failure is relatively uncommon in adults less than 45 years of age, but both the incidence and prevalence increase progressively after age 45.[1] In the Framingham Heart Study, the annual incidence of heart failure in men increased from 0.2% in the 45–54 year age group to 1.4% in individuals 75–84 years of age, and to 5.4% in those aged 85–94 years (Figure 7.1).[1] In women, the rise in incidence at older age was even more dramatic, reaching

8.5% among women 85–94 years of age.[1] Similarly, the prevalence of heart failure in the Framingham population increased from 0.8% in individuals 50–59 years of age, to 9.1% in those over the age of 80 (Figure 7.2).[1] Thus, among individuals over 80 years of age, nearly 1 in 10 has overt heart failure, and the risk of

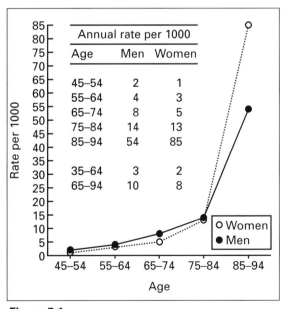

Figure 7.1
Incidence of heart failure by age and sex: 30-year follow-up from the Framingham Heart Study. (From Kannel & Belanger[1] with permission)

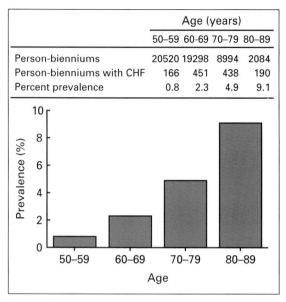

	Age (years)			
	50–59	60–69	70–79	80–89
Person-bienniums	20520	19298	8994	2084
Person-bienniums with CHF	166	451	438	190
Percent prevalence	0.8	2.3	4.9	9.1

Figure 7.2
Prevalence of heart failure by age: 34-year follow-up from the Framingham Heart Study. (From Kannel & Belanger[1] with permission)

developing new heart failure in any given year ranges from 5% in men to over 8% in women after the age of 85. Importantly, although the majority of heart failure patients under age 65 are men, women comprise 60% of all cases after age 65, and the proportion of females continues to rise with advancing age.[2,3]

Consequent to the increasing incidence and prevalence of heart failure at older age, heart failure is now the most common reason for hospitalization in adults over age 65 in the United States. In 1995, there were 872 000 hospital admissions with a primary diagnosis of heart failure.[4] Of these, 698 000 (80%) occurred in individuals over age 65. More-over, hospitalization rates for heart failure increased from 2.6 per 10 000 population in the 15–44 year age group to 208 per 10 000 in individuals over age 65, representing an 80-fold rise.[4] Although precise data on hospitalizations in octogenarians are unavailable, over 50% of all heart failure admissions occur in individuals over age 75,[5] and it is likely that as many as one-third of cases are over the age of 80.

Not only is heart failure a common cause of hospitalization, it is also a major source of chronic disability in the very elderly. Among cardiovascular disorders, heart failure is second only to hypertension as a reason for out-patient clinic visits by older adults, and heart failure accounts for up to 12 million office visits per year in the US.[2] Once again, data specific to octogenarians are unavailable, but it is likely that a sizeable proportion, perhaps one-third, of all office visits for heart failure occur in this age group.

Given the high in-patient and out-patient resource utilization rates by older heart failure patients, it is not surprising that heart failure is the most costly medical disorder in the US, with estimated annual expenditures in excess of $40 billion.[2] Indeed, expenditures for heart failure exceed those for all cancers combined by a factor of 2.4 and for all myocardial infarctions combined by a factor of 1.7.[2]

Finally, as illustrated in Figure 7.3, mortality rates for heart failure increase exponentially with advancing age in all major demographic subgroups of the US population.[6] Thus, annual mortality rates increase from less than 10 per 100 000 individuals 45–49 years of age, to over 150 per 100 000 in octogenarians. In addition, although the prognosis for patients with established heart failure is poor at all ages, with an estimated 5-year survival rate of approximately 50%, the prognosis in very elderly patients is far worse, with fewer

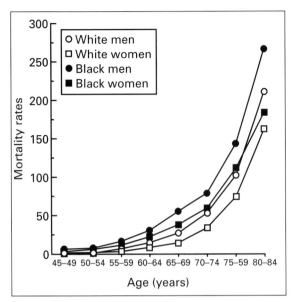

Figure 7.3
Mortality rates for congestive heart failure in the US by age, sex and race: 1990. (Adapted from Gillum[6] with permission)

tion due to reduced compliance of the aorta and other large arteries;
3. Impaired ventricular diastolic relaxation and reduced compliance with a shift in ventricular filling from early to late diastole;
4. Altered myocardial energy metabolism at the mitochondrial level.

Recalling that cardiac output, both at rest and under conditions of stress, is determined by four principal factors—heart rate, preload, afterload and contractility—it is noteworthy that each of these factors is adversely affected by one or more of the age-related changes listed above. In addition, age-related changes in other organs, particularly the kidneys, lungs and neurohumoral system, further predispose very elderly individuals to the development of heart failure (Table 7.1).[8] Finally, superimposed on these intrinsic organ system changes is an increasing prevalence of cardiovascular diseases at older age, particularly hypertension and coronary heart disease, which are major risk factors for the development of heart failure.

than 20% of patients over 80 years of age surviving for more than 5 years.[7]

Pathophysiology

As discussed in Chapters 1–3, aging is associated with extensive changes in cardiovascular structure and function that serve to diminish cardiac reserve and predispose aged individuals to the development of heart failure. From the clinical perspective, the principal effects of cardiovascular aging are as follows:[8]

1. Impaired responsiveness to beta-adrenergic stimulation;
2. Increased impedance to left ventricular ejec-

Heart failure with normal systolic function

In the past, most heart failure has been attributed to impaired left ventricular contractility (i.e. systolic dysfunction), and indeed most heart failure patients under the age of 65 have substantially reduced left ventricular ejection fractions. However, with advancing age an increasing proportion of heart failure occurs in the setting of normal left ventricular systolic function, as evidenced by an ejection fraction of 50% or greater.[9–11] This syndrome, which has been referred to as 'diastolic heart failure', occurs in up to 50% of heart failure cases after the age of 75, and it is also more common in women than in men.[12]

Diastolic heart failure in the elderly is

Kidneys
- Decreased renal blood flow and glomerular filtration rate
- Decreased concentrating and diluting capacity
- Decreased capacity to excrete sodium
- Decreased plasma renin activity and aldosterone
- Decreased responsiveness to antidiuretic hormone

Respiratory system
- Decreased vital capacity
- Decreased forced expiratory volume (FEV_1) and expiratory flow rate
- Increased ventilation/perfusion (V/Q) mismatching
- Increased chest wall stiffness
- Decreased respiratory muscle strength
- Blunted response to hypoxia, hypercapnia and acidosis
- Increased sleep-related breathing disorders

Nervous system
- Impaired thirst mechanism
- Decreased autoregulatory capacity to maintain organ perfusion, especially the central nervous system
- Impaired reflex responsiveness (e.g. baroreceptors)

Altered absorption, distribution, metabolism and excretion of most pharmacological agents

Table 7.1
Age-related changes in organ function

largely attributable to the effects of aging on left ventricular diastolic filling, as detailed in Chapters 1 and 3. Briefly, the aging heart has an impaired capacity to relax at the onset of diastole, which results in prolongation of the isovolumic relaxation period as well as a reduction in the rate of early diastolic filling.[8] In addition, the older heart is 'stiffer' (i.e. less compliant), and this further impairs filling during early and mid-diastole. These changes are compensated by augmented atrial contraction, such that a greater proportion of ventricular filling occurs at the end of diastole.[8] As a result, left ventricular stroke volume and car-diac output are preserved in the resting state. However, this occurs at the expense of an increase in left ventricular end-diastolic pressure and a reduction in cardiac reserve. Thus, older hearts are less able to respond to increased demand by further augmenting left ventricular diastolic volume and stroke volume via the Frank–Starling mechanism.[13] In addition, since the older heart functions on a steeper portion of the pressure–volume curve, modest increases in intravascular volume lead to substantial increases in intraventricular pressure which, in turn, may result in pulmonary congestion. Finally, elevated left ventricular and left atrial pressures in older individuals predispose them to the development of supraventricular arrhythmias, especially atrial fibrillation (see Chapter 21). Atrial fibrillation further reduces stroke volume because the atrial contribution to ventricular filling (atrial 'kick') is lost, and there is also a rate-related shortening of the diastolic filling period.[8] As a result, acute atrial fibrillation is a common precipitant of heart failure in aged individuals.

Diagnosis

Heart failure in octogenarians is both over-diagnosed and underdiagnosed.[14] Overdiagnosis occurs because the cardinal symptoms of heart failure, that is exertional dyspnea, fatigue, orthopnea and dependent edema, are all nonspecific and frequently occur as manifestations of other disease processes common to the elderly. For example, impaired exercise tolerance may be caused by such diverse disorders as anemia, thyroid dysfunction, acute or chronic lung disease, psychological depression, or poor physical conditioning. Similarly, peripheral edema may be due to venous or lymphatic obstruction, liver disease or renal failure. On the other hand, very elderly patients are often sedentary, and may not notice or report exertional symptoms. In addition, atypical manifestations of heart failure are more common at older age, and include restlessness, irritability, altered mental status or confusion, sleep disturbances, anorexia, abdominal discomfort, nausea and diarrhea.[14] Unless the physician maintains a high index of suspicion, the diagnosis of heart failure in older patients may be easily overlooked.

When 'classic' symptoms and signs of heart failure are present (e.g. moist pulmonary rales, elevated jugular venous pressure, an S_3 gallop, pitting edema), the diagnosis of heart failure is not difficult to establish. Frequently, however, the history and physical findings are inconclusive, and additional evaluation is necessary. The chest radiograph remains the simplest and most useful test for confirming the diagnosis. Typical findings include cardiomegaly, pulmonary vascular redistribution to the upper lung fields, bilateral pulmonary infiltrates and pleural effusions.

Once the presence of heart failure has been firmly established, the next step is to determine the primary and secondary etiologies and to identify any contributing or precipitating factors. Heart failure in octogenarians is often multifactorial in origin, with the most common etiologies being hypertension (especially systolic hypertension), coronary heart disease and valvular lesions (especially aortic stenosis and mitral regurgitation). Less common etiologies include nonischemic dilated cardiomyopathy, hypertrophic or restrictive cardiomyopathy (e.g. amyloid), high output failure (e.g. hyperthyroidism, chronic anemia) and pericardial disease. Common precipitants of heart failure include ischemia, uncontrolled hypertension, arrhythmias (especially atrial fibrillation), dietary or medication noncompliance and comorbid illnesses (e.g. pneumonia).[8] Medications and other iatrogenic factors may also contribute to the development of heart failure.[15]

In addition to a chest radiograph, an electrocardiogram and routine laboratory studies are appropriate. All patients with new-onset heart failure or an unexplained deterioration should have an echocardiogram to assess left ventricular function and to identify any valvular or pericardial abnormalities.[16] In octogenarians who are suitable candidates for invasive procedures, a stress test to evaluate for the presence and severity of myocardial ischemia may be appropriate.

Management

The primary goals of heart failure therapy are to maximize quality of life, reduce the frequency of heart failure exacerbations and prolong survival. In octogenarians, optimizing quality of life and maintaining independence are usually of greater importance than increasing longevity.

As in all heart failure patients, appropriate treatment of octogenarians is composed of three principal components: correction of the underlying etiology whenever possible; nonpharmacological measures; and the judicious use of medications. Therapies directed at the underlying etiology of heart failure include: aortic valve replacement for severe aortic stenosis or regurgitation; mitral valve repair or replacement for mitral stenosis or regurgitation; percutaneous transluminal coronary angioplasty (PTCA) or coronary artery bypass surgery for severe obstructive coronary artery disease; pacemaker implantation for severe bradycardia; antiarrhythmic drugs and/or radiofrequency ablation (RFA) for supraventricular or ventricular tachyarrhythmias; antibiotics for infective endocarditis; and correction of anemia, thiamine deficiency or thyroid dysfunction. Although octogenarians are at increased risk for major complications (including death) following percutaneous interventions (e.g. PTCA, RFA) as well as open heart procedures (e.g. coronary bypass graft surgery, valve repair or replacement), there is now good evidence that these procedures can be performed with reasonable safety in appropriately selected patients, and that long-term outcomes, in terms of both quality of life and survival, are significantly improved.[17,18] In particular, aortic valve replacement for severe aortic stenosis, which is the second most frequently performed open heart procedure in octogenarians (after coronary bypass surgery), has been associated with marked symptomatic improvement. In addition, age-adjusted survival rates are comparable to those seen in the general population.[19,20] Based on these considerations, advanced age alone is not a contraindication to invasive interventions.

Nonpharmacological measures

Heart failure in octogenarians virtually never occurs as an isolated disease process, and it is frequently associated with multiple comorbid illnesses. In addition, a variety of other behavioral and psychosocial factors may confound the management of heart failure in the very elderly (Table 7.2). Importantly, these factors contribute to over 50% of heart failure exacerbations,[21] and they are a major reason why 30–50% of all elderly patients hospitalized with heart failure are readmitted within 3–6 months of initial discharge.[22–25] It follows that optimal heart failure management must be undertaken in the context of each individual's unique set of comorbidities and environmental circumstances. To this end, a multidisciplinary approach to patient care is effective in improving clinical outcomes and quality of life, as demonstrated in several recent studies.[26–30]

In the largest of these trials, Rich et al randomized 282 elderly patients (mean age 79 years) hospitalized with heart failure to usual physician-directed care or to usual care supplemented by a nurse-directed multidisciplinary team.[26] During the 90-day period following hospital discharge, patients assigned to the multidisciplinary team experienced a 44% reduction in all-cause readmissions, a 56% reduction in heart failure readmissions and a 29% reduction in readmissions for reasons other than heart failure.[26] In addition, patients in the intervention group reported an improved quality of life, and compliance with both medications and diet was enhanced.[26,31]

Multiple comorbid illnesses and other conditions

Polypharmacy
- Noncompliance
- Drug interactions

Dietary issues

Psychosocial and financial concerns
- Depression
- Social isolation
- Cost of medications

Physical limitations
- Arthritis
- Neuromuscular disorders (e.g. stroke)
- Sensory deficits (e.g. visual, auditory)

Cognitive dysfunction

Table 7.2
Factors confounding heart failure management

The overall cost of medical care was also lower in the intervention group as a result of the marked reduction in readmissions.[26]

In the above study, 137 patients were 80 years of age or older (mean age 84.5 ± 3.7 years, range 80–96, 73% female). In this subgroup, 90-day readmission rates were 42% and 29% in the usual care and intervention groups, respectively, representing a 32% reduction in the risk of readmission. Similarly, total readmissions were reduced by 36% in the intervention group during the 90-day follow-up period. The overall effects in octogenarians were similar to those in patients 70–79 years of age, thus demonstrating the efficacy of this approach even in the very elderly.

The key elements of nonpharmacological therapy that should be provided by the multidisciplinary team are outlined in Table 7.3. Since not all patients will require all of the interventions listed, it is essential to identify a 'team-leader' who is responsible for coordinating all aspects of the patient's care. Although a physician could serve in this capacity, an experienced nurse case manager or advance practice nurse (nurse practitioner) may be a more effective and less costly alternative. Most of the items in Table 7.3 are self-explanatory, but the role of exercise and rehabilitation in elderly heart failure patients requires further comment.

Cardiac rehabilitation

In the past, regular exercise has been viewed as inadvisable and possibly hazardous in heart

Patient education
- Symptoms and signs of heart failure
- Specific information about when and how to contact the nurse or physician if symptoms worsen
- Detailed discussion of all medications
- Emphasize importance of compliance
- Involve family/significant other as much as possible

Dietary consultation
- Individualized and consistent with needs/lifestyle
- Sodium restriction (1.5–2 g/day)
- Weight loss, if appropriate
- Low fat, low cholesterol, if appropriate
- Adequate calorie intake
- Emphasize compliance while allowing flexibility

Medication review
- Eliminate unnecessary medications
- Simplify regimen whenever possible
- Consolidate dosing schedule

Social Services
- Assess social support structure
- Evaluate emotional and financial needs
- Intervene pro-actively when feasible

Daily weight chart
- Specific directions on when to contact nurse or physician for changes in weight

Support stockings to reduce edema

Activity prescription (see text)

Intensive follow-up
- Telephone contacts
- Home visits
- Outpatient clinic

Contact information
- Names and phone numbers of nurse and physician
- 24-hour availability

Table 7.3
Nonpharmacological aspects of heart failure management

failure patients. However, it is now recognized that excessive restriction of physical activity leads to cardiovascular and muscular deconditioning which contributes to the decline in functional capacity that occurs in patients with chronic heart failure. In addition, several small trials have now shown that exercise tolerance can be improved with an appropriately structured exercise program.[32,33] Moreover, the greatest improvements have been seen among patients who were most severely impaired prior to entering the program. As a result, most experts now recommend some form of regular physical activity for the majority of heart failure patients.[34,35]

The validity of the above recommendations in octogenarians is unclear, however, since none of the published trials have included patients of elderly age. None the less, since the very elderly are likely to be the most severely limited, the potential benefit to be derived from an exercise program, in terms of improving functional capacity and maintaining independence, is substantial. In addition, even low intensity exercise, suitable for octogenarians, may be associated with clinically significant benefits.[36] In addition, strength training, an integral component of cardiac rehabilitation, has been shown to improve functional capacity in frail octogenarians and nonagenarians without heart failure.[37,38] On balance, it seems prudent to encourage very elderly heart failure patients to remain active and to engage in appropriate, low-intensity exercise (e.g. walking) on a regular basis in the absence of contraindications.

Exercise guidelines for older *coronary* patients are provided in Chapter 15 and will not be reviewed here. However, several modifications may be necessary for very elderly patients with heart failure. First, until additional data become available, exercise intensity in this population should be maintained in the low to moderate range (e.g. 40–60% of heart rate reserve). Second, since most patients will be unable to engage in prolonged periods of exercise (i.e. more than 10 minutes), the duration of exercise should be tailored to each individual's capacity. Third, patients should be encouraged to exercise daily or even several times daily if possible. For example, if an elderly heart failure patient is only able to walk 25 meters before experiencing discomfort, it is desirable to have the patient walk that distance two or three times every day. Then, over a period of several weeks, the distance may be gradually increased as tolerated. As discussed in Chapter 15, it is important to supplement aerobic activity with flexibility exercises and strength training when feasible.

Medical therapy

In general, the pharmacotherapy of heart failure does not differ substantially between older and younger patients. However, older patients are at greater risk for adverse side-effects, in part due to the presence of comorbid illnesses and polypharmacy. Similarly, patients over age 80 may be less tolerant of standard medication dosages, and the maximum attainable doses may be well below those found to be efficacious in clinical trials involving younger patients.

The first step in designing drug therapy for heart failure patients of all ages is to determine whether heart failure is primarily systolic or diastolic. Although these two forms of heart failure are not mutually exclusive and frequently coexist, the distinction is useful from the therapeutic perspective. Patients with a left ventricular ejection fraction of less than 45%, as determined by echocardiography, radionuclide angiography or contrast ventriculography, may be classified as having predominantly systolic heart failure. Conversely, heart failure patients with normal or near normal systolic function, as defined by an ejection fraction of 45% or greater, may be viewed as having predominantly diastolic heart failure.

Table 7.4 outlines currently available treatment options for patients with systolic heart failure. Each of these options is discussed in more detail below.

Angiotensin-converting enzyme inhibitors
Other vasodilators • Angiotensin II receptor antagonists (e.g. losartan) • Hydralazine/nitrates combination
Diuretics
Digoxin
Beta-adrenergic blocking agents
Calcium channel blockers
Antithrombotic agents • Aspirin • Warfarin

Table 7.4
Treatment options for systolic heart failure

Angiotensin-converting enzyme inhibitors

Angiotensin-converting enzyme (ACE) inhibitors improve quality of life and reduce mortality in a wide range of patients with impaired left ventricular systolic function, including the elderly.[39–44] Although none of the randomized trials included a significant number of octogenarians, data from several trials indicate that ACE inhibitors are as effective in patients over 70 years of age as in younger patients.[39,42,43] Therefore, in the absence of major contraindications (e.g. hypotension or severe renal insufficiency), ACE inhibitors should be considered standard therapy in all elderly patients with reduced left ventricular systolic function, with or without clinical heart failure.

Based on data from randomized trials, appropriate daily dosages of ACE inhibitors are as follows: captopril 150 mg; enalapril and lisinopril 20 mg; and ramipril 10 mg. In general, initial doses should be lower in the very elderly, with gradual titration to the target dose as tolerated. Throughout the titration period, blood pressure, renal function and serum potassium should be carefully monitored. The most common side-effect of ACE inhibitors is a dry, hacking cough, which may require discontinuation of treatment in up to 10% of patients. More serious side-effects include hypotension, renal insufficiency, hyperkalemia and allergic reactions. In addition, ACE inhibitors have important adverse drug interactions with potassium-sparing diuretics (hyperkalemia) and nonsteroidal anti-inflammatory drugs (neutralization of ACE inhibition), and these drug combinations should be avoided whenever possible.

Other vasodilators

At least 10–20% of individuals are unable to take ACE inhibitors due to contraindications or side-effects, and this percentage may be higher in the very elderly. In these patients, the angiotensin II receptor antagonist losartan and the combination of nitrates and hydralazine are suitable alternatives.[45–47] In a recent study involving 722 patients 65 years of age or older with clinical heart failure and a left ventricular ejection fraction of ≤40%, losartan was associated with fewer serious side-effects than captopril and, in addition, hospital admissions and mortality were reduced during a 48-week follow-up period.[45] Although these findings require confirmation in larger studies, which are now ongoing, at present losartan appears to be a rational choice in patients unable to take an ACE inhibitor. The initial dose of losartan in the very elderly is 12.5–25 mg once daily, with gradual titration to 50 mg once daily as tolerated. Hypotension and renal insufficiency are the most important side-effects.

Another alternative to ACE inhibitors is the combination of nitrates and hydralazine. When prescribed together, these agents reduce mortality in heart failure patients.[46,47] The doses used in the clinical trials were isosorbide dinitrate 40 mg and hydralazine 75 mg, each administered four times daily. Common side-effects from this combination include headache, dizziness, fatigue and gastrointestinal disturbances. A small percentage of patients may develop the 'drug lupus syndrome', which may occur when high doses of hydralazine are used.

Diuretics

Although there is no evidence that diuretics improve clinical outcomes in heart failure, diuretics remain a cornerstone of therapy because they are the most effective agents for relieving symptoms of pulmonary congestion and edema. Some patients with mild heart failure may not need maintenance diuretic therapy or may respond to a thiazide diuretic, but most will require a 'loop' diuretic, such as furosemide, bumetanide or torsemide. In patients with acute heart failure, intravenous diuretics are more effective than the corresponding oral agents, and continuous intravenous infusion promotes a more brisk diuresis than intermittent 'boluses'. In patients who fail to respond satisfactorily to appropriate doses of loop diuretics, the addition of metolazone or spironolactone may facilitate diuresis.[48,49]

The most common and important side-effects of diuretics are electrolyte disturbances, including hyponatremia, hypo- or hyperkalemia, hypomagnesemia and metabolic alkalosis. Due to age-related changes in renal function and a higher prevalence of comorbid illnesses such as diabetes, older patients are at increased risk for serious diuretic-induced electrolyte abnormalities. Therefore, electrolytes should be monitored closely while diuretic therapy is being adjusted.

Digoxin

Digoxin exerts a modest positive inotropic effect on left ventricular contractility in individuals of all ages.[50] However, due to changes in lean body mass and renal function, the therapeutic range is lower in older patients.[50] In octogenarians, serum digoxin concentrations of 0.5–1.3 ng/ml are appropriate; higher levels are associated with increased toxicity but no greater efficacy.[51]

Although digoxin is no longer considered first-line therapy for heart failure, it remains a useful agent for managing patients with severe left ventricular systolic dysfunction who remain symptomatic despite optimal doses of ACE inhibitors and diuretics. In the recently completed Digitalis Investigation Group (DIG) trial, digoxin had no effect on overall mortality compared with placebo, but mortality and hospitalizations due to heart failure were reduced.[52] In this study, older age was an independent risk factor both for all-cause mortality and hospital admissions, as well as for heart failure deaths and hospitalizations. However, the beneficial effects of digoxin on heart failure mortality and hospitalizations among 425 patients over 80 years of age were similar to those in younger patients (W. Williford, personal communication).

Side-effects from digoxin include cardiac, neurologic, and gastrointestinal disturbances. In the DIG study, adverse effects which occurred more frequently in patients receiving digoxin included nausea and vomiting, diarrhea, visual disturbances, supraventricular and ventricular arrhythmias, and advanced atrioventricular block. Elderly patients are at increased risk for both cardiac and neurological toxicity from digitalis.

In older patients with normal renal function, a digoxin dose of 0.125 mg daily is usually sufficient to achieve a therapeutic effect. Patients with renal dysfunction or small body habitus may require a lower dose. Routine monitoring of serum digoxin levels is no longer recommended, but clinicians should maintain a high index of suspicion for digoxin toxicity, and blood levels should be obtained when clinically indicated. This is particularly important in the elderly, since 10–20% of older patients will develop symptoms or signs of toxicity, at some time during the course of therapy.[53] Additionally, since diuretic-induced hypokalemia and hypomagnesemia potentiate digoxin's cardiac effects and toxicities, serum levels of these electrolytes should be maintained within the normal range.

Beta-blockers

Although beta-blockers lower cardiac output by decreasing heart rate and contractility, recent studies indicate that beta-blockers may exert long-term beneficial effects in heart failure patients with reduced left ventricular systolic function.[54] In the US Carvedilol Study patients with heart failure and an ejection fraction of 35% or less who were randomized to carvedilol treatment had a 65% lower mortality than placebo-treated patients after a mean follow-up of 6.5 months.[55] In addition, carvedilol was associated with improved quality of life, fewer hospitalizations, and a greater increase in ejection fraction. Moreover, the benefits were similar in patients older or younger than 60 years of age, as well as in patients with ischemic or nonischemic heart failure.[55] Unfortunately, very few patients over 75 years of age were enrolled in the trial. Nonetheless, beta-blockers are a reasonable therapeutic option in elderly patients without contraindications who fail to respond satisfactorily to conventional triple drug therapy (i.e.

an ACE inhibitor or other vasodilator, diuretic and digoxin).

The starting dose of carvedilol is 3.125 mg twice daily, and the dose should be gradually increased at 2-week intervals to a target dose of 25–50 mg twice daily. Therapy should not be initiated in unstable or severely decompensated patients. Other contraindications to beta-blockers include marked bradycardia, hypotension (systolic blood pressure less than 90–100 mmHg), advanced atrioventricular block and bronchospastic lung disease. In addition, the patient's heart rate, blood pressure, cardiorespiratory examination and clinical symptomatology should be monitored closely during the titration phase.

Calcium channel blockers

The first generation calcium antagonists nifedipine, diltiazem, and verapamil have each been associated with adverse outcomes in patients with systolic heart failure. As a result, these drugs are usually contraindicated. In the Prospective Randomized Amlodipine Survival Evaluation (PRAISE), amlodipine was associated with a 16% reduction in mortality compared to placebo ($P = 0.07$),[56] but the benefit was limited to patients with nonischemic dilated cardiomyopathy, a condition that is relatively uncommon in the very elderly. In addition, no patients of advanced age were enrolled in the trial. Based on available evidence, calcium channel blockers are not recommended for routine heart failure management in older patients. However, in those patients who require a calcium antagonist for another reason (e.g. angina control), amlodipine is a suitable choice.

Antithrombotic therapy

Aspirin 75–325 mg daily or every other day is recommended for all patients with proven coronary heart disease regardless of age.[57]

Selected patients with cerebrovascular disease or atrial fibrillation may benefit as well.[57,58] In most other situations, aspirin should probably be avoided, since it may antagonize the beneficial effects of ACE inhibitors or induce bleeding complications.[59]

Warfarin is indicated for patients with chronic or recurrent atrial fibrillation, advanced rheumatic mitral valve disease, prosthetic heart valves or prior thromboembolic events.[60] Its value in other settings is unproven, and elderly patients taking warfarin are at increased risk for serious hemorrhage. When prescribing warfarin, the dosage should be adjusted to maintain the Internal Normalized Ratio (INR) within the range of 2.0–3.5.

Diastolic heart failure

Despite the fact that up to 50% of octogenarians with heart failure have normal or near normal left ventricular systolic function at rest, there have been no large clinical trials evaluating the safety and efficacy of pharmacological agents for treating this condition. As with systolic heart failure, diuretics are appropriate for the relief of congestion and edema. However, overzealous diuresis may decrease left ventricular end-diastolic volume, stroke volume, and cardiac output. This in turn may result in hypotension, reduced exercise tolerance, and prerenal azotemia (i.e. a disproportionate rise in the blood urea nitrogen level relative to the creatinine level). Thus, overly aggressive diuresis of patients with diastolic heart failure should be avoided in most cases.

In the US, ACE inhibitors, beta-blockers and calcium channel blockers are commonly used to treat diastolic heart failure in the elderly. ACE inhibitors may reduce symptoms of diastolic heart failure by improving left ventricular compliance and reducing hypertrophy.[10] In one study involving 21 elderly patients (mean age 80 years) with dias-

tolic heart failure, enalapril was associated with improved diastolic function and left ventricular mass, as well as an increase in exercise capacity.[61]

By slowing heart rate and prolonging the diastolic filling period, beta-blockers may increase stroke volume and reduce symptoms in patients with diastolic heart failure.[10] Beta-blockers are also effective as anti-ischemic agents and they reduce left ventricular hypertrophy. Moreover, in a recent randomized trial involving 158 elderly heart failure patients (average age 81 years) with an ejection fraction of 40% or greater, treatment with propranolol was associated with improved survival compared with nontreatment.[62]

Calcium channel blockers exert a modest beneficial effect on diastolic function, and they also reduce ventricular hypertrophy and ischemia. In addition, verapamil has been associated with improved symptoms, exercise capacity and diastolic function in older patients with heart failure and an ejection fraction of 45% or greater.[63,64]

Additional agents which may be of benefit in selected patients with diastolic heart failure include nitrates and digoxin. Nitrates lower left ventricular diastolic pressure and help relieve pulmonary congestion. However, nitrates have the potential for reducing left ventricular stroke volume and cardiac output. In addition, tolerance to nitrates may occur in up to 50% of patients.[65,66] Digoxin is usually considered contraindicated in patients with heart failure and normal systolic function. However, in the recently completed DIG study (see above), 988 patients with heart failure and an ejection fraction of 45% or greater were enrolled in the trial.[52] In these patients, digoxin had no effect on mortality, but there was an 18% reduction in the combined endpoint of death or hospitalization for heart failure.[52]

In summary, the treatment of diastolic heart failure is largely empirical at the present time. Diuretics provide effective palliation for congestive symptoms and edema, but overdiuresis should be avoided. Patients with a resting heart rate of 75/minute or greater may benefit from a beta-blocker, but ACE inhibitors and calcium channel blockers are also acceptable first-line agents. In patients who fail to respond to initial therapy, adding a second agent or substituting an agent from another class is appropriate. The addition of nitrates or digoxin may be beneficial in selected cases. Finally, since atrial fibrillation is often poorly tolerated in patients with diastolic heart failure who rely on atrial contraction to optimize ventricular filling, maintenance of sinus rhythm is desirable in most cases.

Prevention

Once established, heart failure is associated with substantial morbidity and mortality. Therefore, measures designed to prevent the development of heart failure are highly desirable whenever feasible. Since coronary artery disease and hypertension are the most common etiologies of heart failure in Western countries, aggressive treatment of coronary risk factors and hypertension is appropriate. Although the impact of cholesterol-lowering medications on the incidence of heart failure is unknown, both the Scandinavian Simvastatin Survival Study (4S) and the Cholesterol and Recurrent Events (CARE) Trial showed that both older and younger patients benefit from cholesterol reduction following myocardial infarction.[67,68]

Numerous studies have now documented that treatment of both systolic and diastolic hypertension reduces cerebrovascular and cardiac events in elderly patients.[69] Moreover, the incidence of heart failure is reduced by approximately 50%, and this benefit is most

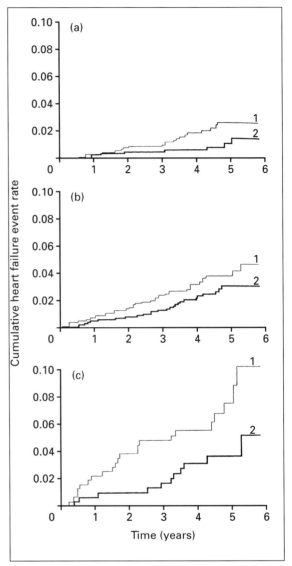

Figure 7.4

Effect of antihypertensive drug therapy on the development of heart failure in the Systolic Hypertension in the Elderly Program (SHEP). (a) Age 60–69 years; (b) age 70–79 years; (c) age 80 years and older. In each panel, line 1 represents placebo and line 2 represents active treatment. (From Kostis et al[71] with permission)

pronounced in the oldest patients.[70] In the Systolic Hypertension in the Elderly Program (SHEP), for example, the absolute reduction in heart failure was greatest in patients over 80 years of age (Figure 7.4).[71] Since at least 20% (and possibly 40%) of octogenarians have systolic hypertension, aggressive treatment of this condition offers tremendous potential for reducing the incidence and prevalence of heart failure in the very elderly.[72]

Finally, ACE inhibitors have been shown to prevent or delay the onset of heart failure in asymptomatic patients with left ventricular systolic dysfunction (ejection fraction ≤40%), and elderly patients benefit to at least as great an extent as younger patients.[41,42] Therefore, ACE inhibitors are appropriate in all patients with reduced left ventricular systolic function, regardless of age.

Ethical issues and end-of-life decisions

Heart failure in octogenarians is associated with an extremely poor prognosis. Indeed, the 5-year survival rate for both men and women is less than 20%, which is worse than for most forms of cancer. In addition, the quality of life for patients with advanced heart failure is often very limited, and all heart failure patients are at risk for sudden arrhythmic death.

For these reasons, the wishes of the patient and family with respect to treatment intensity and end-of-life care should be discussed early in the disease process. The patient should be encouraged to develop a 'living will' and to appoint a durable power-of-attorney to serve as an advocate in the event that the patient is no longer capable of making decisions. In addition, the physician should refrain from recommending overly aggressive or experimental treatments that offer little hope for altering the course of the disease and only serve to prolong the dying process.

As the patient approaches the terminal stages of illness there should be discussions with the patient and family to determine where the patient would like to spend his or her final days. Possible options include the home environment, a reputable hospice, a nursing home or other chronic care facility, and the local hospital, and the patient's wishes should be accommodated whenever possible.

References

1. Kannel WB, Belanger AJ. Epidemiology of heart failure. *Am Heart J* (1991) **121**:951–7.

2. O'Connell JB, Bristow MR. Economic impact of heart failure in the United States: time for a different approach. *J Heart Lung Transplant* (1994) **13**(Suppl 10):S107–12.

3. Ho KKL, Pinsky JL, Kannel WB, Levy D. The epidemiology of heart failure: the Framingham Study. *J Am Coll Cardiol* (1993) **22**(Suppl A):6–13A.

4. Graves EJ, Owings MF. 1995 summary: National Hospital Discharge Survey. Advance data from vital and health statistics; no. 291. (National Center for Health Statistics: Hyattsville, MD, 1997).

5. Graves EJ. National Hospital Discharge Survey: annual summary, 1990. Advance data from vital and health statistics; no. 112. (National Center for Health Statistics: Hyattsville, MD, 1992).

6. Gillum RF. Epidemiology of heart failure in the United States. *Am Heart J* (1993) **126**:1042–7.

7. Ho KKL, Anderson KM, Kannel WB et al. Survival after the onset of congestive heart failure in Framingham Heart Study subjects. *Circulation* (1993) **88**:107–15.

8. Rich MW. Epidemiology, pathophysiology, and etiology of congestive heart failure in older adults. *J Am Geriatr Soc* (1997) **45**:968–74.

9. Wong WF, Gold S, Fukuyama O, Blanchette PL. Diastolic dysfunction in elderly patients with congestive heart failure. *Am J Cardiol* (1989) **63**:1526–8.

10. Tresch DD, McGough MF. Heart failure with normal systolic function: a common disorder in older people. *J Am Geriatr Soc* (1995) **43**:1035–42.

11. Davie AP, Francis CM, Caruana L, Sutherland GR. The prevalence of left ventricular diastolic filling abnormalities in patients with suspected heart failure. *Eur Heart J* (1997) **18**:981–4.

12. Luchi RJ, Snow E, Luchi JM et al. Left ventricular function in hospitalized geriatric patients. *J Am Geriatr Soc* (1982) **30**:700–5.

13. Kitzman DW, Higginbotham MB, Lobb FR et al. Exercise intolerance in patients with heart failure and preserved left ventricular systolic function: failure of the Frank–Starling mechanism. *J Am Coll Cardiol* (1991) **17**:1065–72.

14. Wenger NK, Franciosa JA, Weber KT. Heart failure. 18th Bethesda Conference. Cardiovascular disease in the elderly. *J Am Coll Cardiol* (1987) **10**(Suppl A):73–6A.

15. Rich MW, Shah AS, Vinson JM et al. Iatrogenic congestive heart failure in older adults: clinical course and prognosis. *J Am Geriatr Soc* (1996) **44**:638–43.

16. Aronow WS. Echocardiography should be performed in all elderly patients with congestive heart failure. *J Am Geriatr Soc* (1994) **42**:1300–2.

17. Little T, Milner MR, Lee K et al. Late outcome and quality of life following percutaneous transluminal coronary angioplasty in octogenarians. *Cathet Cardiovasc Diagn* (1993) **29**:261–6.

18. Edmunds LH, Stephenson LW, Edie RN, Ratcliffe MB. Open-heart surgery in octogenarians. *N Engl J Med* (1988) **319**:131–6.

19. Elayda MA, Hall RJ, Reul RM et al. Aortic valve replacement in patients 80 years and older. Operative risks and long-term results. *Circulation* (1993) **88**(Suppl II):11–16.

20. Logeais Y, Roussin R, Langanay T et al. Aortic valve replacement for aortic stenosis in 200 consecutive octogenarians. *J Heart Valve Dis* (1995) **4**(Suppl 1):S64–71.

21. Ghali JK, Kadakia S, Cooper R, Ferlinz J. Precipitating factors leading to decompensation of heart failure: traits among urban blacks. *Arch Intern Med* (1988) **148**:2013–16.

22. Gooding J, Jette AM. Hospital readmissions among the elderly. *J Am Geriatr Soc* (1985) **33**:595–601.

23. Rich MW, Freedland KE. Effect of DRGs on three-month readmission rate of geriatric patients with congestive heart failure. *Am J Public Health* (1988) **78**:680–2.

24. Vinson JM, Rich MW, Sperry JC et al. Early

readmission of elderly patients with congestive heart failure. *J Am Geriatr Soc* (1990) **38:** 1290–5.

25. Krumholz HM, Parent EM, Tu N et al. Readmission after hospitalization for congestive heart failure among Medicare beneficiaries. *Arch Intern Med* (1997) **157:**99–104.

26. Rich MW, Beckham V, Wittenberg C et al. A multidisciplinary intervention to prevent the readmission of elderly patients with congestive heart failure. *N Engl J Med* (1995) **333:** 1190–5.

27. Kostis JB, Rosen RC, Cosgrove NM et al. Nonpharmacologic therapy improves functional and emotional status in congestive heart failure. *Chest* (1994) **106:**996–1001.

28. Kornowski R, Zeeli D, Averbuch M et al. Intensive home-care surveillance prevents hospitalization and improves morbidity rates among elderly patients with severe congestive heart failure. *Am Heart J* (1995) **129:**762–6.

29. West JA, Miller NH, Parker KM et al. A comprehensive management system for heart failure improves clinical outcomes and reduces medical resource utilization. *Am J Cardiol* (1997) **79:**58–63.

30. Fonarow GC, Stevenson LW, Waldon JA et al. Impact of a comprehensive heart failure management program on hospital readmission and functional status of patients with advanced heart failure. *J Am Coll Cardiol* (1997) **30:** 725–32.

31. Rich MW, Gray DB, Beckham V et al. Effect of a multidisciplinary intervention on medication compliance in elderly patients with congestive heart failure. *Am J Med* (1996) **101:** 270–6.

32. McKelvie RS, Teo KK, McCartney N et al. Effects of exercise training in patients with congestive heart failure: a critical review. *J Am Coll Cardiol* (1995) **25:**789–96.

33. Keteyian SJ, Levine AB, Brawner CA et al. Exercise training in patients with heart failure: a randomized, controlled trial. *Ann Intern Med* (1996) **124:**1051–7.

34. Konstam MA, Dracup K, Baker DW et al. Heart failure: evaluation and care of patients with left ventricular systolic dysfunction. Clinical Practice Guideline No. 11 ((AHCPR publication no. 94-0612) Agency for Health Care Policy and Research: Rockville, MD, 1994).

35. ACC/AHA Task Force Report. Guidelines for the evaluation and management of heart failure. *J Am Coll Cardiol* (1995) **26:**1376–98.

36. Belardinelli R, Georgiou D, Scocco V. Low intensity exercise training in patients with chronic heart failure. *J Am Coll Cardiol* (1995) **26:**975–82.

37. Fiatarone MA, Marks EC, Ryan ND et al. High-intensity strength training in octogenarians. Effects on skeletal muscle. *JAMA* (1990) **263:**3029–34.

38. Fiatarone MA, O'Neill EF, Ryan ND et al. Exercise training and nutritional supplementation for physical frailty in very elderly people. *N Engl J Med* (1994) **330:**1769–75.

39. Garg R, Yusuf S, for the Collaborative Group on ACE Inhibitor Trials. Overview of randomized trials of angiotensin-converting enzyme inhibitors on mortality and morbidity in patients with heart failure. *JAMA* (1995) **273:** 1450–6.

40. The SOLVD Investigators. Effect of enalapril on survival in patients with reduced left ventricular ejection fractions and congestive heart failure. *N Engl J Med* (1991) **325:**293–302.

41. The SOLVD Investigators. Effect of enalapril on mortality and the development of heart failure in asymptomatic patients with reduced left ventricular ejection fractions. *N Engl J Med* (1992) **327:**685–91.

42. Pfeffer MA, Braunwald E, Moyé LA et al. Effect of captopril on mortality and morbidity in patients with left ventricular dysfunction after myocardial infarction. *N Engl J Med* (1992) **327:**669–77.

43. The Acute Infarction Ramipril Efficacy (AIRE) Study Investigators. Effect of ramipril on mortality and morbidity of survivors of acute myocardial infarction with clinical evidence of heart failure. *Lancet* (1993) **342:**821–8.

44. Rogers WJ, Johnstone DE, Yusuf S et al. Quality of life among 5025 patients with left ventricular dysfunction randomized between placebo and enalapril: the Studies of Left Ventricular Dysfunction. *J Am Coll Cardiol* (1994) **23:**393–400.

45. Pitt B, Segal R, Martinez FA et al. Randomised trial of losartan versus captopril in patients over 65 with heart failure (Evaluation of Losartan in the Elderly Study, ELITE). *Lancet* (1997) **349:**747–52.

46. Cohn JN, Archibald DG, Ziesche S et al. Effects of vasodilator therapy on mortality in chronic congestive heart failure. Results of a Veterans Administration Cooperative Study. *N Engl J Med* (1986) **314**:1547–52.

47. Cohn JN, Johnson G, Ziesche S et al. A comparison of enalapril with hydralazine-isosorbide dinitrate in the treatment of chronic congestive heart failure. *N Engl J Med* (1991) **325**:303–10.

48. Channer KS, McLean KA, Lawson-Matthew P, Richardson M. Combination diuretic treatment in severe heart failure: a randomised controlled trial. *Br Heart J* (1994) **71**:146–50.

49. van Vliet AA, Donker AJM, Nauta JJP, Verheugt FWA. Spironolactone in congestive heart failure refractory to high-dose loop diuretic and low-dose angiotensin-converting enzyme inhibitor. *Am J Cardiol* (1993) **71**:21–8A.

50. Ware JA, Snow E, Luchi JM, Luchi RJ. Effects of digoxin on ejection fraction in elderly patients with congestive heart failure. *J Am Geriatr Soc* (1984) **32**:631–5.

51. Slatton ML, Irani WN, Hall SA et al. Does digoxin provide additional hemodynamic and autonomic benefit at higher doses in patients with mild to moderate heart failure and normal sinus rhythm? *J Am Coll Cardiol* (1997) **29**:1206–13.

52. The Digitalis Investigation Group. The effect of digoxin on mortality and morbidity in patients with heart failure. *N Engl J Med* (1997) **336**:525–33.

53. Schneeweiss A, Schettler G. Digitalis glycosides. In: *Cardiovascular Drug Therapy in the Elderly* (Martinus Nijhoff Publishing: Boston, 1988) 6–28.

54. Doughty RN, Rodgers A, Sharpe N, MacMahon S. Effects of beta-blocker therapy on mortality in patients with heart failure. A systematic overview of randomized controlled trials. *Eur Heart J* (1997) **18**:560–5.

55. Packer M, Bristow MR, Cohn JN et al. The effect of carvedilol on morbidity and mortality in patients with chronic heart failure. *N Engl J Med* (1996) **334**:1349–55.

56. Packer M, O'Connor CM, Ghali JK et al. Effect of amlodipine on morbidity and mortality in severe chronic heart failure. *N Engl J Med* (1996) **335**:1107–14.

57. Antiplatelet Trialists' Collaboration. Collaborative overview of randomised trials of antiplatelet therapy. I: Prevention of death, myocardial infarction, and stroke by prolonged antiplatelet therapy in various categories of patients. *BMJ* (1994) **308**:81–106.

58. The Atrial Fibrillation Investigators. The efficacy of aspirin in patients with atrial fibrillation. Analysis of pooled data from three randomized trials. *Arch Intern Med* (1997) **157**:1237–40.

59. Cleland JGF, Bulpitt CJ, Falk RH et al. Is aspirin safe for patients with heart failure? *Br Heart J* (1995) **74**:215–19.

60. Fourth American College of Chest Physicians Consensus Conference on Antithrombotic Therapy. *Chest* (1995) **108**(Suppl): 225–522S.

61. Aronow WS, Kronzon I. Effect of enalapril on congestive heart failure treated with diuretics in elderly patients with prior myocardial infarction and normal left ventricular ejection fraction. *Am J Cardiol* (1993) **71**:602–4.

62. Aronow WS, Ahn C, Kronzon I. Effect of propranolol versus no propranolol on total mortality plus nonfatal myocardial infarction in older patients with prior myocardial infarction, congestive heart failure, and left ventricular ejection fraction $\geq 40\%$ treated with diuretics plus angiotensin-converting enzyme inhibitors. *Am J Cardiol* (1997) **80**:207–9.

63. Setaro JF, Zaret BL, Schulman DS et al. Usefulness of verapamil for congestive heart failure associated with abnormal left ventricular diastolic filling and normal left ventricular systolic performance. *Am J Cardiol* (1990) **66**:981–6.

64. Arrighi JA, Dilsizian V, Perrone-Filardi P et al. Improvement of the age-related impairment in left ventricular diastolic filling with verapamil in the normal human heart. *Circulation* (1994) **90**:213–19.

65. Thadani U. Nitrate tolerance, rebound, and their clinical relevance in stable angina pectoris, unstable angina, and heart failure. *Cardiovasc Drugs Ther* (1997) **10**:735–42.

66. Elkayam U. Nitrates in the treatment of congestive heart failure. *Am J Cardiol* (1996) **77**: 41–51C.

67. Scandinavian Simvastatin Survival Study Group. Randomised trial of cholesterol lowering in 4444 patients with coronary heart disease: the Scandinavian Simvastatin Survival

Study (4S). *Lancet* (1994) **344**:1383–9.

68. Sacks FM, Pfeffer MA, Moye LA et al. The effect of pravastatin on coronary events after myocardial infarction in patients with average cholesterol levels. *N Engl J Med* (1996) **335**:1001–9.

69. Mulrow CD, Cornell JA, Herrera CR et al. Hypertension in the elderly. Implications and generalizability of randomized trials. *JAMA* (1994) **272**:1932–8.

70. Moser M, Hebert PR. Prevention of disease progression, left ventricular hypertrophy and congestive heart failure in hypertension treatment trials. *J Am Coll Cardiol* (1996) **27**: 1214–18.

71. Kostis JB, Davis BR, Cutler J et al. Prevention of heart failure by antihypertensive drug treatment in older persons with isolated systolic hypertension. *JAMA* (1997) **278**:212–16.

72. The Sixth Report of the Joint National Committee on Prevention, Detection, Evaluation, and Treatment of High Blood Pressure. *Arch Intern Med* (1997) **157**:2413–46.

8

Syncope in the elderly
Stephen F Schaal

Introduction

Syncope is a common problem in the elderly with an incidence approaching 7% per year in the very old (institutionalized population, mean age 87 years).[1] Presyncope and syncope account for a significant proportion of falls with resultant injuries and fractures. Coexistent age-related diseases or processes such as aortic stenosis, congestive heart failure, angina, hypertension, diabetes, chronic renal disease, cerebrovascular disease and postural hypotension contribute to an increased likelihood for syncope as well as increased mortality. Most elderly patients with syncope have multiple clinical abnormalities contributing to syncope. Of elderly patients admitted for syncope to a medical intensive care unit (45% older than 70 years), the 1-year mortality was 6% in patients with noncardiovascular causes for syncope and 19% in those with cardiovascular causes for syncope.[2]

The various causes for syncope are listed in Table 9.1. While the causes are essentially those of any age group, certain entities such as arrhythmic syncope due to sinoatrial disease or atrioventricular block, hypersensitive carotid sinus syndrome, postprandial syncope and orthostatic hypotension are more likely in the elderly population.

Arrhythmic syncope

A variety of rhythm disturbances may cause syncope in the elderly. Any brady- or tachyarrhythmia may reduce cerebral blood flow sufficient to produce syncope. Syncope with arrhythmia is more likely to occur when the patient is upright, particularly if the individual has difficulty with postural hypotension. Tachyarrhythmias are more likely to produce significant hypotension if the individual is upright or either active or postexercise when the catecholamine levels might effect a faster ventricular response with both supraventricular and ventricular tachycardias.

Bradyarrhythmias

Because the elderly are more likely to have fibrodegenerative involvement of the sinoatrial node and atrioventricular conduction system, sick sinus syndrome manifest by sinoatrial exit block, sinus bradycardia, and brady/tachy syndrome and atrioventricular block are more commonly associated with syncope.[3,4]

Sinoatrial disease is quite common in the elderly because of the gradual replacement of sinus node and sinoatrial region cells by collagen and fibrosis. Sinus bradycardia may be associated with syncope, but usually the bradycardia must be quite profound with episodes of sinoatrial exit block or the event must be in association with changes in posture when the expected rise in heart rate with

Arrhythmic
  Sinoatrial disease
  Atrioventricular block
  Supraventricular tachycardia
  Ventricular tachycardia
  Pacemaker related
    Pacemaker malfunction
    Pacemaker syndrome
    Pacemaker-induced tachycardia
Orthostatic
Vasodepressor
Postprandial
Hypersensitive carotid sinus syndrome
Reflex
  Cough
  Micturition
  Defecation
  Deglutition
Cardiac obstructive
  Aortic stenosis
  Hypertrophic obstructive cardiomyopathy
  Mitral stenosis
  Left atrial myxoma
  Pulmonary hypertension
  Pulmonary emboli
  Pulmonary stenosis
Neurological
  Seizure
  Transient ischemic attack
  Cerebral vascular accident
  Subclavian steal
  Migraine
  Tumor
Metabolic
  Hypoglycemia
  Hyperventilation
  Ethanol/drug
Psychiatric
Unknown origin

Table 8.1
Classification of syncope

standing is nonexistent or markedly blunted. The more common scenario associated with syncope in the elderly in the setting of sinoatrial disease is the presence of supraventricular tachycardia such as atrial fibrillation terminating in sinoatrial pause. An example of a patient with atrial fibrillation converting to sinus rhythm with a prolonged pause is shown in Figure 8.1. The fibrosis also involves the atrial myocardium; this results in various supraventricular tachyarrhythmias, usually atrial fibrillation.

Atrioventricular (AV) conduction disorders responsible for significant bradycardia and ventricular asystole are more common in the elderly. An example of high grade AV block causing near syncope is shown in Figure 8.2. This patient had premature ventricular depolarizations (PVCs) noted on 24-hour ECG Holter monitoring but required an ECG event recorder to witness the AV block responsible for syncope. Atrioventricular block may be quite evanescent; the suspicion level needs to be high in patients with a prolonged PR interval, particularly in the setting of bundle branch block.

A variety of supraventricular tachycardias (SVT) may be associated with a sufficiently rapid ventricular rate to cause syncope in the elderly. Atrial fibrillation is the most common supraventricular arrhythmia to cause syncope although atrial flutter, atrial ectopic or triggered tachycardia are common and AV node re-entry as well as AV re-entry (accessory pathway) tachycardia may not have onset or be more problematic until later years. Because these rhythms generally require a premature beat for the triggering of onset, the increased frequency of premature beats that occurs with the aging process makes these rhythms more likely to occur.

Ventricular tachyarrhythmias of a nonsustained or sustained nature may produce hypotension significant to cause syncope in the

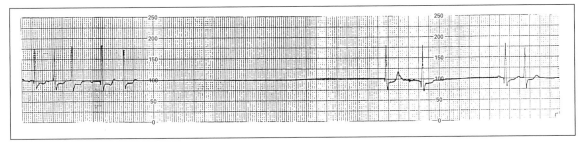

Figure 8.1
A 72-year-old with syncope. ECG lead demonstration of atrial fibrillation converting to escape rhythm with approximate 5s asystole.

elderly. These rhythms usually occur in patients with ventricular myocardial abnormalities, particularly patients who have documented coronary heart disease with previous scar. Catecholamine-sensitive and exercise-provoked ventricular tachycardia are less commonly seen in the elderly compared with a younger population.

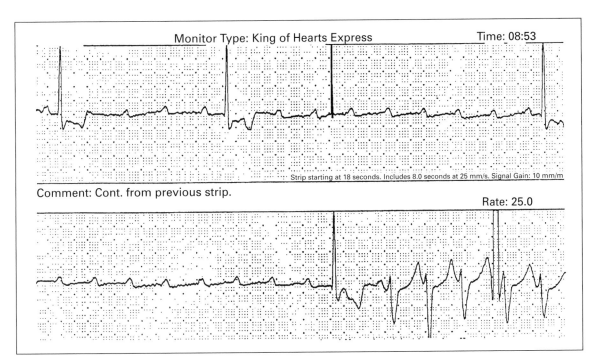

Figure 8.2
A 75-year-old with repeated episodes of syncope resulting in falls and fractures. Holter ECG monitoring had demonstrated isolated PVCs. Continuous ECG strip shows high grade AV block during near-syncopal episode.

Evaluation

The history is usually the most helpful clue to the detection of arrhythmic syncope, but often the bradycardias are not associated with palpitations and sometimes the tachycardia is not sensed in the prodrome to syncope, or a warning prior to the syncopal event does not exist.

The baseline ECG may offer a variety of clues to arrhythmic syncope. The presence of profound sinus bradycardia, sinoatrial exit block, prolonged PR interval or bundle branch block suggests the possibility of bradycardic syncope. Other clues on the 12-lead ECG are markedly abnormal P-waves (implying atrial abnormalities sufficient to cause atrial fibrillation or flutter), short PR interval or delta wave. Premature supraventricular or ventricular depolarizations or short asymptomatic bursts of tachycardia make further ECG long-term recording probably fruitful. The presence of an intraventricular conduction delay, hypertrophy or myocardial infarction all heighten the likelihood for syncope due to ventricular tachycardia. ECG Holter monitoring may provide additional information such as sinus pause or sinus exit block or intermittent AV block with or without symptoms. While the presence of symptoms during an episode of modest bradycardia or tachycardia is most helpful, the absence of symptoms during such rhythms does not suggest that the rhythms noted or more profound rhythms of the same ilk are not responsible for syncope. To cause syncope, the brady- or tachyarrhythmia often occurs when the patient is upright, in a precarious volume state or ill. For example, the finding of sinoatrial exit block on a routine ECG tracing should trigger the use of an ECG event recorder or electrophysiological catheterization studies. The high grade AV block associated with near syncope recorded by ECG event recorder in Figure 8.2 was pro-

found enough to proceed with pacemaker implantation.

If the patient has a history and/or physical examination findings to suggest ventricular myocardial disease, a signal-averaged ECG may be helpful, particularly if the patient has known coronary heart disease. A positive signal-averaged ECG would suggest the need for further evaluation such as electrophysiological study.

If the history and/or physical examination suggest myocardial disease, an echocardiogram is helpful to document the presence and degree of myocardial dysfunction. In general, the worse the ventricular myocardial function, the more likely that syncope is secondary to a ventricular tachyarrhythmia. In the patient with known or suspected coronary heart disease or activity-related syncope, an exercise ECG study should be performed. The production of ventricular or supraventricular tachycardia with or without symptoms associated with the arrhythmia raises significant suspicion for that rhythm as the cause for syncope and the need for long-term ECG monitoring or electrophysiological study. Additionally, the rare elderly patient with exercise-induced hypotension due to profound myocardial ischemia, valvular or other obstructive disease can be identified.

Electrophysiological catheterization study identifies the presence and degree of sinoatrial dysfunction, AV node or distal AV conduction abnormalities. Inducible tachycardias in the electrophysiology laboratory may provide a definitive explanation for syncope. Rapid sustained supraventricular or ventricular tachycardia with associated hypotension in the supine position are such rhythms. Inducible nonsustained tachycardias or tachycardias with modest heart rates (120–150 beats per minute) may reflect rhythms responsible for syncope or may be only potential clinical rhythms probably not the cause for syncope. Production of the tachycardia in an upright position in the electrophysiology laboratory may provide insight to the hemodynamic sequelae of the tachycardia.[5]

Therapy

Bradycardic rhythms responsible for syncope generally require pacemaker therapy. Occasionally, bradycardias may be due to drug therapy, such as digitalis, beta-blocker or calcium channel blocker. Discontinuation of the medication may sufficiently influence the conduction delay such that a pacemaker is not required. The bradycardia–tachycardia syndrome usually requires a pacemaker plus an anti-arrhythmic agent to control the SVT.

The tachyarrhythmias require precise identification to permit appropriate therapy. Any of the tachycardias is more likely to occur in a setting of hypokalemia. Identification of arrhythmia aggravation that might be present with an anti-arrhythmic, tricyclic or long-acting antihistamine drug would necessitate discontinuation of such medication. Specific therapy for some of the tachycardias may include anti-arrhythmic drugs, drugs to slow AV conduction, AV node modification or ablation in the case of uncontrolled atrial fibrillation with a rapid ventricular response or tachycardia ablation.

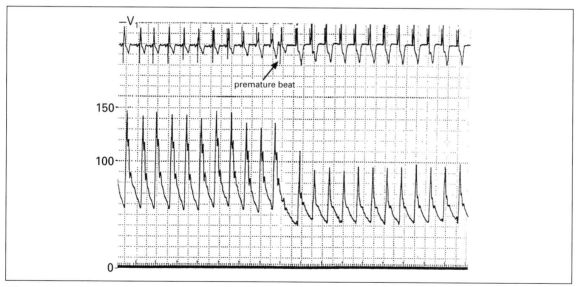

Figure 8.3
ECG and blood pressure recordings in sitting position in an 80-year-old with syncope and near syncope. In normal sinus rhythm, blood pressure is 145 systolic. With ventricular demand pace four beats prior to premature beat, a slight fall in blood pressure is noted. The premature beat is followed by VVI pacing with dramatic decrease in blood pressure.

Pacemaker-associated syncope

The pacemaker syndrome is a constellation of symptoms and signs resulting from an adverse reaction to ventricular demand (VVI) pacing. Orthostatic hypotension, fatigue and near syncope are common while syncope may occur. Figure 8.3 demonstrates a hypotensive episode due to VVI pacing in an 80 year old who had near syncope and syncope. Most symptoms occur because of lack of AV synchrony and because of retrograde conduction. Atrial contraction against closed AV valves results in atrial distention. This, in turn, may lead to reflex vasodepression effects and diuresis mediated by elevated levels of atrial natriuretic peptide.[6]

Other events leading to syncope in the patient with a pacemaker include loss of capture and resultant bradycardia or abnormally rapid paced rates. The latter may occur with DDD pacing with response to atrial tachycardia or pacemaker-mediated tachycardia. Retrograde atrial activity is present during the pacemaker-mediated tachycardia.

Therapy for pacemaker syndrome usually requires upgrade of the system to dual chamber demand (DDD). The rapid pacing rates require definition of the tachycardia and therapy for the tachycardia or a reduction of the upper rate for pacing. The pacemaker-mediated tachycardia is usually prevented by programming to a longer atrial refractory period.

Orthostatic hypotension

A postural fall in blood pressure defined as a decline of 20 mmHg or more in systolic pressure upon assumption of an upright posture is more commonly found in the elderly and may be responsible for syncope and falls. Medical outpatients over the age of 65 years have been found to have a prevalence of orthostatic hypotension as high as 20%,[7] although healthy normotensive elderly persons without risk factors for orthostatic hypotension have a prevalence of less than 7%.[8,9]

A variety of mechanisms account for the increased prevalence of orthostatic hypotension as a cause for syncope. Medications such as anti-anxiety agents, tricyclics, phenothiazines and particularly antihypertensive drugs contribute to orthostasis. Coupled with the drug effects are often disease processes that necessitate bed rest for illness or inactivity and thus increase the postural hypotension. The elevation in systolic blood pressure that occurs with increasing prevalence with aging results in impaired baroreceptor-reflex responsiveness and reduced vascular compliance, thereby making postural hypotension more likely.[10] The normal baroreflex-mediated heart rate response to upright posture tends to be diminished as a function of aging as well.[11] Autonomic insufficiency, probably most common with the peripheral neuropathy of insulin-dependent diabetes mellitus, but also noted with primary autonomic failure such as that seen with inappropriate plasma norepinephrine responses in 'idiopathic orthostatic hypotension' or the Shy–Drager syndrome are entities associated with aging. These entities, not uncommonly, are found to cause lightheadedness or syncope in a setting of a relatively fixed heart-rate response and other dysautonomic features such as incontinence, impotence and inability to sweat. Because the state of hydration is important in the postural responsiveness, elderly patients with decreased fluid intake because of illness or the mechanisms associated with aging such as altered levels of atrial natriuretic hormone or lack of usual thirst mechanisms with water deprivation may be responsible for increased postural hypotension and syncope.

The evaluation for postural hypotension

must include multiple blood pressure checks at various times of the day. The first morning blood pressure (or middle of night after prolonged bed rest) is most likely to demonstrate a greater fall in upright systolic blood pressure than those taken later in the day although the orthostatic pressure remains quite variable during the day. The blood-pressure response may be more profound at peak drug effects as seen commonly 2–3 hours after drug dosing. In addition, the presence of arrhythmia at the time of arising, intercurrent illness and state of hydration are other important factors potentially bearing on the degree of postural hypotension likely to cause syncope.

Evaluation

The diagnosis of orthostatic syncope can be an elusive one. Quite often, the patient may have rather profound orthostatic change whenever checked. The difficulty in making the diagnosis rests with the patient who is only occasionally quite orthostatic and has only minimal or borderline decline in upright blood pressure when seen in the physician's office. Such a patient will require multiple blood pressure checks, particularly the early morning blood pressure after taking additional sleep medication or when feeling poorly with intercedant illness. The patient may be instructed to take her/his blood pressure or a visiting nurse may be required. While symptomatic difficulty present with posture change is helpful, a fall in systolic blood pressure without symptoms is suggestive that orthostasis may be the cause of syncope.

Therapy

Therapy for orthostatic hypotension starts with a drug history. If the patient is receiving antihypertensive medication, an effort to decrease same or switch to medication with less orthostatic effect should be tried. Other medications likely to contribute to orthostatic

hypotension should be discontinued or reduced in dose.

The state of hydration is important. The patient should be encouraged to drink sufficient fluids, even if not thirsty. Using diuretics for cosmetic ankle swelling should be discouraged. Support stockings are often helpful but tend to be poorly tolerated. The patient should be advised to sit for a few minutes before standing and to sit or become supine should they have warnings such as lightheadedness.

Therapies for the dysautonomic causes of orthostatic syncope are quite varied. In addition to the general recommendations, use of midodrine often affords benefit.

Vasodepressor syncope

Vasodepressor or neurocardiogenic syncope is a not uncommon cause for loss of consciousness in the elderly. While passive head-up tilt testing with or without isoproterenol provocation is less likely to cause syncope in the elderly compared with young adults,[12,13] the vasodepressor response remains a most important cause for syncope in the relatively healthy elderly individual. The occurrence of syncope in the upright posture in a patient with a normal ECG and absence of cardiac disease strongly suggests a vasodepressor response.

A remote history of syncope at a young age may be recalled, but often the syncope has occurred only in the later years. Prodromal symptoms, if present, are quite helpful in suggesting the diagnosis. Nausea, warmth, lightheadedness and visual disturbances are some of the more common symptoms heralding a vasodepressor event. However, the elderly in contrast to the younger population with vasodepressor syncope are much less likely to have prodromal symptoms. Syncope usually occurs in the upright posture but may also occur in the sitting position.

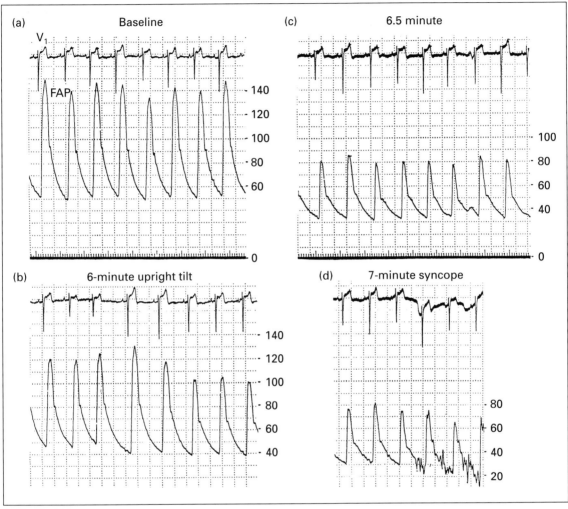

Figure 8.4
Electrocardiogram and femoral artery blood pressure recordings during tilt-study response in a 64-year-old with syncope. No prodromal symptoms had been experienced prior to syncope. The heart rate decreased slightly at 6 min with mild decline in blood pressure (b). Some 20 s later the blood pressure dropped profoundly followed by syncope in (d). No symptoms were mentioned prior to syncope.

Evaluation

The elderly patient with syncope in the upright or sitting position who demonstrates an absence of significant postural change and absence of significant myocardial dysfunction should have tilt-table testing performed. Passive upright tilt is at times more difficult to interpret because of the lack of bradycardia development and symptoms only of near syncope associated with borderline decrease in blood pressure. Passive upright tilt should be performed for 45–60 minutes. If negative, isoproterenol (up to 4 µg/min) should be administered with repeat tilt for 10 minutes. Positive responses are usually dramatic with reproduction of syncope (see Figure 8.4) although near syncope with a 30–40 mmHg blood-pressure decrease while constituting only a borderline response, may be sufficiently diagnostic to warrant therapy toward a vasodepressor response. The specificity of tilt-table testing tends to be much less with use of isoproterenol.[14] Elderly patients have been demonstrated to have reduced blood shift into the lower extremities with lower body negative pressure;[15] this in turn, may produce less baroreceptor stimulation. Coupled with the decreased degree of bradycardia with tilt compared with a younger population, the responses may be blunted.

Use of ECG event recorders in this population may provide helpful information if relative bradycardia and absence of significant arrhythmic abnormality is present at the time of presyncope or syncope. If prodromal symptoms are present, blood pressure Holter recordings may also lend diagnostic information.

Therapy

The mainstay of therapy for vasodepressor syncope is volume expansion with adequate fluid and salt. The elderly are often prone to limiting fluid therapy because of decreased thirst and desire to decrease voiding. Fludrocortisone acetate has been beneficial in some patients although weight gain and ankle edema are sometimes poorly tolerated. Theophylline has been shown to have beneficial effects,[17] although it is not tolerated well in a significant proportion of patients. Theophylline may reverse the isoproterenol resis-

tance to tachycardia noted in the elderly as well as increase the orthostatic rise in plasma renin activity.[17] Other medications deemed to be helpful in vasodepressor syncope are beta-blockers midodrine and disopyramide.[18] Cardiac pacing has been used, although this is a most rare form of therapy because of the lack of significant bradycardia noted at the time of syncope in the elderly.

Postprandial syncope

Postprandial hypotension and syncope occur in the elderly, most often in the setting of multiple illnesses and autonomic insufficiency.[19,20] A prospective study of causes of syncope showed that 8% of syncopal episodes were associated with a postprandial reduction in blood pressure.[21]

Patients usually have orthostatic hypotension with additional postprandial effect sufficient to produce syncope. Patients with postprandial hypotension demonstrate decreases in blood pressure between 15 and 90 minutes post meal. The blood-pressure change is associated with an absence of change in peripheral vascular resistance as seen in the healthy elderly.[22] Even healthy elderly patients have been shown to have a decline in supine blood pressure. However, the healthy elderly individual does not demonstrate a postprandial fall in blood pressure when upright.[23] Somatostatin has been shown to prevent postprandial blood pressure reductions; this suggests that vasoactive peptides may be important in the blood pressure regulation.[20]

Evaluation

The confirmation of potential postprandial syncope primarily involves consideration of same with documented blood pressure measurements supine and standing post meal. Variability in responses has not been evaluated although responses would be predictably quite varied as noted in patients with idiopathic orthostatic hypotension. Exclusion of arrhythmic events with ECG Holter monitoring is often helpful.

Therapy

The approach to the patient with postprandial hypotension and syncope involves education regarding the post-meal period to avoid abrupt or prolonged standing. Antihypertensive medication should be administered between rather than with meals. The state of hydration is to be stressed with encouragement of adequate salt and fluid intake. Smaller meals and reduced carbohydrate content may be helpful. Pharmacological therapy includes the α_1-adrenergic agonist midodrine and fludrocortisone since these have been shown to reduce postprandial hypotension in the elderly and may be of benefit in those with syncope due to postprandial hypotension. For those most symptomatic, the somatostatin analog octreotide may be of benefit due to the demonstrated reduction in postprandial blood pressure in patients with autonomic dysfunction.[24]

Hypersensitive carotid sinus syndrome

Hypersensitive carotid sinus syndrome is an important yet occasionally overlooked cause for syncope in the elderly.[25] Of patients with unexplained syncope, as many as one-quarter may be due to carotid sinus hypersensitivity.[26] Patients often present with syncope without prodrome.[27] Symptoms may be provoked or historically present with head movement or looking upwards in a significant percentage of patients.[27]

Afferent nerve traffic for the carotid sinus reflex originates from baroreceptors located in the wall of the carotid sinus at the bifurcation of the common carotid artery. These fibers join the glossopharyngeal nerve and ascend to the brainstem. Efferent activity is via the vagus and sympathetic chain to the sinoatrial and atrioventricular nodes and peripheral vasculature. The site of abnormality is not known; atropine is known to inhibit the vasodepressor response.

The diagnosis of carotid sinus hypersensitivity is made by applying firm steady massage to each right and left carotid sinus separately for approximately 5 s while monitoring ECG and blood pressure. The maneuver should be performed in the supine state as well as standing or 60–80° upright tilt. A 3 s or greater ventricular asystolic pause constitutes a positive cardio-inhibitory response, while a 50 mmHg blood pressure decline without significant bradycardia is diagnostic of a vasodepressor response. The cardio-inhibitory response is the most common although mixed responses also occur. Figure 8.5 shows the ECG response to carotid sinus massage in a 76 year old with abrupt onset syncope. The reproduction of symptoms with a positive response is reassuring but not essential.

Therapy for the hypersensitive carotid sinus syndrome includes discontinuation of digitalis followed by repeat massage maneuvers because the drug appears to sensitize the reflex. Drug therapy with anticholinergic agents or sympathomimetic drugs is usually poorly tolerated and generally not effective.[28] Cardiac pacing has been shown to be an effective therapy. Dual-chamber pacing is required because of the need to maintain AV synchrony to offset the vasodepressor component.[29] Additionally, the cardio-inhibitory component may include atrioventricular block. Patients with primarily a vasodepressor component may be difficult to render symptom-free. Atrioventricular sequential pacing plus use of α-adrenergic agonists may be useful.[30]

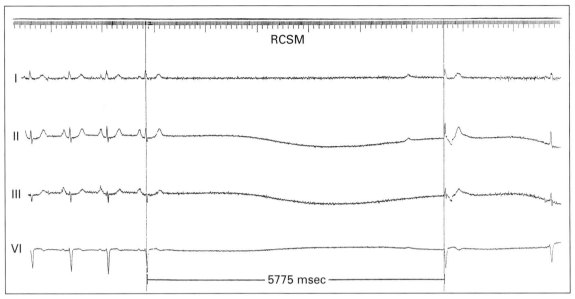

Figure 8.5
ECG recordings in a 76-year-old with abrupt onset syncope. Right carotid sinus massage resulted in a 5.8 s pause with attendant lightheadedness.

Other causes of noncardiac or reflex syncope

Uncommon causes of syncope, particularly in the elderly, include those that are related to the Valsalva maneuver or that trigger vagal events.

Cough syncope occurs with only extremely vigorous and usually protracted paroxysms of cough. A variety of mechanisms have been implicated as causes. The marked increase in intrathoracic pressure reduces cardiac output with purported peripheral vasodilation post cough. A marked increase in cerebrospinal fluid pressure with resultant compression of the intracranial capillary and venous beds may occur. Rhythm abnormalities reflecting a vagomimetic effect contributing to or cause

for syncope include profound sinus bradycardia, sinoatrial pause and atrioventricular block.

An increase in intrathoracic pressure associated with prolonged exhalation against a closed glottis as with the Valsalva maneuver may result in a fall of arterial pressure sufficient to cause syncope. Occasionally, post-Valsalva sinus bradycardia may contribute to the impairment in cerebral blood flow.

Cough and Valsalva-associated syncope require treatment of cough and avoidance of the Valsalva maneuver.

Postmicturition syncope may occur in elderly men, particularly in the setting of nocturia. Syncope occurs suddenly, often without premonitory symptoms.[28] Voiding large volumes or consuming large quantities of alcohol prior to retiring may contribute to the reflex changes that are similar to those of vaso-depressor syncope. Avoidance of alcohol and recommendation of voiding in the sitting position may be required in some instances.

Defecation syncope occurs most commonly in the elderly, most often after arising from bed at night, with strained defecation (Valsalva maneuver may contribute), or during manual disimpaction of the rectum. Vagally mediated sinus bradycardia or atrioventricular block may cause or contribute to the syncope. Avoiding constipation is the most effective approach to therapy.

Cardiac obstructive syncope

Obstructive cardiac disease of a significant degree can cause syncope. Common obstructive lesions such as aortic stenosis, hypertrophic obstructive cardiomyopathy or mitral stenosis often coexist with arrhythmias that may contribute to syncope. Other causes of syncope due to obstruction on the left side of the heart include left atrial myxoma and prosthetic valve dysfunction. On the right side of the heart, pulmonary hypertension, pulmonary emboli and pulmonary stenosis may be associated with obstruction significant to cause syncope.

The elderly individual with a significant obstructive lesion may have syncope with activity or exercise. Syncope with exercise in the setting of aortic stenosis is marked by a lack of increase in cardiac output ultimately resulting in decreased peripheral vascular resistance with syncope due to bradycardia and hypotension much like that noted with vasodepressor syncope. Syncope immediately after effort may occur in patients with hypertrophic obstructive cardiomyopathy. These patients, however, are more likely to have syncope based on an arrhythmic cause.[31]

Evaluation

The patient with obstructive syncope usually has syncope when upright and very often with activity. The physical examination in a patient with exertional syncope is likely to provide the diagnosis. The echocardiogram is most helpful in the definition of most obstructive abnormalities and in assessment of the severity of same. The chest X-ray, arterial blood gases and combined ventilation–perfusion lung scanning or special CT study should provide adequate information regarding pulmonary embolism.

Therapy

The treatment for most of the obstructive causes for syncope is surgery. Patients with hypertrophic obstructive cardiomyopathy may respond to a variety of approaches including pharmacological or pacemaker therapy. The patient with severe pulmonary hypertension due to any cause presents a treatment dilemma since most pharmacological therapies have demonstrated only marginal benefit at most.

Neurological syncope

Neurological disorders are a common cause of falls in the elderly but a less common cause for syncope. Loss of consciousness effects the brainstem reticular formation and its ascending pathways, which project diffusely and bilaterally to the cerebral cortex. Therefore, lack of perfusion to the reticular formation or widespread bilateral perfusion defects are required for syncope to occur. Cerebral transient ischemic attacks are an uncommon cause for syncope. Of 557 episodes of ischemic stroke or transient ischemia, only 6.5% resulted in syncope.[32] Carotid arterial disease is almost always bilaterally significant to cause syncope. Vertebrobasilar disease is more commonly associated with syncope; spells invariably are associated with other brainstem symptoms such as diploplia, vertigo, ataxia, dysarthria, paresthesia and nausea and vomiting.[32]

Seizure disorders rarely cause syncope in the elderly. Less than 2% of the total number of patients presenting with syncope have a seizure identified as the cause for syncope. Series of patients with syncope collected from an emergency room base have a higher incidence of seizure-associated syncope since patients are often seen in an emergency room after seizure and are labeled as syncope.

Seizures responsible for syncope may be primary generalized, simple or complex partial. An increase in heart rate is usually associated with partial seizures; bradyarrhythmia and asystole responsible for syncope have been reported with temporal lobe epilepsy or partial seizures.[33] Since seizure-like activity may frequently be noted with syncope due to any cause, the diagnosis of seizure-induced syncope is at times made without presence of true seizure activity. This has become particularly apparent with observations associated with tilt-induced vasodepressor syncope. While the seizure-like activity is usually different from tonic-clonic activity, electroencephalographic (EEG) recordings permit differentiation of true seizure activity.[34]

Drop attacks refer to a heterogenous syndrome that increases in frequency in the aged and may be confused with syncope. The clinical features as originally described by Sheldon include a sudden, dramatic loss of tone often when walking or standing with abrupt fall and quick recovery in an otherwise healthy individual.[35] The mechanism is probably due to ischemia of the corticospinal tract in the medullary pyramids or basis pontis with sparing of the reticular formation. Atherosclerotic, embolic or mechanical etiologies have been suggested although the cause is often not identified.[36] While not associated with syncope, drop attacks may account for nearly one-quarter of all falls of patients 85 years or older.[36]

The subclavial-steal syndrome is a rare cause of cerebrovascular syncope in the elderly. Obstruction of the subclavian artery proximal to the origin of the vertebral artery results in shunt of blood retrogradely from the circle of Willis to the distal subclavian artery during exercise resulting in potential cerebral ischemia and syncope. A diminished pulse on the affected side with a subclavian bruit and reproduction of symptoms during exercise provides the diagnosis.

Evaluation and therapy

Because cerebrovascular ischemia significant to cause syncope (in the absence of concomitant symptoms due to vertebrobasilar insufficiency) is most unusual, the assessment of carotid flow by noninvasive or invasive methodologies is not recommended for the evaluation of syncope per se. When symptoms of vertebrobasilar insufficiency are present, cerebral angiography is required to confirm the diagnosis.

Therapy is limited for the patient with cerebrovascular insufficiency although reduction of factors compounding the ischemia such as hypotension from postural, postprandial or arrhythmic cause may be helpful.

If seizure activity has been noted or seizure is suspected from the history of postictal or partial seizure behavior, an EEG is required. EEG abnormalities in an elderly population with syncope are common.[32] The likelihood of EEG results affecting the diagnosis and therapy of this population is as low as 1%. Therefore, EEG recording is only recommended when a seizure disorder is strongly suspected. If spells are recurrent, long-term EEG recording may be helpful.[37]

Therapy for seizure-mediated syncope is usually quite effective with drug therapy directed toward the specific seizure abnormality.

Other causes for syncope

A variety of other pathological states or conditions (Table 8.1) may cause syncope but are quite uncommon in the elderly. Hypoglycemia as a cause of syncope in the elderly is usually caused from excessive insulin or hypoglycemia drug. Hyperventilation producing syncope is occasionally the cause in the young individual but a very rare cause for syncope in the elderly. Ethanol or other drug intoxication resulting in syncope is usually suspect from the history and protracted course of the event. Hysterical syncope likewise is an event usually found in the younger individual. After evaluation, a small percentage of patients will have syncope of unexplained cause. These are often multifactorial; continued rhythm analysis, frequent blood pressure checks and general observation are usually fruitful.

Evaluation of syncope

The evaluation of syncope in the elderly starts with a detailed history (Figure 8.6). Often a family member or observer who witnessed a syncopal event may be helpful in supplying additional information about the event. The position of the individual at the onset of syncope is important. Syncope occurring in the supine position effectively excludes vasodepressor syncope. Prodromal symptoms if present are extremely helpful in pointing toward vasodepressor syncope if symptoms are lightheadedness, warmth or nausea, while prodomal palpitations suggest arrhythmic syncope. Witnessed seizure activity signals possible seizure disorder, although syncope due to any cause may be associated with seizure-like activity. Syncope occurring during activity or exercise suggests obstructive cardiac disease or arrhythmic syncope although rarely vasodepressor syncope may occur during or shortly after activity. The history of post-voiding syncope or syncope while coughing or defecating suggests reflex-response syncope.

The physical examination will be diagnostic if cardiac obstructive disease has caused syncope. Abnormal ventricular size and function make arrhythmic syncope much more common; these findings suggest a need for further definition by echocardiography. The finding of significant orthostatic hypotension, particularly if symptomatic difficulty is attendant, suggests orthostatic syncope; therapy can be started based on the possible history of hypertension, drugs used and other influencing factors.

The ECG is done as part of the original evaluation because of the potential to direct the evaluation for suspected arrhythmic syncope or the possibility that arrhythmia may be recorded at the time.

Carotid sinus stimulation is included in the initial evaluation (Figure 8.1) although stimulation is done more readily if two are in attendance such that one can watch the rhythm while massaging and the other takes multiple blood pressure recordings while carotid massage is performed both in the supine and standing (or upright tilt) positions.

Once cardiac disease is either suspected or confirmed by the history, physical examination and ECG, echocardiography provides information that will help direct further study. If cardiac obstructive disease is present, cardiac catheterization is usually warranted. Significant left ventricular dysfunction, particularly if segmental disease is present, suggests a need for coronary angiography usually followed by an electrophysiological catheterization study (EPS). An exercise study is often helpful for the definition of ischemia,

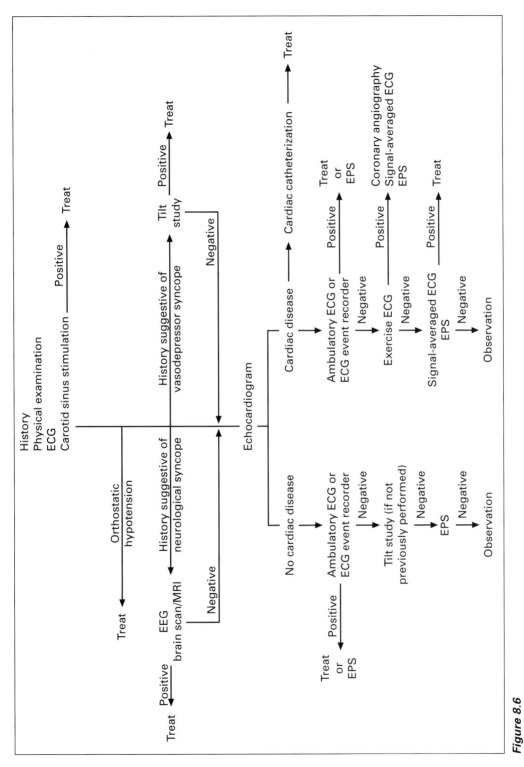

Figure 8.6
Flow chart for evaluation of syncope. See text.

particularly if suggested by history. The signal-averaged ECG may be helpful if positive in directing the need for EPS. A negative examination with confirmation by echocardiography suggests that vasodepressor or hypersensitive carotid sinus syndrome syncope is most likely. Tilt study is to be performed; if negative, EPS may provide clues in a small percentage of patients. If these studies are not diagnostic or sufficiently abnormal to direct therapy, further observation is required, often with the use of an ECG event recorder or an ambulatory blood pressure Holter study for helpful positive or negative information.

References

1. Lipsitz LA, Wei JY, Rowe JW. Syncope in an elderly, institutionalized population: prevalence, incidence and associated risk. *Q J Med* (1985) **55**:45–54.

2. Silverstein MD, Singer DE, Mulley AG et al. Patients with syncope admitted to medical intensive care units. *JAMA* (1982) **248**: 1185–9.

3. Kuga K, Yamaguchi I, Sugishita Y, Ito I. Assessment by autonomic blockade of age-related changes of the sinus node function and autonomic regulation in sick sinus syndrome. *Am J Cardiol* (1988) **61**:361–6.

4. Davies MJ, Pomerance A. Quantitative study of aging changes in the human sinoatrial node and internodal tracts. *Br Heart J* (1972) **34**:150–2.

5. Hermiller JB, Walker SS, Binkley PF et al. The electrophysiologic effects of upright posture. *Am Heart J* (1954) **108**:1250–4.

6. Noll B, Krappe J, Goke B, Maisch B. Influence of pacing mode and rate on peripheral levels of atrial natriuretic peptide (ANP). *Pacing Clin Electrophysiol* (1989) **12**:1763–9.

7. Caird FI, Andrews GR, Kennedy RD. Effect of posture on blood pressure in the elderly. *Br Heart J* (1973) **35**:527–30.

8. Myers MG, Kearns PM, Kennedy DS, Fisher RH. Postural hypotension and diuretic therapy in the elderly. *Can Med Assoc J* (1978) **119**:581–4.

9. Mader SL, Josephson KR, Rubenstein LZ. Low prevalence of postural hypotension among community-dwelling elderly. *JAMA* (1987) **258**:1511–14.

10. Lakatta EG. Do hypertension and aging have a similar effect on the myocardium? *Circulation* (1987) **75**:169–77.

11. Collins KJ, Exton-Smith AN, James MH, Oliver DJ. Functional changes in autonomic nervous responses with aging. *Age Ageing* (1980) **9**:17–24.

12. Sheldon R. Effects of aging on responses to isoproterenol tilt-table testing in patients with syncope. *Am J Cardiol* (1994) **74**:459–63.

13. Lipsitz LA, Marks ER, Koestner J et al. Reduced susceptibility to syncope during postural tilt in old age. Is beta-blockade protective? *Arch Intern Med* (1989) **149**:2709–12.

14. Kapoor W, Brant N. Evaluation of syncope by upright tilt testing with isoproterenol. A nonspecific test. *Ann Intern Med* (1992) **116**: 358–63.

15. Ebert TJ, Hughes CV, Tristani FE et al. Effects of age and coronary heart disease on the circulatory responses to graded lower body negative pressure. *Cardiovasc Res* (1982) **18**:663–9.

16. Nelson SD, Stanley M, Love CJ et al. The autonomic and hemodynamic effects of oral theophylline in patients with vasodepressor syncope. *Arch Intern Med* (1991) **151**:2425–9.

17. Gerber JG, Suteparak S, Andros E, Nies AS. Role of adenosine in promoting cardiac β-adrenergic sensitivity in aging humans. *Clin Res* (1993) **41**:89A (abst).

18. Schaal SF, Nelson SD, Boudoulas H, Lewis RP. Syncope. *Curr Probl Cardiol* (1992) **17**: 207–64.

19. Lipsitz LA, Ryan SM, Parker JA et al. Hemodynamic and autonomic nervous system responses to mixed meal ingestion in healthy young and old subjects and dysautonomic patients with postprandial hypotension. *Circulation* (1993) **87**:391–400.

20. Jansen RWMM, Hoefnagels WHL. Influence of oral and intravenous glucose loading on blood pressure in normotensive and hypertensive elderly subjects. *J Hypertens* (1987) **5**: 5501–3.

21. Lipsitz LA, Pluchino FC, Wei JY, Rowe JW. Syncope in institutionalized elderly: the impact of multiple pathologic conditions and situational stress. *J Chronic Dis* (1986) **39**: 619–30.

22. Robertson D, Wade D, Robertson RM. Postprandial alterations in cardiovascular hemodynamics in autonomic dysfunctional status. *Am J Cardiol* (1981) **48**:1048–52.

23. Mader SL. Effects of meals and time of day on

postural blood pressure responses in young and elderly subjects. *Arch Intern Med* (1989) 49:2757–60.

24. Hoeldtke RD, O'Dorisio TM, Boden G. Treatment of autonomic neuropathy with a somatostatin analogue SMS-201-995. *Lancet* (1986) ii: 602–5.

25. Kenny RA, Traynor G. Carotid sinus syndrome clinical characteristics on elderly patients. *Age Ageing* (1991) 20:449–54.

26. Huang SKS, Ezri MD, Hanser RG, Denes P. Carotid sinus hypersensitivity in patients with unexplained syncope: clinical electrophysiologic, and long-term follow-up observations. *Am Heart J* (1988) 116:989–96.

27. McIntosh SJ, Lawson J, Kenny RA. Clinical characteristics of vasodepressor, cardio-inhibitory, and mixed carotid sinus syndrome in the elderly. *Am J Med* (1993) 95:203–8.

28. Boudoulas H, Nelson SD, Schaal SF, Lewis R. Diagnosis and management of syncope. In: Hurst WJ, ed., *The Heart*, 9th edn (McGraw-Hill: New York, 1998) 1059–80.

29. Madigan NP, Flaker GC, Curtis JC et al. Carotid sinus hypersensitivity: beneficial effects of dual-chamber pacing. *Am J Cardiol* (1984) 53:1034–40.

30. Katritsis D, Ward DE, Camm AJ. Can we treat carotid sinus syndrome? *Pacing Clin Electrophysiol* (1991) 14:1367–74.

31. Fananapazir L, Tracy CM, Leon MB et al. Electrophysiologic abnormalities in patients with hypertrophic cardiomyopathy. *Circulation* (1989) 80:1259–68.

32. Bousser MG, Dubois B, Castaigne P. Transient loss of consciousness in cerebral ischemic events: a study of 557 ischemic strokes and transient ischemic attacks. *Ann Intern Med* (1980) 132:300–5.

33. Constantin L, Martins JB, Fincham RW, Daqli RD. Bradycardia and syncope as manifestation of partial epilepsy. *J Am Coll Cardiol* (1990) 15:900–5.

34. Grubb BP, Gerard G, Roush K et al. Differentiation of convulsive syncope and epilepsy with head-up tilt testing. *Ann Intern Med* (1991) 115:871–6.

35. Sheldon JH. On the natural history of falls in old age. *BMJ* (1960) ii:1685.

36. Lipsitz LA. The drop attack: a common geriatric symptom. *J Am Geriatr Soc* (1983) 31: 617–20.

37. Lai C-W, Ziegler DK. Syncope problem solved by continuous ambulatory simultaneous EEG/ECG recording. *Neurology* (1981) 31: 1152–4.

9

Cardiovascular evaluation for noncardiac surgery: the role of advanced age

Douglas C Morris

The scope of the problem

Of the 25 million patients who undergo non-cardiac surgery yearly in the United States, 4 million are older than 65 years of age.[1] Furthermore, the number of elderly patients undergoing surgical procedures is on the rise reflecting both an aging of the population of the United States and the readiness of this elderly cohort of our society to accept risks in order to maintain their quality of life. Currently, 13% of the US population is older than 65 years of age and 3% (over 7 million people) is aged 80 or older. By the year 2010, these subsets of the elderly will increase to 21% (35 million people) and 4.3% (12 million people) respectively.[2] Many of these elderly patients continue at remunerative work or participate in an active retirement. They are pleased with the fact that they live independently and are committed to continue to do so.

Relative surgical risk in the elderly

Thirty years ago Warren Cole pointed out that surgical mortalities are two to five times higher in the elderly.[3] Half of these postoperative deaths are directly related to cardiac complications. Subsequent studies by Goldman and associates in 1977,[4] and by Larsen and associates in 1987,[5] found that these differences between the elderly and younger persons in major nonfatal and fatal postoperative cardiac complications have not been diminished during the subsequent three decades. The challenge for the physician rendering a pre-operative evaluation of the elderly patient is to segregate the low-risk patient from the patients requiring further assessment or special management because their risk is intermediate or high. The elderly population is a more heterogeneous group with respect to severity of cardiac illness, coexisting medical problems and functional capabilities than their younger cohorts.

Pre-operative assessment

The role of the cardiovascular consultant in evaluating the pre-operative status of the patient is not to merely 'clear' the patient for surgery, but instead to define the patient's pre-existing cardiovascular conditions and assess their potential impact on the chances for acceptable surgical recovery; to outline the pre-operative management of these conditions; and to provide counsel as to the influence the surgical procedure will have upon the expected prognosis for the cardiac conditions that have surfaced. The consultant must remain mindful that the prognosis of advanced coronary artery disease and severe symptomatic left ventricular dysfunction is worse than some malignancies.[6]

Several multivariate indices of risk have been formulated in an attempt to quantify the operative risk. The first of these was the Dripps–American Society of Anesthesiologists classification of physical status proposed in 1963 (Table 9.1).[7] While this index is still used by the American Society of Anesthesiology, it is subjective and probably less applicable to certain subsets of patients such as the elderly. In 1977, Goldman and associates constructed a more elaborate 'point scale' system derived from a multivariate analysis of 39 variables and arrived at nine independent predictors of peri-operative cardiac events[4] (Table 9.2). By altering several features of the Goldman index including defining the severity of coronary artery disease on the basis of the Canadian Heart Association angina class and considering the type of surgery in the pretest probability of cardiac complications, Detsky and associates in 1986 proposed a modified multifactorial index (Table 9.3).[8] None of these cardiac risk indices have proven to be generally applicable because of institution-specific variables and confounding factors specific for a given patient and are, therefore, not widely utilized.[9]

Probably more important than the index of cardiac risk defined by these studies are the variables they established as worthy of pre-operative recognition. The three cardiac conditions identified in these studies as most critical of pre-operative identification are heart failure, myocardial ischemia and aortic stenosis. The first two of these conditions are responsible for the majority of peri-operative cardiac morbidity and mortality.[10]

Heart failure evident on physical examination by persistent pulmonary rales, S_3 gallop, or jugular venous distention or on chest X-ray by interstitial or alveolar pulmonary edema places the patient at substantial operative risk. The presence of any of the above findings

1. A normal healthy patient
2. A patient with a mild systemic disease
3. A patient with a severe systemic disease that limits activity, but is not incapacitating
4. A patient with an incapacitating systemic disease that is a constant threat to life
5. A moribund patient not expected to survive 24 hours with or without operation

Note: in the event of emergency operation, precede the number with an E.

Reprinted with permission.[7]

Table 9.1
The Dripps–ASA classification of physical status

except for the third heart sound would warrant delay of all but emergency surgery. More than 25% of patients with clinically manifest congestive heart failure develop pulmonary edema peri-operatively as opposed to 6% of patients without signs of heart failure.[11]

If evidence for latent heart failure exists but is not conclusive, an assessment of left ventricular systolic function is warranted. The evaluation of left ventricular function can be provided by radionuclide ventriculography, echocardiography or contrast ventriculography (appropriate if coronary arteriography is also indicated). Radionuclide ventriculography quantifies the ejection fraction and allows for analysis of regional wall motion but does not define valvular anatomy and function or wall thickness. Conversely, echocardiography demonstrates cardiac anatomy and function, but the assessment of the ejection fraction is

Criteria	Multivariate discriminant-function coefficient	Points
1. History		
Age > 70 yr	0.191	5
MI in previous 6 months	0.384	10
2. Physical examination		
S₃ gallop or JVD	0.451	11
Important VAS	0.119	3
3. Electrocardiogram		
Rhythm other than sinus or PACs on last pre-operative ECG	0.283	7
>5 PVCs/min documented at any time before operation	0.278	7
4. General status		
P_{O_2} < 60 or P_{CO_2} > 50 mmHg, K < 3.0 or HCO_3 < 20 mEq/l, BUN > 50 or Cr > 3.0 mg/dl, abnormal SGOT, signs of chronic liver disease, or patient bedridden from noncardiac causes	0.132	3
5. Operation		
Intraperitoneal, intrathoracic, or aortic operation	0.123	3
Emergency room	0.167	4
Total		53

MI, myocardial infarction; JVD, jugular-vein distension; VAS, valvular aortic stenosis; PAC, premature atrial contractions; ECG, electrocardiogram; PVC, premature ventricular contractions; P_{O_2}, partial pressure of oxygen; P_{CO_2}, partial pressure of carbon dioxide; K, potassium; HCO_3, bicarbonate; BUN, blood urea nitrogen; Cr, creatinine; SGOT, serum glutamic oxalacetic transaminase.
Reprinted from Goldman et al [4] with permission.

Table 9.2
The Goldman multifactorial cardiac risk index

more subjective. Moreover, echocardiography is more technologist-dependent and inadequate studies will be obtained in 10–15% of the population.[6]

Patients determined to have an ejection fraction of 35% or less will be likely candi-dates for the development of heart failure without careful peri-operative monitoring and management. An ejection fraction over 40%, however, should not be viewed as assurance that the patient will not develop heart failure. Heart failure can occur as a consequence of

Variables	Points
CAD	
MI within 6 months	10
MI more than 6 months	5
Canadian Cardiovascular Society angina	
Class 3	10
Class 4	20
Unstable angina within 3 months	10
Alveolar pulmonary edema	
Within 1 week	10
Ever	5
Valvular disease	
Suspected critical aortic stenosis	20
Arrhythmias	
Sinus plus atrial premature beats or rhythm other than sinus on last pre-operative ECG	5
More than five ventricular premature beats at any one time before surgery	5
Poor general medical status*	5
Age over 70 years	5
Emergency operation	10

* Oxygen pressure < 60 mmHg; carbon dioxide pressure > 50 mmHg; serum potassium < 3.0 mEq/l (<3.0 mmol/l); serum bicarbonate < 20 mEq/l (<20 mmol/l); serum urea nitrogen > 50 mg/dl (>18 mmol/l); serum creatinine > 3 signs of chronic liver disease; and/or bedridden because of noncardiac causes.
Reprinted from Detsky et al[8] with permission.

Table 9.3
The modified multifactorial cardiac risk index

disturbed diastolic filling of the left ventricle in the absence of systolic dysfunction. Whether an analysis of ventricular function by ventriculography is superior to clinical variables in predicting peri-operative cardiac outcomes is debatable. Larsen and associates found that radionuclide ventriculography added little information to clinical parameters for predicting peri-operative risk,[5] while Foster and associates found more disturbed ventricular function correlated independently with operative mortality and cardiovascular morbidity.[12] While a depressed left ventricular ejection fraction may predict postoperative heart failure, it is a relatively unreliable marker for peri-operative myocardial infarction or death. Pasternack and associates found the resting ejection fraction was a good discriminator between those patients who would and would not experience a peri-operative infarction.[13]

Subsequent studies, however, failed to confirm this correlation between resting ejection fraction and the development of peri-operative infarction.[9,14,15]

Myocardial ischemia is a particular threat in the octogenarians. This segment of our society has the highest prevalence of coronary atherosclerotic heart disease which, in turn, is responsible for half of all deaths in people over 85 years of age.[16] Since myocardial ischemia in the elderly often has an atypical presentation, coronary artery disease can easily go unrecognized in these patients. Furthermore, the propensity for the elderly patient to be more sedentary makes it less likely that exertional symptoms reflecting heart failure or myocardial ischemia will be apparent. A history of previous myocardial infarction increases the chance of sustaining a peri-operative myocardial infarction from less than 1% to approximately 6%.[17,18] This risk of peri-operative infarction is inversely related to the interval between the previous myocardial infarction and surgery.[19] The myocardial infarction rate is 27% when the interval is less than 3 months, 11% when the interval is 3–6 months, and 4–5% when over 6 months.[19] It should be recognized that these studies occurred prior to the widespread use of coronary arteriography. Presently, the appropriate pre-operative approach in any patient with previous myocardial infarction is to assess for other myocardial regions in jeopardy of ischemia with a noninvasive function test ('stress test'). The testing possibilities include exercise testing, exercise radionuclide testing, pharmacological radionuclide testing, or exercise or pharmacological echocardiography. The exercise may be treadmill or bicycle ergometry; and the pharmacological stress may be produced by dobutamine, adenosine or dipyridamole. Since optimal pre-operative assessment should not only define the presence or absence of myocardial ischemia but the extent of the ischemia (number of ventricular segments involved), some form of radionuclide testing or stress echocardiography is preferable to simple exercise ECG testing. Assessment of the exercise capacity, however, has been documented to be an important predictor of cardiac outcome following noncardiac surgery. McPhail and associates found that patients who achieved 85% of their predicted maximum heart rate during exercise testing had a cardiac complication rate of 6% compared with a 24% complication rate in those patients unable to reach this target heart rate.[20] Gerson and associates noted that an inability to perform 2 minutes of supine bicycle exercise testing was a good predictor of peri-operative cardiac complications.[21] Consequently, when possible, exercise seems preferable to pharmacological 'stress'. Nevertheless, dipyridamole myocardial perfusion scintigraphy has been established to have negative predictive value for myocardial infarction or death following noncardiac surgery of approximately 99%. The positive predictive value is relatively low at 4–20%.[22] While dobutamine stress echocardiography has not been as extensively tested, the available data substantiate that it is a reliable risk-stratification modality.[9] The patient with stable angina pectoris might also be most appropriately evaluated by a 'stress test'. If the diagnosis of angina pectoris is definite and, particularly if the patient has had a previous myocardial infarction; a more appropriate and expedient approach would be to proceed directly to coronary arteriography. Uncertainty about the etiology of chest pain should usually be resolved by a 'stress test'.

Valvular aortic stenosis was established in the Goldman study to be associated with a significant increase in peri-operative cardiac death.[4] Since about 60% of patients over 65 years of age have systolic murmurs[23] and since the physical findings of aortic stenosis in the elderly may be quite atypical, severe aortic stenosis in the geriatric population could be overlooked by the inattentive physician. Aortic stenosis in the elderly may present with a musical systolic murmur, equally as intense at the apex as at the base, accompanied by a normalized carotid pulse contour.[24] Furthermore, the symptoms of chest pain, dyspnea or syncope are often inappropriately attributed to coronary artery disease, conduction system dysfunction or postural effects; while in the more sedentary patients the lack of activity precludes the manifestation of exertional symptoms. Any patient 65 years of age or older with a grade 2/6 or greater systolic murmur, particularly when accompanied by any of the above symptoms or left ventricular hypertrophy on the electrocardiogram, should have a pre-operative echocardiogram with Doppler studies to evaluate for aortic stenosis.

Mitral stenosis may predispose a patient to peri-operative congestive heart failure. The natural history of rheumatic valvular disease makes it very unlikely, however, that an octogenarian would present with uncorrected severe mitral stenosis. Severe aortic or mitral regurgitation is generally well tolerated during the peri-operative period, unless there is depressed left ventricular function.

The study by Goldman and associates also found that a cardiac rhythm other than sinus and greater than five premature ventricular contractions per minute were risk factors for cardiac complications,[4] whereas the study by Larsen and associates could not confirm that abnormal rhythms or premature beats were risk factors.[5] The increased prevalence of ventricular ectopy in the elderly patient (27–60% depending on the study)[25,26] argues against the presence of isolated (even though frequent) ventricular ectopic beats being a significant predictor of peri-operative events in this age group. Potentially life-threatening ventricular tachyarrhythmias in the geriatric population are usually associated with extensive coronary artery disease, previous myocardial infarction or heart failure. Ventricular ectopy in the absence of one of these conditions merits only peri-operative monitoring. Bradyarrhythmias are less common, particularly if the sinus pauses which may appear during sleeping hours are ignored.[26]

In assessing the peri-operative cardiac risk of a patient, the consultant must consider comorbid factors particularly respiratory insufficiency, renal insufficiency, diabetes mellitus and electrolyte abnormalities. Each of these conditions increases the chances of peri-operative cardiac complications and makes the complications more difficult to treat.

Pre-operative management

Effective pre-operative management of congestive heart failure with vasodilator drugs, diuretics, and digoxin if necessary can contribute to a satisfactory surgical outcome.[27] Historical evidence of previous heart failure should be noted and should alert the physicians that the stress of surgery may cause a recurrence. Monitoring of pulmonary artery and pulmonary artery occlusion pressures is appropriate in selected high-risk patients. In those patients with pulmonary edema secondary to severely dilated cardiomyopathy, hypertrophic cardiomyopathy or regurgitant valvular lesions, the pulmonary artery catheter will facilitate pre-operative optimization of the preload of the left ventricle and the cardiac output. In the elderly patient, central venous pressures are an unreliable reflection of left ventricular filling pressures.

The correct management of patients with potentially ischemic myocardium can be debated. Generally, those patients with evidence of reversible ischemia are referred for coronary arteriography prior to their surgery. The expectation would be that (when appropriate) coronary angioplasty or coronary bypass surgery would reduce the likelihood of myocardial infarction and cardiac death after noncardiac surgery.[11,28] Coronary angioplasty has rapidly emerged as an effective and relatively safe means of addressing this life-threatening situation in the octogenarian. At the Emory Heart Center, the proportion of patients undergoing coronary angioplasty in 1994–96 who were older than 75 years was 14% versus only 3% in 1988–90. These same data confirm an equivalency in angiographic and clinical success rates until age 80, when the success rate trend is downward. A review of the data reveals that even after age 80, age alone does not play a significant role in the success of coronary angioplasty. The octogenarians in the Emory data were a higher risk subgroup with more females, more patients with unstable angina, more patients with depressed left ventricular function and patients with generally more extensive coronary disease. Coronary artery bypass surgery has also been found to have an acceptable 2.7–6% hospital mortality in the octogenarian.[29–31] While this mortality rate is higher than in younger cohorts, the excellent long-term survival in this age group argues for consideration of surgical revascularization despite their advanced age.[31] Foster and associates concluded, based upon an analysis of 1600 patients from the CASS registry, that the use of coronary artery bypass surgery was advisable in patients with significant coronary artery disease prior to their undergoing a major noncardiac operation.[11] In this analysis, the operative mortality for the noncardiac procedure was 0.9% in those patients with prior coronary artery bypass surgery compared with a mortality of

2.4% in those patients with unbypassed coronary disease.

It would be a mistake, however, to adopt the stance that every patient with reversible myocardial ischemia must be revascularized prior to noncardiac surgery. The potential benefits of an added margin of safety must be measured against the risk of an additional intervention or delay in the performance of the required noncardiac surgery. It is worth noting that, in the CASS registry, the patients' cumulative operative mortality (2.3%) for elective coronary artery bypass surgery (1.4%) plus the noncardiac procedure (0.9%) was little different from the 2.4% mortality for the noncardiac procedure in the unbypassed patients.[12] The higher operative risk for elective coronary bypass surgery in the octogenarian makes this conundrum particularly relevant to this age group. Clearly, each decision regarding prophylactic myocardial revascularization prior to noncardiac surgery must be appropriate for the individual based upon the extent of myocardium in jeopardy of ischemia, the assessment of left ventricular function, the patient's comorbid conditions and the type of noncardiac surgery to be performed. Vascular operations impose the stress of blood loss, the possibility of intra-operative hypotension and fluid shifts. Thoracic surgery is accompanied by all of the above plus the stress of prolonged mechanical ventilation. Orthopedic procedures are often quite long and, likewise, associated with major fluid shifts. Head and neck, prostate and ophthalmologic surgery is less stressful and generally better tolerated.

Aortic valve replacement in the geriatric population, including octogenarians, offers excellent symptomatic and hemodynamic improvement with acceptable operative mortality.[32] In those patients in whom aortic valve surgery is inadvisable prior to their previously planned noncardiac surgery, percutaneous balloon aortic valvuloplasty can be considered for palliation.[33]

In patients with severe aortic or mitral regurgitation, instances of increase in afterload can hopefully be avoided but, if not, should be treated aggressively with vasodilators. Patients with symptomatic bradyarrhythmias are usually candidates for permanent pacemakers and, consequently, should be considered for temporary pacemaker insertion prior to urgent surgery. Patients with asymptomatic bradyarrhythmias or conduction system disease (including trifascicular block) do not require prophylactic pacemaker insertion[34] but benefit from intra-operative and postoperative rhythm monitoring.

The presence of atrial fibrillation will not only demand attention to ventricular rate control during the peri-operative period but should also alert the physician to preclinical left ventricular dysfunction. While advanced age of the patient is the most important predisposing factor for atrial fibrillation, an enlargement of the left atrium makes the patient's atria even more prone to fibrillate. If unexplained atrial fibrillation is present preoperatively and unassociated with left ventricular hypertrophy on electrocardiogram or clinical heart failure, an echocardiographic–Doppler evaluation of wall thickness and systolic and diastolic left ventricular function seems warranted. Hyperthyroidism should also be excluded. The need for anticoagulation must also be addressed.

Physiological changes unique to the geriatric patient

The cardiovascular consultant must be knowledgeable enough to foresee possible cardiac consequences of the surgery that are unique to the geriatric patient and to manage the patient accordingly. The physiological changes with aging most likely to result in cardiovascular sequelae are a decrease in diastolic compliance of the left ventricle, increased vascular stiffness, decreased baroreceptor responsiveness and a predisposition for developing atrial fibrillation. (See also Chapter 23.) Aging also reduces the functional reserve of other organ systems particularly the lungs, kidneys and liver.

Aging of the heart primarily reduces left ventricular distensibility and increases wall thickness. The structural changes in the heart as a consequence of aging are fibrosis and an increase in collagenous tissue between myocytes. It is probably these degenerative changes rather than an increase in afterload that account for the increased wall thickness.[35] This decrease in left ventricular compliance makes the octogenarian heart less capable of handling excess fluid volume or tachycardia.

Age-related vascular changes include an increase in vascular stiffness of the large arteries secondary to a decrease in the elastic tissue and an increase in collagen in the arterial media.[2] Consequently, 10–40% of elderly patients are hypertensive. The age-related rise in diastolic blood pressure levels off about age 55 years but systolic blood pressure continues to rise.[36] These elevated pressures impose an increased afterload on the heart. Elderly hypertensive patients can be expected to respond appropriately to antihypertensive therapy without significant adverse reactions. The medications should be started at low doses and increased gradually.[37]

Aging of the heart is also characterized by an increase in left atrial size as a likely consequence of reduced distensibility of the left ventricle (Figure 9.1).[35] This increase in left atrial size and the age-related loss of sinus node pacemaker cells predispose the patient to the

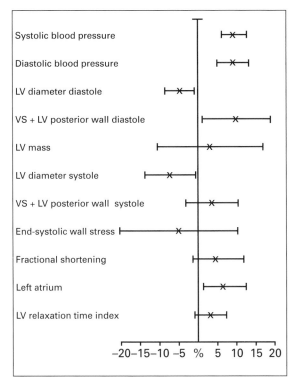

Figure 9.1
Blood pressure, left ventricular (LV) morphology and function. Mean changes during a 4–year period (%), and 95% confidence levels. V5 = ventricular septal. Reproduced from Lernfelt[35] with permission.

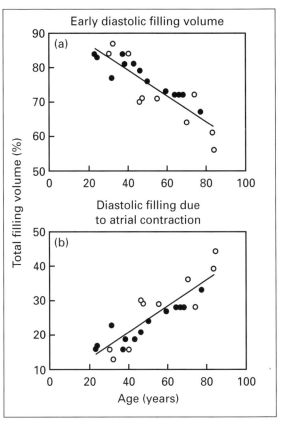

Figure 9.2
The relative contribution of early distolic filling (top) and atrial contraction (bottom) to left ventricular filling as assessed by echocardiographic Doppler technique in healthy men (●) and women (○) ranging from 20 to 80 years of age. Reproduced from Geokas[39] with permission.

development of atrial fibrillation.[38] The elderly patient, therefore, has a greater likelihood of developing atrial fibrillation postoperatively. The development of atrial fibrillation is likely to have more pronounced consequences in terms of decreased cardiac output in the elderly patient because of the relatively greater contribution of atrial contraction to ventricular filling in this age group (Figure 9.2).[39]

The decrease in baroreceptor responsiveness with aging exaggerates the propensity for pos-

tural hypotension. Decreases in intravascular volume are likely to have greater adverse effects in the geriatric population because of the decreased baroreceptor responsiveness coupled with the other effects of aging; namely, decreased circulating blood volume and increased vascular stiffness.[2]

Aging also diminishes the functional reserve of other organ systems. Both the glomerular filtration rate and the tubular secretion rates decline with aging. The glomerular filtration rate decreases by 40–50% as renal blood flow falls by a half. The decline in creatinine clearance (generally about 30%) associated with aging may be obscured by a normal serum creatinine due to a decrease in lean body mass.[2] Further decreases in renal perfusion due to diuresis, ACE inhibitors or hypotension will produce rises in serum creatinine. Hepatic mass and hepatic blood flow both decline with aging. Consequently, the clearance of drugs metabolized slowly in the liver is reduced. Drugs with significant hepatic first-pass metabolism must also be given cautiously in the elderly due to a reduction in hepatic blood flow. These drugs include most major tranquilizers, tricyclic antidepressants, and anti-arrhythmic agents (see Chapter 10).[40]

Another area of possible impairment in the geriatric population that should not be ignored is psychological function. Decreased cognitive efficiency and increased prevalence of psychiatric symptoms have been noted in the elderly. Disturbances of mood are also common in the geriatric population.[41] Shaw and associates found minor neuropsychological impairment in 31% of patients undergoing peripheral vascular surgery but no severe intellectual dysfunction in any patient.[42] Pre-existing or induced neuropsychological impairments may be aggravated by sedatives, analgesics, anti-arrhythmics, sleep deprivation, fever or hypoxia.

Peri-operative management of the geriatric patient is also unique due to pharmacotherapeutic considerations. Drug selection and dosing will often need to be altered due to changes in lean body mass, reduced hepatic and renal functional reserve, impaired chronotropy and previous drug reactions. Adverse drug reactions are two to three times higher in the elderly compared with younger adults.[41]

The patient's pre-operative drug therapy should be reviewed and the appropriate peri-operative usage of these drugs outlined. Patients receiving a beta-blocker for treatment of coronary artery disease should continue the drug until the morning of surgery. Myocardial ischemia is less frequent in patients undergoing coronary artery bypass surgery who are receiving beta-blockers than those receiving a calcium channel blocker alone or on no medications. Patients on antihypertensive medications should have their medications continued because uncontrolled hypertension increases the peri-operative risk. The premature cessation of most antihypertensive drugs means that the blood pressure is untreated during the stress imposed by surgery; also, with the cessation of clonidine, rebound hypertension can develop. Digitalis and nitrates can be continued up to the day of surgery, while diuretics might be discontinued or reduced for a few days before surgery to prevent volume depletion.

Conclusion

The evaluation of the elderly patient prior to noncardiac surgery requires an appraisal of the patient's peri-operative risk based upon clinical parameters, a decision on whether adequate risk appraisal requires further testing, an assessment of the possible complications attendant to the planned surgical procedure, and a design of monitoring techniques necessary to detect these complications (Figures 9.3–9.7). The cardiovascular consultant must be cognisant of the costs and quality of the testing modalities available. The consultant should also be alert throughout the peri-operative period to adverse cardiovascular changes, so that such changes will trigger appropriate actions. The majority of cardiovascular complications occur during the first 2–3 post-

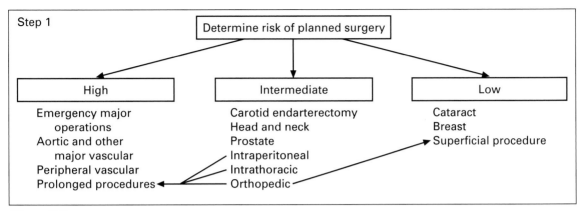

Figure 9.3
Source: ACC/AHA Guidelines for Perioperative Cardiovascular Evaluation for Noncardiac Surgery[22]

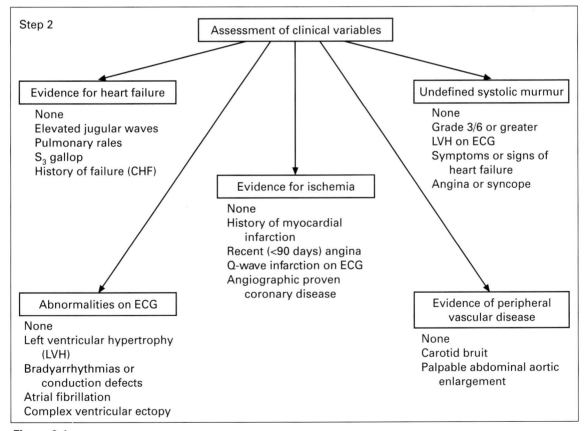

Figure 9.4
Source: ACC/AHA Guidelines for Perioperative Cardiovascular Evaluation for Noncardiac Surgery[22]

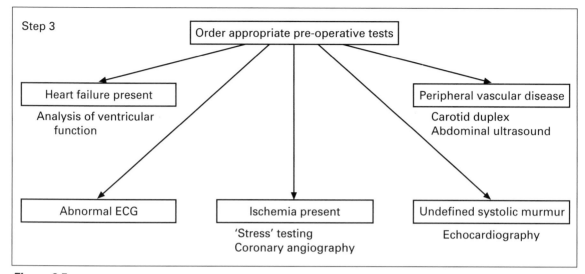

Figure 9.5
Source: ACC/AHA Guidelines for Perioperative Cardiovascular Evaluation for Noncardiac Surgery [22]

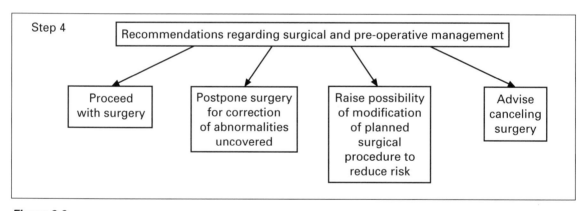

Figure 9.6
Source: ACC/AHA Guidelines for Perioperative Cardiovascular Evaluation for Noncardiac Surgery [22]

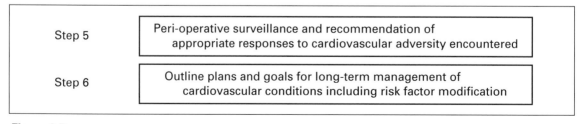

Figure 9.7
Source: ACC/AHA Guidelines for Perioperative Cardiovascular Evaluation for Noncardiac Surgery [22]

operative days. Finally, the consultant must realize that, for some patients, the pre-operative evaluation represents their first opportunity for cardiovascular evaluation. In these cases, it will be imperative for the cardiovascular consultant to outline long-term therapy of the cardiovascular conditions and risk factor modification.

References

1. Hollenberg M, Mangano DT, Browner WS, London MJ, Tubau JF, Tateo IM. Predictors of postoperative myocardial ischemia in patients undergoing noncardiac surgery. *JAMA* (1992) **268**:205–9.
2. Wenger N. Cardiovascular disease in the elderly. *Curr Probl Cardiol* (1992) **17**:611–90.
3. Del Guercio LRM, Cohn JD. Monitoring operative risk in the elderly. *JAMA* (1980) **243**:1350–5.
4. Goldman L, Caldera DL, Nussbaum SR et al. Multifactorial index of cardiac risk in noncardiac surgical procedures. *N Engl J Med* (1977) **297**:845–50.
5. Larsen SF, Olesen KH, Jacobsen E. Prediction of cardiac risk in non-cardiac surgery. *Eur Heart J* (1987) **8**:179–85.
6. Blaustein AS. Preoperative and perioperative management of cardiac patients undergoing noncardiac surgery. *Cardiol Clin* (1995) **13**: 149–61.
7. American Society of Anesthesiologists. New classification of physical status. *Anesthesiology* (1963) **24**:111.
8. Detsky AS, Abrams HB, Forbath N et al. Cardiac assessment for patients undergoing noncardiac surgery: a multifactorial clinical risk index. *Arch Int Med* (1986) **146**:2131–4.
9. Cohen MC, Eagle KA. The role of the cardiology consultant. In: Topol EJ, ed, *Comprehensive Cardiovascular Medicine* (Lippincott-Raven: Philadelphia, 1998) 1007–31.
10. Goldman L. Cardiac risk in noncardiac surgery, an update. *Anesth Analg* (1995) **80**:810–20.
11. Goldman L. Multifactorial index of cardiac risk in noncardiac surgery. Ten years status report. *J Cardiothorac Anesth* (1987) **1**: 237–42.
12. Foster ED, Davis KB, Carpenter JA et al. Risk of noncardiac operation in patients with defined coronary disease: the coronary artery surgery study (CASS) registry experience. *Am Thorac Surg* (1986) **41**:42–50.
13. Pasternack PF, Imparato AM, Riles TS et al. The value of the radionuclide angiogram in the prediction of perioperative myocardial infarction in patients undergoing lower extremity revascularization procedures. *Circulation* (1985) **72**:1113–17.
14. Kazmers A, Cerquiera MD, Zierler RE. Perioperative and late outcome in patients with left ventricular ejection fraction of 35% or less who require major vascular surgery. *J Vasc Surg* (1988) **8**:307–15.
15. Franco CD, Goldsmith J, Veith FJ et al. Resting gated pool ejection fraction: a poor predictor of perioperative myocardial infarction in patients undergoing vascular surgery for infrainguinal bypass grafting. *J Vasc Surg* (1989) **10**:656–61.
16. Abrams J, Coulas DB, Malhota D et al. Coronary risk factors and their modification: lipids, smoking, hypertension, estrogen, and the elderly. *Curr Probl Cardiol* (1995) **20**: 535–610.
17. Abraham SA, Coles NA, Coley CM et al. Coronary risk of noncardiac surgery. *Prog Cardiovasc Dis* (1991) **3**:205–34.
18. Tarhan S, Moffitt EA, Taylor WF, Giuliani ER. Myocardial infarction after general anesthesia. *JAMA* (1972) **220**:1451–4.
19. Steen PA, Tinker JH, Tarhan S. Myocardial reinfarction after anesthesia and surgery. *JAMA* (1978) **239**:2566–70.
20. McPhail N, Calvin JE, Shariatmadar A et al. The use of preoperative exercise testing to predict cardiac complications after arterial reconstruction. *J Vasc Surg* (1988) **7**:60–8.
21. Gerson MC, Hurst JM, Hertzbert VS et al. Prediction of cardiac and pulmonary complications related to elective abdominal and noncardiac thoracic surgery in geriatric patients. *Am J Med* (1990) **88**:101–7.
22. Eagle KA, Brundage BH, Chaitman BR et al. Guidelines for perioperative cardiovascular evaluation for noncardiac surgery. Report of the American College of Cardiology/American

Heart Association Task Force on Practice Guidelines (Committee on Perioperative Cardiovascular Evaluation for Noncardiac Surgery). *J Am Coll Cardiol* (1996) **27**:910–48.

23. Davison ET, Friedman SA. Significance of systolic murmurs in the aged. *N Engl J Med* (1968) **279**:226–30.

24. Roberts WC, Perloff JK, Costantino T. Severe valvular aortic stenosis in patients over 65 years of age. *Am J Cardiol* (1971) **27**:497–506.

25. Martin A, Benbow LJ, Buhous GS et al. Five-year follow-up of 101 elderly subjects by means of long-term ambulatory cardiac monitoring. *Eur Heart J* (1984) **5**:592–6.

26. Kantelip JP, Sage E, Duchere-Marallaz P. Findings on ambulatory electrocardiographic monitoring in subjects older than 80 years. *Am J Cardiol* (1986) **57**:398–401.

27. Babu SC, Pathanjali S, Raciti A et al. Monitor-guided responses: operability with safety is increased in patients with peripheral vascular disease. *Arch Surg* (1980) **115**:1384–90.

28. Tool KW, Jacocks MA, Elkins RC. Preoperative coronary artery bypass grafting in patients undergoing abdominal aortic reconstruction. *JAMA* (1984) **148**:825–9.

29. Ko W, Gold JP, Lazars R et al. Survival analysis of octogenarian patients with coronary artery disease managed by elective coronary artery bypass surgery versus conventional medical treatment. *Circulation* (1992) **86**(Supp II): 191–7.

30. Mick MJ, Simpfendorfer C, Arnold AZ et al. Early and late results of coronary angioplasty and bypass in octogenarians. *Am J Cardiol* (1991) **68**:1316–20.

31. Kaul TK, Fields BL, Wyatt DA et al. Angioplasty versus coronary bypass in octogenarians. *Am Thoracic Surg* (1994) **58**:1419–26.

32. Craver JM, Weintraub WS, Jones EJ et al. Predictors of mortality, complications, and length of stay in aortic valve replacement for aortic stenosis. *Circulation* (1988) **78**(Suppl I): 85–90.

33. Rodriguez AR, Kleiman NS, Minor ST et al. Factors influencing the outcome of balloon aortic valvuloplasty in the elderly. *Am Heart J* (1990) **120**:373–80.

34. Pastore JO, Yourchok PM, Janis KM et al. The risk of advanced heart block in surgical patients with right bundle branch block and left axis deviation. *Circulation* (1978) **57**: 677–80.

35. Lernfelt B, Wikstrand J, Svanborg A, Landahl S. Aging and left ventricular function in elderly healthy people. *Am J Cardiol* (1991) **68**:547–9.

36. Applegate WB. Hypertension in elderly patients. *Ann Intern Med* (1989) **110**:901–15.

37. Moser M. Are the hemodynamic changes in elderly hypertensive patients of clinical importance? Do they influence the choice of medication? *Am J Geriatric Cardiol* (1996) **5**:44–9.

38. Davies MJ. Pathology of the conduction system. In: Caird FL, Dall LC, Kennedy RD, eds, *Cardiology in Old Age.* (Plenum: New York, 1976) 57–9.

39. Geokas MC, Lakatta EG, Makinodon T et al. The aging process. *Ann Intern Med* (1990) **113**:455–66.

40. Montamat SC, Cusack BJ, Vestal RE. Management of drug therapy in the elderly. *N Engl J Med* (1989) **321**:303–8.

41. Blumenthal JA, Emery CF, Madden DJ et al. Cardiovascular and behavioral effects of aerobic exercise training in healthy older men and women. *J Gerontol* (1989) **44**:M147–M157.

42. Shaw PJ, Bates D, Cartlidge NEF et al. Neurologic and neuropsychological morbidity following major surgery: comparison of coronary artery bypass and peripheral vascular surgery. *Stroke* (1987) **18**:700–7.

10

Principles of cardiovascular pharmacology at advanced age

Paula M Podrazik and Janice B Schwartz

Introduction

Current understanding of cardiovascular pharmacology in the very old (age 85 and over) is limited due to a lack of drug investigations in this age group. The prevalence of cardiovascular disease in the elderly, however, makes prescription of cardiovascular drugs common. With the expected growth of the very old population, optimal use of cardiovascular drugs in patients in this age group will present a challenge. Information relevant to optimal drug therapy in the elderly includes understanding: the physiology of aging; the distribution, modification and elimination of drugs (pharmacokinetics); and the physiological effects of drugs (pharmacodynamics). However, most of the currently available data have been gathered from 'young' elderly patients (60–75 years of age), leaving unanswered many questions about pharmacotherapy in the very old. Specific concerns include determining: the appropriate dose and dosing intervals for a cardiovascular drug in the very old; the therapeutic goals in this population; the risk and types of adverse reactions with cardiovascular drugs in the very old; and the impact of drug–drug interactions in those patients with multiple chronic illnesses and the resultant multiple therapeutic prescriptions. Despite the limitations of current information, the elderly patient with cardiovascular disease clearly benefits from pharmacological treatment of hypertension, coronary artery disease, congestive heart failure, peripheral vascular disease and atrial arrhythmias. This chapter provides an overview of cardiovascular pharmacology in the oldest old based on extrapolation of data from study of the elderly (age 65 and over) to the very old. The physiology of aging and aging effects on drug pharmacokinetics and pharmacodynamics and principles of drug interactions are reviewed. The goal is to provide a framework for the choice of cardiovascular drugs, route of administration, dose and dosage interval, and avoidance of adverse drug interactions in the oldest old patients with cardiovascular disease.

Pharmacokinetics

Pharmacokinetics encompasses the handling of a drug from absorption to distribution, metabolism and elimination. These factors determine the concentration and duration of drug delivered to the target site within the body. The major pharmacokinetic parameters that are clinically relevant are: *clearance* (CL), *volume of distribution* (Vd) and *elimination half life* ($t_{\frac{1}{2}}$). Past emphasis has been on understanding age-related changes in drug pharmacokinetics because differences are easy to measure and interpret in contrast to those seen in drug pharmacodynamics.

Absorption

Absorption refers to the delivery of a drug from its point of administration into the circulation. Of the available routes for drug administration, the oral route is the most commonly used. Most medications are absorbed by passive diffusion in the proximal small bowel rather than by the active transport required to absorb nutrients such as thiamine and iron. Factors that affect absorption from the gastrointestinal tract in the nondiseased state include gastric pH, gastric emptying time, gastrointestinal transit time, mucosal absorptive capacity and blood flow. Although the anatomic and physiological changes that occur in normal aging include a decrease in acid secretion, reduced blood flow and delayed gastric emptying, clinically significant decreases in oral absorption of drugs are not usually detected in the geriatric patient.[1–4] The data on age-related absorption of drugs through sublingual or transdermal routes are too limited to arrive at any conclusions on dose adjustment based on absorption by these routes.

The parameter that quantifies differences between the amount of drug that reaches the systemic circulation after administration by differing routes is the *bioavailability* of a drug. Bioavailability is expressed as the fraction of drug administered that reaches the systemic circulation compared with the amount that reaches the circulation after intravenous administration (which is by definition equal to 100%). The area under the plasma drug concentration versus time curve (AUC) after drug administration is a useful quantitative measure of the amount of drug that reaches the systemic circulation. After extravascular administration, this is usually less than after intravascular administration.[5] The AUC after extravascular dosing divided by the AUC after the same drug dose given intravascularly is the relative bioavailability. The clinical consequence is that for a drug with low bioavailability such as propranolol, the clinically administered oral dose is many times greater than the intravascular dose. Factors that influence drug bioavailability after oral administration are solubility and chemical stability of the drug, intestinal metabolism, the drug vehicle or formulation, and first-pass hepatic metabolism. Cardiovascular drugs with low oral bioavailability include the calcium channel blockers, lidocaine and propranolol.[6]

> **Clinical considerations**
> - Clinically significant decreases in oral absorption of drugs do not usually occur in the older patient

Distribution

Distribution of a drug refers to the movement of a drug from the systemic circulation to the extracellular and intracellular spaces.

The measure of drug distribution to these other compartments is called volume of distribution (Vd) and is a mathematically quantifiable measure:

$$Vd = D/C$$

where:
D = amount of drug administered;
C = plasma concentration of administered drug.

Factors that affect distribution to peripheral compartments include blood flow, capillary permeability and drug binding to plasma proteins. Albumin is the major drug binding protein for acidic drugs and alpha acid glycoprotein is the major binding protein for basic drugs.

The Vd may vary widely depending on whether distribution is limited to the plasma compartment, extracellular fluid compartment or intracellular space. This 'hypothetical' Vd is an estimate of the fluid volume required to distribute drug evenly throughout the body. While this assumption may not accurately reflect drug distribution in tissues, the clinical utility of this measure includes the ability to calculate a loading dose needed to reach a desired plasma concentration.[5]

With senescence, there is a decrease in lean body mass and total body water.[7] These changes in body composition tend to decrease the Vd of drugs. For digoxin, which distributes into and is highly bound to muscle with a large Vd, the dose should be based on lean body weight, since higher serum concentrations of digoxin are seen in the elderly given the same loading dose as younger individuals.[8] Diuretics can further reduce Vd by decreasing extracellular fluid volume and thus indirectly decrease Vd of other drugs.

A major factor that can affect Vd is a change in protein binding of drugs, particularly binding to serum albumin. If highly protein bound, the Vd of a drug is small and the amount of drug that is 'free' to produce an effect on the target organ is small. If drug is displaced from albumin, more drug is 'free' and a greater effect from even the same total systemic concentration is seen. In the presence of disease, serum albumin decreases.[9,10] But this decrease is partially counterbalanced by the increase in alpha-1 acid glycoprotein with illnesses.[11,12] Alpha-1 acid glycoprotein is an important binding protein with sites for lidocaine, quinidine and propranolol. The physiological significance of the reported age-related decrease in albumin in hospitalized elderly patients is therefore probably of minor impact. The major exception is in the setting of renal failure or other protein-wasting disorders in which all plasma binding protein concentrations are decreased. While age-related changes in binding of the highly protein bound drugs

phenytoin and warfarin are minor and variable, concomitant administration of other highly bound drugs causes competition for binding sites on albumin and alpha-1 acid glycoprotein and can result in drug displacement from the binding site and greater unbound or free drug concentrations. Most drug interactions with warfarin, which is at least 98% protein bound, are due to alterations in its binding. These interactions should be anticipated with such drugs as amiodarone, rifampin, phenytoin, ketoconazole, intraconazole, fluconazole, and sulfonamides.[13] As a clinical rule, warfarin effect should be clinically reassessed after all drug additions or drug discontinuations in patients.

> **Clinical considerations**
> - Vd of drugs may be decreased in the elderly and loading doses may need to be reduced
> - Changes in protein binding with age or disease may be important for highly protein bound drugs with narrow therapeutic to toxic ratios, for example warfarin and phenytoin

Elimination

The kidney and liver serve as the major sites of drug elimination or *clearance* of a drug. Clearance can be defined as the volume of biological fluid per unit of time that is cleared of drug. The clearance of a drug by various organ systems is additive. The liver plays a major role in the biotransformation of many drugs by enzymatic processes that lead either to a biologically inactive compound or a hydrophilic, polar compound that can be renally excreted. Although the liver remains the major site for drug metabolism, this process can occur elsewhere. For example, adenosine's effects are very short lived because it is rapidly metabolized by an esterase in the blood. Some drugs may also be metabolized in the gut wall where enzymes similar to those in the liver have been isolated. Nonetheless, for orally prescribed cardiovascular drugs, extra-hepatic sites currently play a clinically insignificant role for biotransformation.[14]

Biotransformation

The ability of the liver to biotransform drugs depends on hepatic blood flow and liver enzyme content and activity. Hepatic blood flow and liver size decline with age. Data on age-related changes in enzymatic function are mixed. Glucuronidation pathways are unchanged with aging, while oxidation pathways have shown both preserved and decreased action. In general, there are age-related decreases in metabolism by the liver which are most marked for 'high' clearance drugs.[15-17] High clearance drugs are those for which hepatic clearance is limited mainly by drug delivery to the liver or hepatic blood flow. Hepatic blood flow is reduced by 35% or more in the elderly.[18,19] Decreases in the metabolism of high hepatic clearance of drugs thus can be anticipated from this decline in blood flow. These drugs include alprenolol, amitriptyline, labetalol, lidocaine, propranolol and verapamil.

Liver metabolism consists of phase I and phase II reactions. Phase I reactions represent oxidative pathways of cytochrome P450 located in the endoplasmic reticulum. Phase II conjugation includes glucuronidation, sulfation and acetylation and occurs in the cytosolic portion of the cell. Cytochrome P450 is a multigene family of approximately 100 variations of enzymes, responsible for metabolizing drugs, food, chemicals, toxins and hormones. The cytochrome P450 (CYP) system in the human liver is largely derived from three distinct groups, the CYP1, CYP2 and CYP3 (most common) families.[20,21] In the aging patient, activity of several oxidative pathways of the CYP system appears to decrease. Examples of cardiovascular drugs metabolized by the CYP system that demonstrate age-related decreases in metabolism include propranolol and calcium channel blockers from all three classifications: phenylalkylamine (verapamil), benzothiazepine (diltiazem) and dihydropyridine (amlodipine, felodipine, isradipine, nicardipine, nifedipine, nitrendipine). Phase II metabolic pathways do not appear to be markedly affected by age.[22-24] Examples of cardiovascular drugs metabolized by phase II acetylation include procainamide and hydralazine. Additional factors that influence drug biotransformation include: induction or inhibition of hepatic enzyme systems by drugs, diet, the environment or other factors; genetic polymorphism in enzyme content or activity; disease; and gender. It is the multifactorial influences on hepatic metabolizing systems that have thwarted attempts to develop reliable formulas to estimate hepatic drug clearance.

The CYP system can be inhibited and induced by various drugs. Cimetidine, ketaconazole, macrolide antibiotics (e.g. erythromycin) and quinidine are compounds that are inhibitors of the CYP system. Recently, it has been shown that grapefruit juice can also inhibit CYP3A metabolism.[25] Drugs such as rifampin, glucocorticoids and phenytoin induce the CYP3A form which metabolizes more than 60% of clinically prescribed drugs, including warfarin, quinidine, verapamil and nifedipine. Ethanol and isoniazid induce the CYP2(E1) enzyme. Thus, drug-induced alterations in hepatic clearance can be anticipated in the elderly patient given these drugs. Environmental factors such as industrial pollutants, cigarette smoke and caffeine are potent inducers of CYP1A.[26] The effects of cigarette smoke and ethanol use do not diminish in the geriatric population and can be factors in drug metabolism. Cigarette smoking decreases the clearance of propranolol through inhibition of hepatic enzymes and enhances that of theophylline through increased induction of hepatic enzymes, even in those of advanced age.[27]

In addition, inter-individual differences in genetically determined CYP content or activity can also exist. The most common genetic polymorphisms associated with the CYP system are those involving mutations in the CYP2D6 enzyme system. A 5–10% incidence of the slow metabolizer phenotype is seen in caucasians with a 1% incidence in Asians. Impaired metabolism of encainide, flecainide and metoprolol can result.[28,29]

Additional considerations that can affect drug biotransformation are underlying diseases. Liver disease and congestive heart failure produce deleterious effects on hepatic parenchymal enzyme systems and diminish blood flow due to decreased cardiac output. Finally, older populations are predominantly women, yet most of the studies of age-related changes in drug pharmacokinetics to date have been in men. Gender differences in drug metabolism point to another area with information deficits that is very pertinent to therapeutics of the very old.[30] Even fewer data are available regarding the effects of hormone replacement therapy on drug concentrations or effects in women.

Renal clearance

The renal clearance of a drug and metabolites involves the processes of glomerular filtration, active tubular secretion and passive tubular reabsorption. Decreases in renal size, glomerular filtration rate (GFR), and renal blood flow

---

Clinical considerations

- Drugs that depend on hepatic metabolism show a general decline in clearance with aging
- No reliable formula for estimates of hepatic drug clearance exists; so general recommendations are to decrease initial doses by half and then increase doses in smaller increments than in younger patients
- Drug and environmental inhibition and induction of drug metabolism may occur. Amiodarone, cimetidine, ketaconazole and erythromycin and grapefruit juice can increase other drug levels while rifampin can lower other drug concentrations.

---

occur with aging.[31,32] The age-related decline in renal function after age 40 is approximately 1% per year. Creatinine, a product of muscle breakdown is not an adequate measure of renal function in the old, due to the loss of lean body muscle mass. For drugs renally excreted, dosage adjustments can be estimated by the age-adjusted creatinine clearance.[33,34]

$$\text{Creatinine clearance} = \frac{(140 - \text{age}) \text{ weight (kg)}}{72 \times \text{creatinine (serum)}} (\times 0.85 \text{ in women})$$

Creatinine clearance is a rough estimate of GFR, until GFR is substantially reduced (less than 25 ml/min). Many drugs such as aminoglycosides and digoxin are eliminated by simple glomerular filtration. Therefore, as glomerular filtration decreases with age, doses should be reduced to parallel this decline. Lithium, chlorpropramide, tetracycline, penicillins and procainamide are other drugs that may accumulate due to the decline in renal function.

Two classes of drugs commonly used by the

geriatric patient deserve mention because of potentially adverse effects on the aging kidney. These classes of drugs are the angiotensin-converting enzyme (ACE) inhibitors/angiotensin receptor blocking agents and the nonsteroidal anti-inflammatory agents (NSAIDs). ACE inhibitors decrease peripheral vascular resistance thereby lowering blood pressure. The mechanism of action involves decreasing the formation of angiotensin II—a potent vasoconstrictor in combination with increasing levels of bradykinin—a potent vasodilator, leading to reduction in peripheral vascular resistance. The effects of angiotensin II on the afferent and efferent arterioles influence GFR and can be variable depending on the physiological state.[35] With blockade of the renin–angiotensin system by an ACE inhibitor, angiotensin II's control over the efferent arterioles is inhibited and renal failure can ensue in those with renal artery stenosis. The reduction in angiotensin II also results in decreased aldosterone secretion with small increases in potassium levels, sodium loss and volume contraction. With advancing age and decreasing GFR, dose reduction may be required for the renally excreted active moiety of the ACE inhibitors. Care has to be given not only to dose adjustment but monitoring of serum potassium levels. Study is underway on the use of angiotensin II receptor antagonists in elderly patients with hypertension and congestive heart failure. The use of losartan versus captopril in elderly patients with congestive heart failure[36] however was not associated with less renal dysfunction in this over 65 year-old study population. Further study is needed in the aging population on efficacy, safety and therapeutic utility.

NSAIDs are commonly prescribed in the elderly for their anti-inflammatory and analgesic effects. Most NSAIDs act by inhibiting the synthesis of prostaglandins responsible in part for renal blood flow. These renal prostaglandins are of increasing importance in maintaining renal blood flow in patients with borderline renal function, congestive heart failure, liver disease and the reduction in GFR with aging. Indomethacin, naproxen and ketoprofen can reduce renal clearance in older patients. In the elderly, further decreases in GFR can cause hyperkalemia, or frank renal failure from acute tubular necrosis or interstitial nephritis. Lower doses of NSAIDs for geriatric patients should be initiated and renal function and potassium monitored.[37–39]

Clinical considerations
- In older patients, serum creatinine alone does not predict renal clearance
- Renal clearance decreases with age in a predictable manner. Dose calculations should be based on formulas
- Renal function and potassium levels should be monitored in patients taking ACE inhibitors and NSAIDs

---

Elimination half-life

Elimination half-life or $t_{\frac{1}{2}}$ is the time required to decrease the amount of a drug in the body by half after drug distribution is complete. The terminal elimination $t_{\frac{1}{2}}$ is directly related to the drug volume of distribution and inversely proportional to drug clearance:

$$t_{\frac{1}{2}} = 0.693\, Vd/CL$$

Clinical situations in which the half-life would increase include those that decrease the clearance of a drug and/or increase the volume of distribution of a drug. The drug half-life determines the amount of time to eliminate drug from the body and the time to reach the steady-state concentrations of drug in the body. A simplified estimate of the time to reach 90% of the steady state or 90% drug removal is 3.3 times the terminal half-life. This remains true even if the drug given is an extended release form. Because the clearance of many drugs is decreased with aging, the $t_{\frac{1}{2}}$ is usually increased with aging.[13]

> **Clinical considerations**
> - Steady-state effects of drugs should be assessed after a longer time interval than in younger patients, and dosage changes should be made after longer treatment intervals than in younger patients

Pharmacodynamics

The pharmacodynamics of a drug describes the effects of the drug on its target cell or receptor. The study of the dynamic properties of drugs is based on the theory of drug receptors. Pharmacodynamics attempts to quantify the drug properties of maximum effect and sensitivity. In the receptor-agonist model, as a dose of medication is gradually increased a response will be seen in direct proportion to the increasing dose. This occurs until a plateau approaching the maximal effect is reached after which increasing doses will cause only minimal increases in responses. In therapeutic dosing, the concentration-effect relationship often takes a slightly different form. Often, no effect is seen until a threshold is reached, then effects increase in relation to the concentration, and maximal effects are not reached. Most therapeutic effects are usually seen in the 20–80% range of maximal effect. In the clinical setting, maximal effects are often undesirable (e.g. reducing blood pressure or heart rate to zero). As a corollary, the most potent drugs

may afford less therapeutic range and dosing flexibility in the elderly patient.

Age-related pharmacodynamic changes have been found consistently in all species. Changes especially pertinent to the older cardiovascular patient are in the sympathetic system, parasympathetic system, baroreceptor responses and calcium channels. Decrease in beta-adrenergic responsiveness occurs with aging and is probably due to a decrease in receptors. Isoproterenol infusions in older patients result in less tachycardic response compared with younger patients. Similarly less bradycardia is seen in aging human subjects given beta-1 adrenergic blocking agents.[40] The baroreceptor response also is attenuated with aging.[41,42] The blunted baroreceptor response is probably responsible for the exaggerated hypotensive effects of vasodilators and nitrates in older patients. Another contributor to hypotension is the decrease with age in beta-1 adrenergic responsiveness and lessened reflex tachycardia. Studies using potent vasodilators with differing mechanisms of action support the conclusion that age-related blunting of the baroreceptor response is the primary cause of the longer duration and greater hypotension for most vasodilators seen in the elderly when compared with a younger population.[43] Diminished cardiac parasympathetic responsiveness also is seen with aging. In contrast, bladder and CNS parasympathetic effects appear more pronounced in older individuals compared with younger individuals. Thus, differences exist between age-related changes in peripheral versus central receptors.

Sensitivity to the effects of a number of calcium channel blockers appears increased in the elderly patient. Heart rate and blood pressure are decreased to a greater degree in the older patient compared with a younger patient with the same concentrations of verapamil.[44] Similar age-related differences in heart rate suppression are seen after intravenous diltiazem.[45] Oral nifedipine and slow-release nicardipine resulted in greater blood pressure lowering in older compared with younger hypertensive patients.[46] Warfarin sensitivity also increases with aging.[47]

Clinical considerations
- Age-related changes in receptor systems and reflex responses predispose the older patient to postural hypotension when vasodilators, especially potent vasodilators, are given to the elderly patient.

Adverse drug reactions

Adverse drug reactions in the elderly patient may be an extension of the normal pharmacological drug effect and typically are dose dependent. The altered pharmacokinetics and pharmacodynamics of aging, increased numbers of underlying medical illnesses and administered medications play a prominent role in these adverse drug reactions.

With advancing age, a rise in the number of adverse drug reactions has been reported. It is estimated that reactions occur in 25% of older patients and are responsible for as many as 3–10% of all hospital admissions in the elderly patient.[48–50] Altered pharmacokinetics and pharmacodynamics, underlying medical illnesses and increased numbers of prescribed medications all have been implicated in the rise in adverse drug reactions in the elderly. Recently, it has been shown that the number of medications is the most important risk factor for adverse drug reactions.[51,52] With the chronic administration of two drugs, the risk of an adverse drug reaction is about 15%, but this risk rises sharply to 50–60% with use of six drugs daily. Older community-dwelling North Americans take an average of two to three medications daily. Institutionalized geriatric patients are prescribed three to eight medications daily.[53–56] A decrease in the incidence of adverse drug reactions can be achieved with a reduction in the number of medications prescribed.[57]

Thus, the more medications used, the greater the chance of drug–drug interactions, particularly with medications that have a narrow toxic–therapeutic range. Drug–drug interactions fall into categories of adverse drug effects based on pharmacokinetic or pharmacodynamic mechanisms. A drug can change the concentration of another drug by altering pharmacokinetic parameters (clearance, distribution and half-life are most often affected). Similarly, a drug can change the pharmacodynamic properties (magnitude of the physiological response) to a coadministered drug either by enhancing or antagonizing the drug effect. The cardiovascular drugs commonly associated with drug–drug interactions include digoxin, warfarin, lidocaine, quinidine and amiodarone. Common noncardiac drugs with high potential for drug–drug interactions include: cimetidine, rifampin, NSAIDs, azole antifungal agents (ketoconazole) and macrolide antibiotics (erythromycin). See Table 10.1 for the specifics of the more commonly encountered drug–drug interactions in the geriatric patient.

It is important to recognize that the clinical presentation of adverse drug reactions in the very old may be quite subtle or easily confused with other diagnostic possibilities. Common presentations include: delirium ranging from somnolence to agitation; nausea; frequent falls; and a change in bowel patterns or urinary incontinence.

Type of change	Change	Drugs causing change	Drugs affected or effects
Pharmacokinetic	Decreased clearance leading to increased concentrations	Amiodarone	All drugs, including digoxin and warfarin
		Cimetidine	Hepatically metabolized drugs
		Erythromycin	CYP3A4 metabolized drugs
		Ketaconazole, intracomazole	Effects similar to erythromycin
		Synthetic steroids	CYP3A4 metabolized drugs
	Increased clearance leading to decreased concentrations of hepatically metabolized drugs	Anticonvulsants especially phenytoin, phenobarbital or ethanol or glucocorticoids or rifampin	Quinidine and warfarin, Many ß-blockers Calcium channel blockers HMG CoA reductase inhibitors
Pharmacodynamic		α-Blockers + nitrates or vasodilators or β-blockers	Postural hypotension
		NSAID + ACE inhibitors	Hyperkalemia, renal failure
		NSAIDs + potassium sparing diuretic	Hyperkalemia
		Tricyclic antidepressants + vasodilators	Postural hypotension
		Verapamil + digoxin or ß-blocker or amiodarone	Bradycardia

Table 10.1
Drug–drug interactions between cardiovascular and other commonly prescribed drugs in the elderly patient

---

Clinical considerations
- Adverse drug reactions are a consequence of 'polypharmacy' seen in the very old. Reducing the number of drugs administered will reduce the number of adverse drug effects
- Adverse drug reactions may present atypically in the older patient

Summary

Most studies of cardiovascular drugs have excluded the old and very old. The rapid and continued growth of this segment of the population underscores the need to define the best therapeutic regimens for these patients. Future study needs include the development of pharmacokinetic and pharmacodynamic models that can determine the influences of aging, gender, and multiple illnesses and multiple medications administered in this patient population.[58,59] The pharmacokinetic properties of bioavailability, volume of distribution, clearance and half-life can be altered with aging. The most consistent decline with aging is that of renal elimination. Age-related pharmacodynamic changes also occur but currently are less well described. The risk of drug–drug interactions and adverse drug reactions are increased with the increasing numbers of medications taken by the geriatric population. The clinical caveats for cardiovascular pharmacology in the very old are:

1. Give reduced initial doses of medications;
2. Increase doses slowly, in smaller increments and at longer intervals than in younger patients;
3. Prescribe the smallest number of medications. Discontinue unnecessary medications;
4. Anticipate drug–drug interactions particularly when prescribing warfarin, digoxin, amiodarone and rifampin, azole antifungals, macrolide antibiotics and cimetidine;
5. Monitor for drug–drug interactions;
6. Monitor drugs with a narrow toxic–therapeutic range;
7. Recognize the sometimes subtle and atypical presentations of adverse drug effects in the elderly.

Finally, and most important, remember that administration of drugs to very old patients is often a new experiment. Select, prescribe and monitor with care.

References

1. Kupfer RM, Heppell M, Haggith JW et al. Gastric emptying and small-bowel transit rate in the elderly. *J Am Geriatr Soc* (1985) **33**:340–3.

2. Evans MA, Triggs EJ, Cheung M et al. Gastric emptying rate in the elderly: implications for drug therapy. *J Am Geriatr Soc* (1981) **29**: 201–5.

3. Castleden CM, Volans CN, Raymond K. The effect of ageing on drug absorption from the gut. *Age Ageing* (1977) **6**:138–43.

4. Kekki M, Samloff IM, Ihamaki T et al. Age- and sex-related behavior of gastric acid secretion at the population level. *Scand J Gastroenterol* (1982) **17**:737–43.

5. Schwartz JB. Clinical pharmacology. In: Hazzard WR, Bierman EL, Blass JP, Ettinger WH, Halter JF, eds, *Principles of Geriatric Medicine and Gerontology*, 3rd edn. (McGraw-Hill: New York, 1993) 259–75.

6. Benet LZ, Oie S, Schwartz JB. Design and optimization of dosage regimens; pharmacokinetic data. Appendix II. In: Hardman JG, Limbird LE, Molinoff PB, eds, *Goodman and Gilman's The Pharmacological Basis of Therapeutics*, 9th edn. (McGraw-Hill: New York, 1996) 1712–92.

7. Fulop T, Worum I, Csongor J et al. Body composition in elderly people. *Gerontology* (1985) **31**:6–14.

8. Cusack B, Kelly J, O'Malley K et al. Digoxin in the elderly: pharmacokinetic consequences of old age. *Clin Pharmacol Ther* (1979) **25**: 772–6.

9. Greenblatt DJ. Reduced serum albumin concentration in the elderly: a report from the Boston collaborative drug surveillance program. *J Am Geriatr Soc* (1979) **27**:20–22.

10. Campion EW, deLabry LO, Glynn RJ. The effect of age on serum albumin in healthy males: report from the normative aging study. *J Gerontol* (1988) **43**:M18–20.

11. Abernethy DR, Kerzner L. Age effects on alpha-1-acid glycoprotein concentration and imipramine plasma protein binding. *J Am Geriatr Soc* (1984) **32**:705–8.

12. Veering BT, Burm AG, Souverijin JH et al. The effect of age on serum concentrations of albumin and alpha-1-acid glycoprotein. *Br J Clin Pharmacol* (1990) **29**:201–6.

13. Schwartz JB. Geriatric clinical pharmacology. In: Kelley WN, ed., *Textbook of Internal Medicine*, 3rd edn. (Lippincott-Raven: Philadelphia, 1997) 2547–54.

14. Benet LZ, Kroetz DL, Sheiner LB. Pharmacokinetics. In: Hardman JG, Limbird LE, eds, *Goodman and Gilman's The Pharmacologic Basis of Therapeutics*, 9th edn. (McGraw Hill: New York, 1996) 3–27.

15. Woodhouse KW, James OF. Hepatic drug metabolism and ageing. *Br Med Bull* (1990) **46**:22–35.

16. Salem SA, Rajjayabun P, Shepherd AM et al. Reduced induction of drug metabolism in the elderly. *Age Ageing* (1978) **7**:68–73.

17. Vestal RE. Aging and determinants of hepatic drug clearance. *Hepatology* (1989) **9**:331–4.

18. Wynne HA, Cope LH, Mulch E et al. The effect of age upon liver volume and apparent blood flow in healthy man. *Hepatology* (1989) **9**: 297–301.

19. Geokas MC, Haverback BJ. The aging gastrointestinal tract. *Am J Surg* (1969) **117**: 881–92.

20. Nelson DR, Kamataki T, Waxman DJ et al. The P450 superfamily: update on sequences, gene mapping, accession numbers, early trivial names, and nomenclature. *DNA Cell Biol* (1993) **12**:1–51.

21. Wrighton SA, Stevens JC. The human hepatic cytochromes P450 involved in drug metabolism. *Crit Rev Toxicol* (1992) **22**:1–21.

22. Schwartz JB. Calcium antagonists in the elderly: a risk benefit analysis. *Drugs Aging* (1996) **9**:24–36.

23. Tateishi T, Fujimura A, Shiga T et al. Influence of aging on the oxidative and conjugative metabolism of propranolol. *Int J Clin Pharmacol Res* (1995) **15**:95–101.

24. Murray M. P450 enzymes: inhibition mechanisms, genetic regulation and effects of liver disease. *Clin Pharmacokinet* (1992) **23**: 132–46.

25. Spence J. Drug interactions with grapefruit juice: whose responsibility is it to warn the public? *Clin Pharmacol Ther* (1997) **61**: 395–400.

26. Vestal RE, Norris AH, Tobin JD et al. Antipurine metabolism in man: influence of age, alcohol, caffeine, and smoking. *Clin Pharmacol Ther* (1975) **18**:425–32.

27. Vestal RE, Wood MB, Branch RA et al. Effects of age and cigarette smoking on propranolol disposition. *Clin Pharmacol Ther* (1979) **26**: 8–15.

28. Lennard MS. Genetically determined adverse drug reactions involving metabolism. *Drug Safety* (1993) **9**:60–77.

29. Shimada T, Yamazaki H, Mimura M et al. Interindividual variations in human liver cytochrome P-450 enzymes involved in the oxidation of drugs, carcinogens and toxic chemicals: studies with liver microsomes of 30 Japanese and 30 Caucasians. *J Pharmacol Exp Ther* (1994) **270**:414–23.

30. Harris RZ, Benet LZ, Schwartz JB. Gender effects in pharmacokinetics and pharmacodynamics. *Drugs* (1995) **50**:222–39.

31. Lindeman RD. Changes in renal function with aging. *Drugs Aging* (1992) **2**:423–31.

32. Rowe JW, Andres R, Tobin JD et al. The effect of age on creatinine clearance in men: a cross-sectional and longitudinal study. *J Gerontol* (1976) **31**:155–63.

33. Rowe JW, Andres R, Tobin JD. Letter: Age-adjusted standards for creatinine clearance. *Ann Intern Med* (1976) **84**:567–9.

34. Cockcroft DW, Gault MH. Prediction of creatinine clearance from serum creatinine. *Nephron* (1976) **16**:31–41.

35. Kastner PR, Hall JE, Guyton AC. Control of glomerular filtration rate: role of intrarenally formed angiotensin II. *Am J Physiol* (1984) **246**:F897–F906.

36. Pitt B, Segal R, Martinez FA et al. Randomised trial of losartan versus captopril in patients over 65 with heart failure (Evaluation of Losartan in the Elderly Study, ELITE). *Lancet* (1997) **349**:747–52.

37. Orme M. Pharmacokinetics of non-steroidal anti-inflammatory drugs in the elderly. *Agents Actions* (1985) **17**(Suppl S):135–40.

38. Clive DM, Stoff JS. Renal syndromes associated with non-steroidal antiinflammatory drugs. *N Engl J Med* (1984) **310**:563–72.

39. Lamy PP. Renal effects of nonsteroidal anti-inflammatory drugs: heightened risk to the elderly? *J Am Geriatr Soc* (1986) **34**:361–7.

40. Vestal RE, Wood AJJ, Shand DG. Reduced beta-adrenoreceptor sensitivity in the elderly. *Clin Pharmacol Ther* (1979) **26**:181–6.

41. McGarry K, Laker M, Fitzgerald D et al. Baroreflex function in elderly hypertensives. *Hypertension* (1975) **5**:763–6.

42. Gribbin B, Pickering TG, Sleight P et al. Effect of age and high blood pressure on baroreflex sensitivity in man. *Circ Res* (1971) **29**:424–31.

43. Pan HY, Hoffman BB, Pershe RA, Blaschke TF. Decline in beta adrenergic receptor-mediated vascular relaxation with aging in man. *J Pharmacol Exp Ther* (1986) **239**: 802–7.

44. Schwartz JB. Aging alters verapamil elimination and dynamics: single dose and steady-state responses. *J Pharmacol Exp Ther* (1990) **255**: 364–73.

45. Schwartz JB, Abernethy D. Responses to intravenous and oral diltiazem in elderly and younger patients with systemic hypertension. *Am J Cardiol* (1987) **59**:1111–17.

46. Porchet HC, Loew F, Gauthey L et al. Serum concentration-effect relationship of (+/−)-nicardipine and nifedipine in elderly hypertensive patients. *Eur J Clin Pharmacol* (1992) **43**:551–3.

47. Shepherd AM, Hewick DS, Moreland TA, Stevenson IH. Age as a determinant of sensitivity to warfarin. *Br J Clin Pharmacol* (1977) **4**:315–20.

48. Vestal RF. Pharmacology of aging. *J Am Geriatr Soc* (1982) **30**:191–200.

49. Williamson J, Chopin JM. Adverse reactions to prescribing drugs in the elderly: a multicenter investigation. *Age Ageing* (1980) **9**:73–80.

50. Chrischilles EA, Segar ET, Wallace RB. Self-reported adverse drug reactions and related resource use: a study of community-dwelling persons 65 years and older. *Ann Intern Med* (1992) **117**:634–40.

51. Chutka DS, Evans JM, Fleming KC, Mikkelson KG. Drug prescribing for elderly patients. *Mayo Clin Proc* (1995) **70**:685–93.

52. Gurwitz JH, Avorn J. The ambiguous relation between aging and adverse drug reactions. *Ann Intern Med* (1991) **114**:956–66.

53. Beers MH, Ouslander JG. Risk factors in geriatric drug prescribing: a practical guide to avoiding problems. *Drugs* (1989) **37**:105–12.

54. Nolan L, O'Malley K. The need for a more rational approach to drug prescribing for elderly people in nursing homes. *Age Ageing* (1989) **18**:52–6.

55. Johnson RE, Vollmer WM. Comparing sources of drug data in the elderly. *J Am Geriatr Soc* (1991) **39**:1079–84.

56. Gurwitz JH, Soumerai SB, Avorn J. Improving medication prescribing and utilization in the nursing home. *J Am Geriatr Soc* (1990) **38**: 542–52.

57. Lamy PP. Adverse drug effects. *Clin Geriatr Med* (1990) **6**:293–307.

58. Committee on Pharmacokinetics and Drug Interactions in the Elderly. Conclusions and future directions. *Pharmacokinetics and drug interactions in the elderly and special issues in elderly African-American populations.* (National Academy Press: Washington DC, 1997) 35–42.

59. Schwartz JB. Areas of needed information regarding drug therapy in the elderly population. In: Wenger NK, ed., *Inclusion of Elderly Individuals in Clinical Trials.* (Marion Merrell Dow: Kansas City, MO, 1993) 261–82.

11

Coronary risk factors and coronary prevention in octogenarians

William B Kannel, Peter WF Wilson, Martin G Larson and Jane C Evans

Introduction

Epidemiological studies have shown that the major modifiable cardiovascular risk factors applicable in middle age remain relevant in the elderly.[1-3] However, their importance in the octogenarian is not well documented. The likelihood of disability and death from atherosclerotic cardiovascular disease in general remains a serious concern in the elderly as mortality attributed to cardiovascular disease reaches 58% in persons aged 85 years or older. There has been a world-wide increase in the proportion of the population age 80 years and older in affluent countries.[4] Given the large burden of cardiovascular disease in this segment of the population, the predominance of coronary disease as a cause of death and disability in the oldest of the old, and the limited amount of information available to guide physicians in the cost-effective preventive care of coronary disease in this age group, there is a need to examine the evidence available. Many practitioners question whether decades of exposure to cardiovascular risk factors can be countered by measures imposed so late in life. However coronary heart disease (CHD) ranks high among the chronic conditions that take the joy out of reaching a venerable stage in life. This is an important consideration because the average life expectancy after attaining age 80 years is about 8 years.

Interpretation of prospective epidemiological data in the elderly must take into account the high prevalence of cardiovascular disease in this age group, other comorbidity, the high mortality rate, natural selection and the measure of association employed. The coexistence of other diseases increases with advancing age and may modify the association between risk factors and coronary disease. There are at present no satisfactory procedures for dealing with this comorbidity. Exclusion of persons with other major chronic diseases at baseline is no solution because the remaining subgroup is no longer representative of the general elderly population. Also, since underlying undiagnosed severe coronary artery disease is very common in the elderly, the distinction between primary and secondary prevention in this age group is uncertain. Advanced coronary atherosclerosis is estimated to afflict half the elderly of industrialized countries.[5] Examination of the relationship of risk factors in the development of coronary heart disease in octogenarians in reality must deal with factors that predispose to the onset of clinically overt manifestations of CHD in persons, most of whom already have moderate to severe coronary artery atherosclerosis. In this age group, factors that promote the progression of atherosclerosis or precipitate events may be particularly important.

Comortality can be partly taken into account by using Cox's proportional hazard analysis, which includes persons who are censored due to death from causes other than coronary heart disease. However, with the exception of all-cause mortality, the relative risks for cause specific mortality endpoints retain the assumption of no competing risks. Thus, in prospective studies of coronary morbidity and mortality, it is not possible to eliminate or to account for competing causes of death. Also, the progressive decline in the associations of some risk factors with development of coronary disease observed in many studies may be a consequence of selective survival—a progressive elimination of susceptible persons with elevated risk factor levels from the population—with the remaining individuals less susceptible to coronary disease or the risk factors that predispose to it.[6]

Furthermore, the level of a particular risk factor measured in the very old may not represent the lifetime exposure, making interpretation of the results difficult.[7] This possible risk factor misclassification of elders attenuates the observed association between risk factors and coronary disease. Age-related physiological changes in risk factors, independent of health status, may also reduce risk factor–coronary disease relations. The pathogenesis and clinical manifestations of coronary disease may change with advancing age and influence the risk factors and their impact on the occurrence of clinical events. Thus it is necessary to know whether risk factors tend to change with age. Finally it is important to consider whether risk factors may have long-term or short-term influences on the risk of coronary disease.

There is also a prevailing notion that the strength of the association of cardiovascular risk factors with the development of coronary heart disease (CHD) diminishes with advancing age. Such a situation is evident for relative risks of some risk factors, but absolute risk tends to increase with age, and the risk differences between those with and without risk factors are also larger in the elderly. As a consequence, risk-factor control is potentially at least as cost-effective in the elderly as in the middle aged.

Prevalence

The prevalence of cardiovascular disease in the Framingham cohort age 75–84 years was 44% in men and only 28% in women. In the age group 85–94 years the prevalence increased slightly to 48% in men and substantially to 43% in women (Table 11.1). Thus, about 45% of octogenarians in the general population have some clinical manifestation of atherosclerotic cardiovascular disease, such as coronary heart disease, stroke, heart failure or peripheral arterial disease.

The prevalence of CHD in the US has been estimated from health interviews by NHANES III, combining reported myocardial infarction and angina pectoris (Figure 11.1). This indicates a steep rise with age with a male predominance that persists into the octogenarian age range. In the segment of the population age 80 years and older, about 27% of men and 17% of some women have overt coronary disease.[8] In the Framingham Study the prevalence of CHD in this segment of the elderly population was similarly estimated to be 28% in men and 19% in women. In subjects age 65–74 years of age, 64% of cardiovascular events in men and 60% in women were CHD events. In the 75–94 year age group, this remains at 64% in men, whereas in women it declines slightly to 56%. Only the proportion of initial atherosclerotic cardiovascular events presenting as strokes tends to increase with further advance in age in the elderly (Table 11.2). Among the elderly under age 75 years, 11% of the CHD events in men and 7% in women were sudden deaths, whereas over age

	Men			Women	
Age	*Number*	*CVD (%)*	*Age*	*Number*	*CVD (%)*
65–74	1328	37	65–74	1880	22
75–84	1121	44	75–84	1988	28
85–94	243	48	85–94	598	43
65–94	2692	41	65–94	4466	28

Number: number of person-exams; CVD: coronary disease, stroke, heart failure, or peripheral artery disease.

Table 11.1
Cardiovascular disease prevalence in the elderly by sex and age: Framingham Study subjects age 65–94 years, biennial examinations 18–22

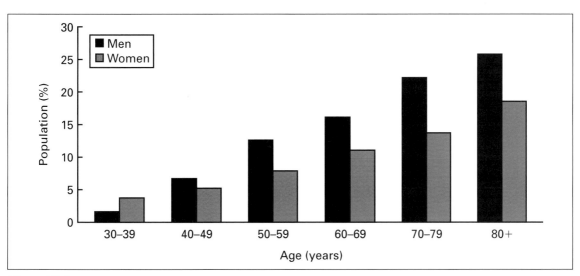

Figure 11.1
Prevalence of CHD by age and sex, NHANES III, US, 1988–91.

	Ages	Number	CHD (%)	Stroke (%)	CHF (%)	PVD (%)
Men	65–74	491	64	15	3	18
	75–84	493	65	18	2	14
	85–94	116	62	18	4	16
Women	65–74	420	60	16	8	16
	75–84	566	56	22	6	17
	85–94	256	55	29	9	7

* Percentage in rows add to 100%.
Number: number of person-exams.

Table 11.2
Initial atherosclerotic events in the elderly: Framingham Study, biennial examinations 18–22
(proportion of the events as specified*)

75 years this rose to 17% and 15% in the two sexes respectively.

Incidence

The annual incidence of initial CHD events is substantial in the elderly, increasing in men from 26 per 1000 in the 65–74 year age group to 39 per 1000 for those age 85–94 years. In women, the rates increased from 12 per 1000 to 24 per 1000 (Table 11.3). In this elderly segment of the population this disease remained male dominant although the sex ratio decreased from 2.2 to 1.6.

In the elderly more than a third of all myocardial infarctions are unrecognized either because they are completely silent or so atypical that neither the patients nor their physicians consider the possibility.[9] These unrecognized infarctions are particularly common in men with diabetes and in hypertensive elderly of both sexes. Fully half of all myocardial infarctions in elderly hypertensive women are silent or unrecognized.[9]

Mortality

Cardiovascular disease, of which CHD is the most common, constitutes the major cause of death in the majority of industrialized countries and 80% of all these deaths occur in the segment of the population over 65 years of age.[4] National data for the US indicate that CHD mortality increases steeply with advancing age, is about twice as high in men as in women and higher in blacks than whites. This higher CHD mortality in black men is noted up to age 70 years, after which the mortality rates are higher in white men.[8] In women, the CHD mortality rates remain higher in blacks than in whites until age 85 years. In octogenarians the CHD mortality rates remain sub-

	Average annual rate per 1000		
Age	Men	Women	Sex ratio (M/F)
65–74	26	12	2.2
75–84	33	15	2.1
85–94	39	24	1.6

Based on 18 incident cases of CHD among 4740 person-exams of subjects free of CHD at cycles 18–21, with 2-year follow-up after each exam.

Table 11.3
Incidence of coronary heart disease in the elderly by sex and age: Framingham Study, biennial examinations 18–22

stantially higher in men than women of either race (Figure 11.2).

Thus, in octogenarians, coronary disease is the most common and most lethal of the cardiovascular manifestations of atherosclerosis, equaling in incidence all the others combined.

Coronary events remain the predominant atherosclerotic feature of cardiovascular disease in this age group even though its incidence as a fraction of all cardiovascular events diminishes slightly with advancing age. The gender gap in CHD incidence narrows

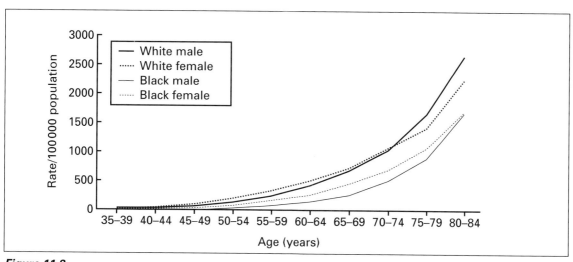

Figure 11.2
Death rates for CHD by age, race and sex in the US, 1993.

with advancing age as women lose their relative protection after undergoing the menopause, but even in octogenarians there is a 60% male predominance. Unrecognized myocardial infarction constitutes a major problem in the elderly population because of its poor prognosis despite lack of alarming symptoms.[9]

After adjustment for the major risk factors, each decade of advancing age confers a two- to three-fold increase in cardiovascular mortality. Multivariate adjustment for associated cardiovascular risk factors has little effect on the steepness of the age gradient of risk. This may indicate an influence of aging itself or reflect the time-dose of exposure to risk factors.

CHD mortality has been declining since 1970 with white men and women experiencing steeper declines than black men and women.[8] Declines in CHD mortality tend to be greater in younger age groups but have included the elderly segment of the population (Figure 11.3). In white men and women, octo-

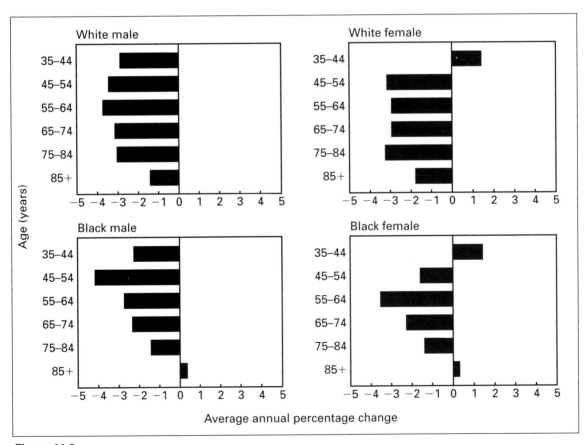

Figure 11.3
Average annual percentage change in death rates for CHD by age, race and sex, US, 1989–93.

				Myocardial							
	10–year percentage probability of another cardiovascular event										
		CHD		*infarction*		*Angina*		*Stroke*		*CHF*	
Age	*Men*	*Women*	*Men*	*Women*	*Men*	*Women*	*Men*	*Women*	*Men*	*Women*	
35–64	67	57	48	41	30	25	12	18	21	24	
65–79	61	70	51	62	22	15	22	21	36	38	
80–94	89	57	85	53	25	4	9	19	70	54	

Table 11.4
Probability of other cardiovascular events following initial myocardial infarction by age and sex: Framingham Study, 42-year follow-up.

genarians have also experienced declines along with the other elderly, albeit not to the same degree. In the black segment of the population, those over age 85 years do not appear to have shared in the decline.[8]

Prognosis after myocardial infarction

Mortality beyond age 65 years is high following a myocardial infarction. About 8% will die annually and half will experience a coronary death within 10 years.[10] The risk of additional cardiovascular events is also high beyond age 65 years and 89% of octogenarian men and 57% of women of this age will experience another event during the last 10 years of their life (Table 11.4). About 85% of men of this age who survive a first myocardial infarction will experience a recurrence within 10 years and 25% of them will develop angina, 9% a stroke and 70% heart failure. For women in this age group, 53% will have a recurrence over the ensuing 10 years, 4% angina, 19% a

stroke and 54% heart failure. In men over age 65 years, the risk of further cardiovascular events after an initial myocardial infarction increases substantially as they enter the octogenarian age group, whereas in women this only applies for the occurrence of heart failure (Table 11.4). The lower postinfarction angina rates compared with the middle-aged may be due to the lower level of physical activity in the elderly. Recurrent myocardial infarction and angina pectoris in the octogenarian age group appear to be substantially higher in men than women. Odds ratios (relative risks) for overall, cardiovascular and coronary mortality following a myocardial infarction actually decrease substantially with advancing age in women, whereas in men they tend to increase (Table 11.5).

Risk factor trends

There is a tendency for some, but not all, risk factors to rise with age. Diabetes, hypertension and left ventricular hypertrophy on ECG

	Odds ratios					
	All causes		Cardiovascular		Coronary	
Age	Men	Women	Men	Women	Men	Women
35–64	4.0	8.7	7.1	20.4	9.6	49.0
65–74	4.0	6.0	6.9	12.1	12.6	34.0
75–84	4.3	3.0	8.7	8.3	17.7	27.7

Table 11.5
Risk of death within 2 years comparing subjects with and without myocardial infarction: Framingham Study, 42-year follow-up

(ECG-LVH) in particular, rise sharply with age into the octogenarian age group (Table 11.6). The rise in body mass index tends to cease at age 65 years and then declines in both sexes. Cigarette smoking declines in prevalence steadily with advancing age from age 35 years on in both sexes. In octogenarians, no more than 18% of men and 6% of women smoke. In this advanced age group the prevalence of hypertension, dyslipidemia and ECG-LVH is greater in women than men, whereas cigarette smoking is greater in men. The average body mass index (BMI) is similar in men and women in this advanced age group. The changes in the level of these risk factors with advancing age do not appear to be inevitable since they can be altered by exercise, weight control and diet.

After age 50 the rise in serum cholesterol with age tends to level off and then declines steadily with advancing age in men. On the other hand, serum cholesterol continues to rise in women until age 65 after which it declines. Despite declines in advanced age, the values in

octogenarian women are substantially higher than those in comparably aged men. Age trends for low-density lipoprotein (LDL) cholesterol are similar to those for total cholesterol in both sexes (Figure 11.4). High-density lipoprotein (HDL) cholesterol remains fairly constant into the octogenarian age group in men and is consistently higher in women than men despite a modest decline from age 50 years on. Subjects in the Framingham Study who attained 80 years of age without developing cardiovascular disease were exceedingly unlikely to have reduced HDL cholesterol levels compared with subjects of similar age who developed cardiovascular disease or died.[11] The total to HDL-cholesterol ratio declines steadily with advancing age in men but rises just as steadily in women, so that in the 80 year old age group this ratio is approximately equal in the two sexes (Figure 11.4). This, to a large extent, accounts for the narrowing gap in CHD incidence between the sexes. These declining trends in blood lipids still leave a substantial proportion of the

Age	Definite ECG-LVH		Definite diabetes		Cigarette smoking		Definite hypertension	
	Men	Women	Men	Women	Men	Women	Men	Women
55–64	2.7	1.7	5.5	4.2	55.9	31.6	26.8	31.5
65–74	3.6	3.2	10.9	7.2	39.0	18.9	38.0	47.6
75–84	4.2	4.9	13.2	10.2	24.2	7.9	48.4	59.9
85–94	5.9	9.4	14.2	11.1	17.9	3.2	47.8	65.6

Age	Body mass index (kg/m²)		Systolic blood pressure (mmHg)		Total cholesterol (mg/dl)	
	Men	Women	Men	Women	Men	Women
55–64	26.6	26.3	138.1	140.8	230.9	255.2
65–74	26.5	26.5	141.5	145.5	223.8	251.5
75–84	25.8	26.0	143.0	149.2	206.5	234.2
85–94	24.6	24.5	140.8	147.6	188.1	206.0

ECG-LVH: Electrocardiographic evidence of left ventricular hypertrophy; diabetes: treated for diabetes or blood sugar 200 mg/dl or greater; definite hypertension: 160/95 mmHg or greater.

Table 11.6
Prevalence or means of risk factors by sex and age: Framingham Study, biennial examinations 1–20.

elderly who require investigation and possible treatment for dyslipidemia according to national guidelines.

About 43% of male and 64% of female octogenarians have hypertension. Isolated systolic hypertension accounts for 60% of this hypertension. It results from the disproportionate rise in the systolic blood pressure with advancing age because of diminished arterial compliance. A wide pulse pressure is produced that has an impact on the rate of development of CHD in the elderly. Combined systolic and diastolic blood pressure elevation occurs in about 30% of the elderly and only about 10% have isolated diastolic elevations. The prevalence of ECG-LVH, which is largely determined by the prevalence of predisposing hypertension, obesity and diabetes in the elderly, rises steeply with age and reaches a prevalence of about 9% in the octogenarian age group. Only in the octogenarian age group is the prevalence of this harbinger of cardiovascular disease more common in women than men (Table 11.6).

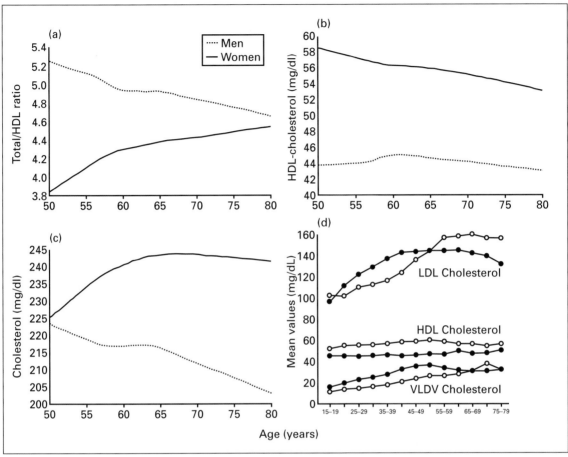

Figure 11.4
Age trends in lipoprotein cholesterol fractions: Framingham Study. (a) Average total/HDL cholesterol ratio by age in men and women, examination 11. (b) Average HDL-cholesterol by age in men and women, examination 11. (c) Average cholesterol by age in men and women, examination 11. (d) Mean values for LDL-, HDL- and VLDL-cholesterol by age group in men (●) and women (○) .

The preponderance of the prevalent diabetes in the elderly is of the noninsulin-dependent variety. About 14% of male and 11% of female Framingham Study octogenarians had diabetes. The prevalence of diabetes has also been increasing over time and is now about three times as common as it was three decades ago.

Fibrinogen values also tend to increase slightly with age and are slightly higher in women than men. They are also higher in persons with hypertension, diabetes or obesity, which are all common in the very old. Elders who continue to smoke also have higher fibrinogen levels in their blood.

The rise in blood pressure, blood lipids,

blood glucose, ECG-LVH and physical indo-lence that occurs with advancing age is not inevitable and can be curbed by a lifestyle characterized by a greater amount of daily exercise, a less fatty diet, not smoking, weight control and adequate amounts of fruits and vegetables in the diet.

Risk factor disease relationships

Hypertension, dyslipidemia, diabetes and obe-sity are responsible for most of the coronary disease afflicting octogenarians. The relative impact of each of the major risk factors tends to diminish in the most advanced age groups but this is offset by a greater absolute risk (Table 11.7).

There is a perception that the influence of hypertension on coronary heart disease occur-rence diminishes with advancing age and that in the very old hypertension may actually be protective. This has made many physicians reluctant to treat hypertension vigorously in the aged. Because mortality has been reported to vary inversely with the blood pressure in this age group, the benefit of treating hyper-tension in elders has been questioned. A recent meta-analysis of the efficacy of antihyperten-sive therapy in this age group has concluded that treatment significantly reduces overall mortality and cardiovascular morbidity and mortality.[12] However, it suggested that ther-apy offered less benefit to those in the 75 year and over age group.

Hypertension is a common and powerful

| | Age 35–64 years | | | | Age 65–94 years | | | |
| | Age-adjusted biennial rate per 1000 | | Age-adjusted relative risk | | Age adjusted biennial rate per 1000 | | Age adjusted relative risk | |
Risk factors	Men	Women	Men	Women	Men	Women	Men	Women
Cholesterol > 240 mg/dl	34	15	1.9**	1.8**	59	39	1.2*	2.0**
High blood pressure	45	21	2.0**	2.2**	73	44	1.6**	1.9**
Diabetes	39	42	1.5**	3.7**	79	62	1.6**	2.1**
ECG-LVH	79	55	3.0**	4.6**	134	94	2.7**	3.0**
Smoking	33	13	1.5**	1.1	53	38	1.0	1.2

Hypercholesterolemia: >240 mg/dl compared with <200 mg/dl. * *P* < 0.05; ** *P* < 0.001.
Risk factors reassessed every 2 years.

Table 11.7
Risk of coronary heart disease in each sex by standard risk factors according to age group: Framingham Study, 36-year follow-up

				Odds ratio for incident cardiovascular disease						
Age	HBP (%)		Risk ratio HBP (y/n)		Systolic BP (20 mmHg)		Diastolic BP (10 mmHg)		Attributable risk	
	Men	Women	Men	Women	Men	Women	Men	Women	Men	Women
35–44	11	6	3.1	2.5	1.6	1.2	1.6	1.2	0.19	0.09
45–54	18	17	2.2	1.8	1.4	1.3	1.3	1.2	0.18	0.11
55–64	25	29	1.9	2.2	1.4	1.5	1.3	1.3	0.17	0.25
65–74	33	43	1.8	1.9	1.4	1.3	1.1	1.2	0.20	0.27
75–84	42	56	1.3	1.1	1.2	1.1	1.0	0.9	0.11	0.06
85–94	42	63	0.7	1.4	1.3	0.9	1.1	0.9	***	0.19

HBP: high blood pressure, ≤160/95 mmHg or treated for hypertension.

Table 11.8
Cardiovascular disease risk associated with hypertension and increments in blood pressure:
Framingham Study, Population at risk examinations 1–20.

promoter of cardiovascular disease in general and coronary disease in particular, in the old and very old. The risk ratio, comparing persons with and without hypertension, and the incremental risk per unit increase in pressure diminish with age in the 65 year and greater age group, but the attributable risk does not (Table 11.8). This is because the prevalence of hypertension and the absolute risk of cardiovascular disease is so much greater in the elderly. The absolute risk of cardiovascular disease imposed by any degree of hypertension continues to increase with age in women from age 65 to 94 years. In men, it also increases but levels off beyond age 75 years. The risk ratio is greatest for stroke but coronary disease is the most common and lethal sequela of hypertension in this advanced age group. Isolated systolic hypertension is the predominant variety of hypertension in this age group. This

variety of hypertension is far from innocuous and predisposes to myocardial infarction at all ages, including the elderly (Figure 11.5). A wide pulse pressure is produced by this variety of hypertension and the risk of CHD increases the greater the pulse pressure.

Low blood pressure in the very old may be a consequence of disease and not a precipitant of it, creating a false perception that the excess mortality observed at low blood pressures in the old is a consequence of the reduced pressure. In the Framingham Study this excess mortality at low blood pressures is only observed in the segment of the population already afflicted with overt CHD.[13] A fall in blood pressure is often observed in the elderly after sustaining a myocardial infarction.[14]

Hypertension in this age group frequently occurs in conjunction with already overt cardiovascular disease and other major risk factors

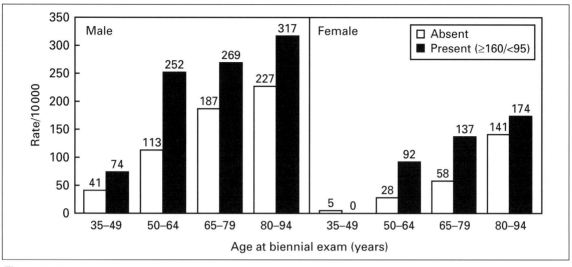

Figure 11.5
Average annual incidence of myocardial infarction with isolated systolic hypertension; Framingham Study, examinations 1–22.

which greatly influence the risk of the hypertension and must be taken into account in treatment decisions. High-risk hypertension is accompanied by dyslipidemia, diabetes or left ventricular hypertrophy. Only 20% of hypertension occurs in the absence of one or more of these associated risk factors.

Blood lipid values measured after attaining age 65 years or greater have not been consistently found to be related to the rate of development of coronary disease.[15,16] However, when the lipoprotein-cholesterol fractions were assessed rather than the serum total cholesterol, a preponderance of investigations have found a positive relationship between dyslipidemia and the development of CHD in the elderly.[17] Recent Framingham Study data indicate that the risk of CHD in those elderly who have attained age 80 years or older is still related to the total/HDL-cholesterol ratio, the

most efficient lipid profile for predicting the occurrence of CHD (Table 11.9). Cholesterol and LDL values measured late in life may differ from the values to which the elderly were exposed most of their adult life, particularly if they have lost weight. Nevertheless, the total/HDL cholesterol ratio continues to predict coronary disease well in the octogenarian age group, whereas the total cholesterol loses its predictive value in men after age 70 years. The total cholesterol continues to predict CHD well in women into the ninth decade of age (Table 11.9). Because the number of coronary events associated with any degree of dyslipidemia in the elderly is so much greater than in the middle aged, substantial risk can be attributed to dyslipidemia in the elderly, making treatment justifiable in the aged.[15,17] It is important to recognize that the majority of CHD events in the old occur in those with

Total/HDL Q5/Q1 hazard ratio					Total cholesterol >240/<200 mg/dl hazard ratio				
Age	50–59	60–69	70–79	80–89	Age	50–59	60–69	70–79	80–89
Men	2.5	1.7	2.3	5.6	Men	1.2	1.3	1.1	1.0
P<	0.001	0.01	0.004	0.05	P<	0.25	0.05	0.56	0.96
Women	3.1	3.5	2.8	4.8	Women	1.4	1.9	1.1	3.3
P<	0.0001	0.0001	0.001	0.024	P<	0.07	0.0001	0.58	0.007

Complete lipids available at one of examinations 10, 11, 12 (1968–73) and examination 15 (1977–79).
Mean follow-up was 9 years, range 0–24 years.

Table 11.9
Risk of coronary heart disease by total and total/HDL cholesterol ratio in each sex according to age. Framingham Study.

only mild to moderate dyslipidemia.[15] Also, it is important to take into account the fact that dyslipidemia usually clusters with diabetes, hypertension, obesity and elevated fibrinogen in the aged CHD candidate. Risk of CHD events in dyslipidemic elderly varies widely depending on the burden of these associated risk factors.[17] Thus, dyslipidemia continues to have relevance in the aged, particularly when partitioned into the LDL and HDL components, and when conceptualized as ingredients of a cardiovascular risk profile.

Electrocardiographic abnormalities such as left ventricular hypertrophy, blocked intraventricular conduction and nonspecific repolarization abnormalities commonly encountered in the elderly, often signify an ischemic or otherwise damaged myocardium. Compared with elderly without such ECG abnormalities, those with ECG-LVH have about a four-fold increase in risk of having a cardiovascular event, those with intraventricular block a two-fold increase and those with other abnormalities (predominantly nonspecific ST and T-wave abnormalities) a 1.5- to 1.7-fold increase (Table 11.10).

Although obesity is not a well demonstrated risk factor for development of CHD in the elderly, unrestrained weight gain and abdominal obesity continue to adversely influence all the major risk factors. A substantial body of evidence links abdominal obesity to insulin resistance, deteriorating glucose tolerance, dyslipidemia and hypertension, all of which independently predispose to the occurrence of coronary disease.[18]

Elevated fibrinogen and leukocyte counts, within the range of values often regarded as within normal limits, have been found to be associated with an excess occurrence of

	Age-adjusted annual incidence		Age-adjusted risk ratio	
ECG Abnormality	Men	Women	Men	Women
None	54	36	1.0	1.0
ECG-LVH	148	132	3.6	4.3
IV Block	82	69	1.7	2.1
Other	88	53	1.7	1.5

Incidence per 1000 person-exams; odds ratio from logistic regression.
Based on 1569 incident cases of CVD among 15 284 person-exams of subjects free of CVD at examination cycles 1–20 with 2 years of follow-up after each examination.

Table 11.10
Risk of cardiovascular events associated with ECG abnormalities in the elderly: Framingham Study Subjects Ages 65–94 Years

CHD.[19] Both may indicate the presence of unstable atherosclerotic plaques that are undergoing fissuring, inflammatory changes or subintimal hemorrhage. Fibrinogen is also thrombogenic.

Framingham Study data indicate that undergoing the menopause promptly escalates the risk of CHD three-fold over that of women who remain premenopausal at the same age.[20] Although hormone replacement therapy with low-dose estrogen has been shown to be protective, it is not clear how long therapy should be continued after the menopause and whether the protection extends into advanced age. The role of an early menopause on vulnerability to CHD in women who reach advanced age is unknown and the efficacy of hormone replacement in the very old needs further investigation because of conflicting effects on hormone-dependent cancers that may offset benefits for CHD and osteoporosis.

Although there is not much data available to document the benefits of altering lifestyles in the very old, the living habits that predispose to accelerated atherosclerosis in the middle-aged individual also promote it in the elderly. Elderly persons also react adversely to excessive calories, saturated fat and cholesterol in the diet. The benefits of exercise are also found at advanced age and unrestrained weight gain and cigarette smoking still adversely affect health.

Even moderate amounts of exercise have now been found to protect against CHD in both middle-aged and old men in the Framingham Study and elsewhere.[21] Daily exercise appears to be a helpful component of a comprehensive risk reduction regimen because it helps lower blood pressure, raise HDL-cholesterol, control obesity and reduce insulin resistance.[22] It also affords some independent protection against CHD. However, more information is needed concerning the benefits of exercise in the very old to determine the optimal frequency and duration of exercise indicated and the minimal threshold for cardiovascular benefit in this advanced age group.

Prospective and case-control studies have shown an association of sleep disturbance with the occurrence of CHD.[23,24] Disordered breathing during sleep, characterized by snoring, has been linked to the occurrence of coronary disease, hypertension and stroke.[24] Snoring is correlated with sleep apnea, a condition that has been reported to occur in 30% of the elderly and 22–60% of hypertensive persons.[24]

New and candidate risk factors

In addition to the established risk factors for CHD, there are a number of other candidate causal risk factors under investigation. There is very little information regarding their influence on CHD incidence in the elderly. It is not clear whether the apolipoproteins are independent risk factors in either the middle aged or elderly. There is still no agreement on desirable levels of these protein components of the lipoproteins. Among the lipoprotein subclasses, small-dense LDL and HDL_2 appear to be most closely related to the occurrence of CHD, but the determinants of these subclasses in the general population are not well understood and controlled trials of the effects of modifying these lipoprotein subclasses are underway. Lp(a) has been found to be an independent risk factor for the occurrence of CHD in many studies, but more information is needed on its interaction with the established risk factors.[25,26]

Homocysteine is a newly discovered risk factor for the development of CHD, that is promoted by a diet deficient in folate, B12 and B6 vitamins.[27,28] The elderly, because of low intakes of leafy vegetables, cereals, wheat products and oranges, are often deficient in these vitamins. The resultant increase in homocysteinemia appears to stimulate growth of smooth muscle, impair endothelial regeneration and enhance thrombogenesis. Framingham Study data indicate that higher concentrations of homocysteine are found in 29% of the elderly, that about 10% of cardiovascular disease may be attributable to elevated homocysteine and that two-thirds of the elderly with such elevations have reduced intake of the B vitamins.[29]

There is a large body of information incriminating hyperinsulinemia and insulin resistance in coronary atherogenesis.[18] Abdominal obesity appears to promote an insulin resistance syndrome comprised of hypertriglyceridemia, low HDL-cholesterol, small-dense LDL, hyperinsulinemia and hypertension.[18] Whether this also operates in the very old and whether correcting this condition by weight reduction or medications such as metformin or acarbose will reduce the risk of CHD is not known.

Several reports have incriminated various infections such as chlamydia in the development of myocardial infarction. However, smoking is associated with chlamydia infection and may be a possible confounder.

Vascular reactivity is under intensive investigation and high levels of LDL-cholesterol have been found to increase vasoconstriction and impair vasodilation. The relationship between dyslipidemia, lipoprotein peroxidation and vascular reactivity is also under scrutiny.

Further investigation is needed to determine whether dietary anti-oxidants such as vitamins E, C, and A, carotenoid, flavinoids and selenium can help prevent CHD. More investigation of the influence of intake of fruit and vegetables on plasma levels of these anti-oxidants and CHD incidence is needed, particularly in the elderly. Countries with a very low incidence of CHD have a higher consumption of vitamin E, mostly from olive oil, cereals and citrus fruits. The evidence that low levels of anti-oxidants are associated with a high incidence of CHD is persuasive. The scientific basis for recommending increased intake of vitamins E and C in the elderly is sound because it has been shown to reduce oxidation of LDL and platelet-related thrombosis as well as to stabilize endothelial function. However, two controlled trials recently published failed to show any benefit of carotenoid anti-oxidants on vascular disease.[30]

Post-CHD risk factors

All the major CHD risk factors continue to predispose to future CHD events and fatalities after the initial event in the elderly. Dyslipidemia, hypertension, diabetes or glucose intolerance, cigarette smoking, fibrinogen and ECG-LVH are all predictive of excess occurrence of further coronary events.[31] A spontaneous fall in the arterial blood pressure level with a recent coronary event is associated with a poor prognosis. However, the protection of exercise against CHD appears to apply in the elderly as well as in the middle aged; moderate exercise, such as a brisk walk for 30 minutes each day, appears to afford significant protection against initial and recurrent events.[21,22]

Preclinical signs

Otherwise unexplained ECG abnormalities in the elderly, such as ECG-LVH, blocked intraventricular conduction, or nonspecific repolarization abnormalities, often signify a

compromised coronary arterial circulation and are associated with an increased risk of developing CHD (Table 11.10). Left ventricular hypertrophy, whether detected by ECG, chest X-ray or echocardiogram is associated with an increased risk of CHD (Table 11.10). The risk is proportional to the severity of the abnormality on the ECG or echocardiogram and reversion toward normal is associated with a reduction in risk.[32]

Vascular bruits in the carotid or femoral arteries in the elderly are also associated with an increased risk of coronary disease, as well as stroke and intermittent claudication, because they usually indicate the presence of diffuse atherosclerosis.[33]

A combination of left ventricular hypertrophy, low vital capacity, cardiac enlargement on X-ray and a rapid resting heart rate in an elderly patient with hypertension or coronary disease is a strong indication of impaired left ventricular function and impending heart failure (Figure 11.6).[34]

Preventive opportunities

Proof of the efficacy of modifying risk factors in the octogenarian age group is meager. However, declines in CHD mortality in the US population have included the elderly in this age group, justifying some optimism.[8] Risk factors respond to treatment in the elderly as well as they do in the middle aged. Preventive treatment appears justified despite lack of proof of efficacy in this extreme age group. More concrete evidence of the efficacy of modifying specific risk factors in this age group is sorely needed, but it seems likely that the demonstrated benefits of lipid and blood pressure lowering in the middle aged and 65–74 year age group can be extrapolated to the octogenarian age group.

Most of the octogenarian population are

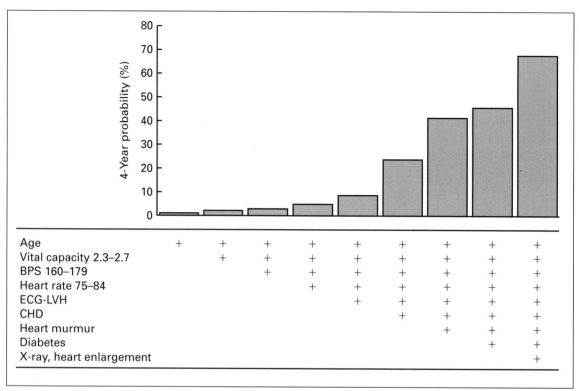

Age	+	+	+	+	+	+	+	+	+
Vital capacity 2.3–2.7		+	+	+	+	+	+	+	+
BPS 160–179			+	+	+	+	+	+	+
Heart rate 75–84				+	+	+	+	+	+
ECG-LVH					+	+	+	+	+
CHD						+	+	+	+
Heart murmur							+	+	+
Diabetes								+	+
X-ray, heart enlargement									+

Figure 11.6
Estimated probability of heart failure at ages 80–84 years according to risk factor profile

women. Extrapolation from available data for men to women would also appear to be justified. CHD is the leading cause of death in women as well as men and its incidence in women is substantial.[10] Also, once women develop CHD they have lost their advantage over men. Vigorous preventive measures are warranted with particular attention to dyslipidemia, glucose intolerance and hypertension associated with left ventricular hypertrophy. These prevalent risk factors tend to eliminate the elderly women's advantage over men.

High-risk elderly candidates can be effi-ciently targeted for treatment using multivariate risk profiles for coronary disease so that needless overtreatment can be avoided and high-risk candidates for CHD with multiple marginal abnormalities are not overlooked. Recent declines in CHD mortality in the elderly justify extrapolation of data on prevention from the elderly under age 80 years of age until data on the efficacy of risk-factor modification in this octogenarian age group become available. The hardy old should not be neglected simply because of their age.

A preponderance of evidence indicates a

relationship of dyslipidemia to the development of CHD in the elderly, particularly when the total/HDL ratio is used to characterize the dyslipidemia. In evaluating blood lipids in the elderly it is important to recognize that the bulk of coronary events occur in those with only moderate dyslipidemia accompanied by other risk factors. This makes it important to assess the need for treatment based on the total/HDL cholesterol ratio and multivariate risk assessment.[17] Lipid-modifying medications have been shown to be safe, well tolerated and effective in correcting dyslipidemia in the aged.[35] Attention to the lipid profile may be important. When triglycerides are elevated and HDL reduced, a fibrate drug or nicotinic acid may be required in addition to an HMG-CoA

reductase inhibitor to optimize the lipid profile in the obese diabetic elderly. In those who have already sustained a CHD event, it is often necessary to use a combination of medications with different modes of action if levels of lipids shown to be maximally effective are to be achieved.[36] Diet therapy, weight control and exercise can help to minimize the amount of drug treatment needed. Controlled clinical trials now indicate that treatment of both moderate and severe elevations of serum total and LDL-cholesterol reduces the risk of recurrent myocardial infarctions in the elderly as well as the middle aged, although data on the efficacy over age 80 is lacking (Figure 11.7).[37,38]

Although there is good evidence that

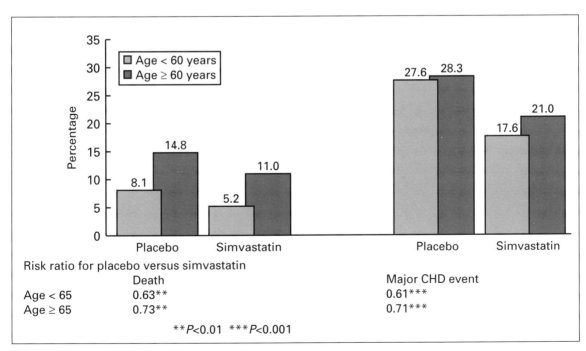

Figure 11.7
Mortality and major CHD events: placebo versus simvastatin in patients with CHD by age: 4S study. (From the 4S Group[37] with permission.)

treatment of dyslipidemia in the middle aged prevents initial CHD events, comparable data for the elderly do not exist.[39,40] However, the distinction between primary and secondary prevention is less clear in the very old than in the middle aged because, despite lack of symptoms, they often have advanced atherosclerotic lesions and a risk of a CHD event comparable to that of the middle aged who have already sustained an event. Some deliberative bodies have recommended against treating the elderly on the grounds that it is of unproven benefit and not cost-effective.[41] Nevertheless, there appears to be evidence to support treatment of the hardy elderly who have already sustained an event, and those whose dyslipidemia is accompanied by a poor CHD risk profile may also be considered for treatment.

Recommendations for treating hypertension in the octogenarian age group are clouded by an inverse relation to mortality observed in the very old.[42] However, the excess mortality reported in this segment of the population appears to reflect the influence of overt cardiovascular disease on the blood pressure and is not attributable to the low blood pressure itself. Hypertension is one of the most modifiable risk factors and treatment has been shown to benefit both middle aged and elderly patients.[42] However, the very old have been underrepresented in controlled trials and questions have been raised about the risk/benefit ratio of treating hypertension in the frail elderly.[43] A recent meta-analysis concluded that, overall, treatment of hypertension in the elderly produces a significant benefit in cardiovascular morbidity and mortality but suggested that the benefit may be reduced in the oldest age groups studied.[12] Data from the Framingham Study showed that elevated blood pressure is detrimental in the octogenarian age group who are free of cardiovascular disease and that the reported excess mortality

at low blood pressures reported is confined to those with overt cardiovascular disease.[13] The benefit or hazard of lowering blood pressure in this age group must await further clinical trials, but the Systolic Hypertension in the Elderly Program (SHEP) trial of treatment of isolated systolic hypertension strongly suggests that such treatment in those elderly who are free of overt cardiovascular disease is warranted.[44] For those who already have cardiovascular disease, rigorous blood pressure lowering should be undertaken with caution.

There is, at the present time, no basis for recommendations about treating lipoprotein (a), or subclasses of HDL or LDL. High triglycerides when accompanied by a low HDL may be a marker for insulin resistance or small-dense LDL and hence warrant attention to weight and associated dyslipidemia. Intervention studies will be required to evaluate whether lowering plasma insulin by weight control, a low carbohydrate diet or medications such as metformin or acarbose reduce CHD risk. Similarly, no specific recommendations can be made concerning the advisability of lowering fibrinogen or PAI-1, but treatment of known risk factors such as dyslipidemia, hypertension or obesity may provide the bonus of lowering these thrombogenic risk factors. There are no controlled trials to support recommendations to lower plasma homocysteine, but ensuring adequate intake of folic acid and vitamins B12 and B6 in this age group would appear to be prudent. The relationship between lipid levels, lipoprotein peroxidation and vascular reactivity requires additional investigation before recommendations about treatments to improve vascular reactivity can be made. There is also insufficient information about the efficacy of antioxidant therapy to make confident recommendations, although ensuring adequate intake of vitamin E and flavinoids would seem reasonable. Whether hormone replacement therapy should be continued or initiated in the very old is not clear and one must weigh the possible benefits for CHD and osteoporosis against the hazards of uterine and breast cancer. The benefits of keeping physically active in this advanced age group are not well documented, but recommending a half-hour walk each day would appear reasonable.

Thus, although data to support recommendations for risk factor modification in octogenarians are sparse, there is no reason to neglect the hardy elderly in this age group. They have a very high risk of CHD events and there is no reason to believe that this is an unmodifiable consequence of their having reached this venerable stage in life. The elderly, like the middle aged, are heterogeneous in their risk factor make-up and CHD risk. Multivariate risk assessment can identify among the elderly those who are truly at increased risk without needlessly alarming or falsely reassuring those who are candidates for lethal or disabling coronary events. Studies are needed to assess the effectiveness of multifactorial risk factor management in this age group.

Acknowledgements

Supported by NIH Grants NO1-HV-92922 and NO1-HV-52971 and the Framingham Visiting Scientist Program, ASTRA-USA, Servier and Hoechst Pharmaceuticals.

References

1. Harris TB, Cook EF, Kannel WB, Goldman L. Proportional hazards analysis of risk factors for coronary heart disease in individuals aged 65 or older. *J Am Geriatr Soc* (1988) **36:** 1023–8.

2. Benfante R, Reed D, Frank J. Do coronary heart disease risk factors measured in the elderly have the same predictive roles as in the middle aged? Comparisons of relative and attributable risks. *Ann Epidemiol* (1992) **2:** 273–82.

3. Cupples LA, D'Agostino RB. The Framingham Study. An epidemiological investigation of cardiovascular disease. Section 23: some risk factors related to the annual incidence of cardiovascular disease and death using pooled repeated biennial measurements: Framingham Heart Study, 30 year follow-up. (US Department of Commerce: Springfield, VA, 1987).

4. WHO Study Group on Epidemiology and Prevention of Cardiovascular Disease in the Elderly. Epidemiology and prevention of cardiovascular disease in elderly people. Report of WHO study Group. WHO Technical Report Series No. 853. (WHO: Geneva, 1995).

5. Harlan WR, Manolio TA. Coronary heart disease in the elderly. In: Marmot MG, Elliot P, eds, *Coronary Heart Disease Epidemiology: From Aetiology to Public Health.* (Oxford University Press: New York, 1992) 114–26.

6. Kaplan GA, Haas MV, Cohen RD. Risk factors and the study of prevention in the elderly. In: Wallace RB, Woolsen RF, eds, *The Epidemiologic Study of the Elderly.* (Oxford University Press: New York, 1992) 20–36.

7. Denke MA, Winker MA. Cholesterol and coronary heart disease in older adults. No easy answers. *JAMA* (1995) **274:** 575–7.

8. Anonymous. Morbidity and Mortality: 1996. Chartbook on cardiovascular, lung and blood diseases. (US Department of Health and Human Services: Bethesda, MD, 1996).

9. Kannel WB, Dannenberg AL, Abbott RD. Unrecognized myocardial infarction and hypertension. The Framingham Study. *Am Heart J* (1985) **109:** 581–5.

10. Kannel WB, Vokonas PS. Demographics of the prevalence, incidence and management of coronary heart disease in the elderly and women. *Ann Epidemiol* (1992) **2:** 5–14.

11. Schaefer EJ, Moussa PB, Wilson PWF et al. Plasma lipoproteins in healthy octogenarians: lack of reduced high density lipoprotein cholesterol levels: results from the Framingham Heart Study. *Metabolism* (1989) **38:** 293–6.

12. Insua JT, Sacks HS, Lau TS et al. Drug treatment of hypertension in the elderly: a meta-analysis. *Ann Intern Med* (1994) **121:** 355–62.

13. Kannel WB, D'Agostino RB, Silberschatz H. Blood pressure and cardiovascular morbidity and mortality in the elderly. *Am Heart J* (1997) **134:** 758–63.

14. Langer RD, Criqui MH, Barrett-Connor EL et al. Blood pressure change and survival after age 75. *Hypertension* (1993) **22:** 551–9.

15. LaRosa JC. Should high lipid levels in very old patients be lowered? *Drugs Aging* (1995) **6:** 85–90.

16. Havel RJ, Rappoport E. Management of primary hyperlipidemia. *N Engl J Med* (1995) **332:** 1491–8.

17. Wilson PWF, Kannel WB. Hypercholesterolemia and coronary risk in the elderly: The Framingham Study. *Am J Geriatr Cardiol* (1993) **2:** 52–6.

18. Reaven GM. Banting Lecture, 1988: role of insulin resistance in human disease. *Diabetes* (1988) **37:** 1595–607.

19. Ernst E, Resch KL. Fibrinogen as a cardiovascular risk factor: a meta-analysis and review of the literature. *Ann Intern Med* (1993) **118:** 956–63.

20. Kannel WB, Hjortland MC, McNamara PM, Gorden T. Menopause and risk of cardiovascular disease. The Framingham Study. *Ann Intern Med* (1976) **85:** 447–52.

21. Kannel WB, Sorley PD. Some health benefits of

physical activity. The Framingham Study. *Arch Intern Med* (1979) **139**:857–61.

22. Haskell WL, Leon AS, Casperson CJ et al. Cardiovascular benefits and assessment of physical activity and physical fitness in adults. *Med Sci Sports Med* (1992) **24**:S201–20.

23. D'Allessandro R, Magelli C, Gamberini G et al. Snoring every night as a risk factor for myocardial infarction: a case-control study. *BMJ* (1990) **300**:1557–8.

24. Hung J, Whitford EG, Parsons RW et al. Association of sleep apnea with myocardial infarction in men. *Lancet* (1990) **336**:261–4.

25. Ridker PM, Hennekens CH. Lipoprotein (a) and risks of cardiovascular disease. *Ann Epidemiol* (1994) **4**:360–2.

26. Schaefer EJ, Lamon-Fava S, Jenner JL et al. Lipoprotein (a) levels and risk of coronary heart disease in men: the Lipid Research Clinics Coronary Primary Prevention Trial. *JAMA* (1994) **271**:999–1003.

27. Selhub J, Jacques PF, Wilson PWF et al. Vitamin status and intake as primary determinants of homocysteinemia in the elderly. *JAMA* (1993) **270**:2693–8.

28. Genest JJ, Malinow MR. Homocysteine and coronary artery disease. *Curr Opin Lipid* (1992) **3**:295–9.

29. Kannel WB, Wilson PWF. Comparison of risk profiles for cardiovascular events: implications for prevention. *Adv Intern Med* (1997) **42**: 39–66.

30. Hennekens CH, Buring JE, Peto R. Antioxidant vitamins: benefits not yet proved (editorial). *N Engl J Med* (1994) **330**:1080–1.

31. Wong ND, Cupples LA, Ostfeld AM et al. Risk factors for long-term coronary prognosis after initial myocardial infarction: the Framingham Study. *Am J Epidemiol* (1989) **130**:469–80.

32. Levy D, Salomon MN, D'Agostino RB et al. Prognostic implication of baseline electrocardiographic features of and their serial changes in subjects with left ventricular hypertrophy. *Circulation* (1994) **90**:1786–93.

33. Kannel WB, D'Agostino RB. The importance of cardiovascular risk factors in the elderly. *Am J Geriatr Cardiol* (1995) **4**:10–23.

34. Kannel WB, Belanger AJ. Epidemiology of heart failure. *Am Heart J* (1991) **121**:951–7.

35. D'Agostino RB, Kannel WB, Stepanians MN, D'Agostino LC. Efficacy and tolerability of lovastatin in the hypercholesterolemic women. *Clin Ther* (1992) **14**:390–5.

36. Pasternak RC, Brown LE, Stone PH et al. Effect of combination therapy with lipid-reducing drugs in patients with coronary heart disease and 'normal' cholesterol levels. A randomized, placebo controlled trial. Havard Atherosclerosis Reversibility Project (HARP) Study Group. *Ann Intern Med* (1996) **125**:529–40.

37. The 4S Group. Randomized trial of cholesterol lowering in 4444 patients with coronary heart disease: the Scandinavian Simvastatin Survival Study (4S). *Lancet* (1996) **344**:1383–9.

38. Sacks FM, Pfeffer MA, Moye LA et al. The effect of pravastatin on coronary events after myocardial infarction in patients with average cholesterol levels. Cholesterol and Recurrent Events Trial Investigators. *N Engl J Med* (1996) **335**:1001–9.

39. Shepherd J, Cobbe SM, Ford I et al. Prevention of coronary heart disease in men with hypercholesterolemia. West of Scotland Coronary Prevention Study Group. *N Engl J Med* (1995) **333**:1301–7.

40. Holme I. Cholesterol reduction and its impact on coronary artery disease and mortality. *Am J Cardiol* (1995) **76**:10–17C.

41. Anonymous. Guidelines for using serum cholesterol, high-density lipoprotein cholesterol and triglyceride levels as screening tests for preventing coronary heart disease in adults. American College of Physicians. Part 1. *Ann Intern Med* (1996) **124**:515–17.

42. Bulpitt CJ, Fletcher AE. Prognostic significance of blood pressure in the very old. Implications for treatment decision. *Drugs Aging* (1994) **5**:184–91.

43. Applegate WB. Hypertension in elderly patients. *Ann Intern Med* (1989) **110**:901–15.

44. Systolic Hypertension in the Elderly Program Cooperative Research Group. Prevention of stroke by antihypertensive drug treatment in older persons with isolated systolic hypertension: Final results of the Systolic Hypertension in the Elderly Program (SHEP). *JAMA* (1991) **265**:3255–64.

12

Noninvasive and invasive diagnostic cardiovascular procedures at very elderly age

Douglas G Ebersole and Ronald E Vlietstra

Introduction

Diagnostic testing for coronary disease in the very elderly involves some issues that are unique to that age group. The patient's ability to complete the test may be impaired and its interpretation may be less certain. Age also impacts on test cost-effectiveness. This chapter focuses on current knowledge and areas for future investigation.

There has been a marked increase in the use of diagnostic testing for coronary disease in the elderly. This is illustrated by the study of Gehlbach and co-workers[1] that showed a dramatic increase in the use of cardiovascular diagnostic testing in Medicare patients from 1985 to 1990. For patients with acute myocardial infarction and congestive heart failure, the use of coronary arteriography tripled and the use of echocardiography doubled. There was also a greater than 50% increase in the use of stress testing. This escalation in testing was seen in rural as well as in urban hospitals and in community hospitals as well as in academic centers.

Obviously only a small part of this increase can be explained by the growing number of elderly patients. Furthermore, life expectancy in the very elderly has lengthened minimally over the last century.[2] It seems more likely that the expectations of the very elderly and their

doctors are changing rapidly. Both parties see benefits from more vigorous testing. So far, however, few studies have critically evaluated whether there is advantage to this.

Noninvasive testing in the elderly

The presenting symptoms of coronary artery disease in the elderly may be atypical and, therefore, accurate diagnosis often requires additional testing. The 12-lead electrocardiogram (ECG) can be helpful although it may be abnormal in approximately 50% of elderly subjects.[3] ECG abnormalities that are found with increased frequency in the elderly are first degree AV block, left axis deviation, left ventricular hypertrophy, bundle branch block, ST-T wave changes, atrial fibrillation, and premature atrial and ventricular contractions.

Exercise ECG testing

Samek et al[4] evaluated exercise testing in patients over 65 years of age in comparison with patients below 65 years and found that older patients have lower heart rates during submaximal exercise than younger patients. At rest and during submaximal exercise elderly patients also have a higher systolic blood pressure while the increase in blood pressure following exercise is the same as in younger patients. The amount of ST segment depression was the most reliable diagnostic indicator for the prediction of either one, two or three vessel coronary disease.

A number of cross-sectional studies have shown that the VO_2max declines at a rate of approximately 10% per decade after the age of 25.[5,6] This decline is not solely the direct effect of aging per se; roughly half of the decrease is more appropriately attributed to decreasing physical activity and the weight gain that is also generally observed with aging. The result of this loss of VO_2max is that VO_2max in a relatively lean male aged 25 would be expected to be 50 ml/kg/min while in a 70 year old healthy male the VO_2max will be roughly half of this value, or 25 ml/kg/min. Thus, on the treadmill, the older man would be able to achieve a maximum work level that is only half that of the younger man.

The most frequently used treadmill exercise test for diagnostic exercise testing is the Bruce protocol (see Table 12.1).[7] A major drawback of the Bruce protocol when exercise testing elderly populations is that the initial stage of the standard Bruce protocol requires an estimated VO_2 of 16 ml/kg/min, which would require 65–80% of a healthy 70 year old's VO_2max. A more appropriate test at elderly age is that described by Naughton.[8] The major benefit of this protocol is that a slower speed (2 miles per hour) is used for the majority of the test and the first stage is on a level grade. Hence, the required VO_2 is markedly lower in the initial stages than is the case in the Bruce protocol. The expected duration of a Naughton protocol treadmill test in a healthy 70 year old male is 15 minutes.

A second frequently used alternative to the Bruce protocol is that described by Balke and Ware.[9] This protocol uses 2-minute stages and a constant speed of 3.4 miles per hour. The

combination of a higher speed and a first stage treadmill grade of 2.5% results in a substantial VO_2 requirement during the initial minutes of exercise, so that the average 70 year old man can be expected to complete about 8 minutes of exercise. Perhaps the most appropriate treadmill protocol for exercise testing in the elderly is a modified Balke protocol[10] in which the first stage is on a level grade and the treadmill speed is kept constant at 2 rather than 3 miles per hour. This protocol results in treadmill test duration in a healthy 70 year old male of 12 minutes, and even a 70 year old with cardiovascular disease, arthritis or obesity should be able to exercise for 6 minutes. Thus, because of the physiological responses that can be measured during graded submaximal levels of exercise, an appropriate exercise prescription can be derived.

There is general consensus that when interpreting the exercise ECG in the elderly, one must consider other factors such as symptoms, arrhythmias, exercise capacity and chronotropic and inotropic responses. One difference in interpreting an exercise test in an elderly population is the finding of a short (less than 3 minute) duration of exercise. In a younger population, this would suggest advanced coronary artery disease, but in an elderly population, a short duration of exercise is not necessarily an ominous sign unless there are associated ST segment changes.[11]

Several studies have found that the significance of ST depression in the elderly may be altered compared with younger subjects due to a high incidence of false-positive findings.[12–14] False-positive exercise ECG responses in the elderly tend to reflect the increased incidence of diseases affecting left ventricular compliance, such as hypertension, valvular heart disease and intraventricular conduction defects. In addition, elderly patients are more likely than middle-aged patients with similar severity

Stage	1	2	3	4	5	6	7
Bruce							
Speed (mph)	1.7	2.5	3.4	4.2	5.0	5.5	6.0
Grade (%)	10	12	14	16	18	20	22
Duration (min)	3	3	3	3	3	3	3
Naughton							
Speed (mph)	1	2	2	2	2	2	2
Grade (%)	0	0	3.5	7.0	10.5	14	17.5
Duration (min)	2	2	2	2	2	2	2
Balke							
Speed (mph)	3.4	3.4	3.4	3.4	3.4	3.4	3.4
Grade (%)	0	1	2	3	4	5	6
Duration (min)	2	2	2	2	2	2	2
Modified Balke							
Speed (mph)	2	2	2	2	2	2	2
Grade (%)	0	1	2	3	4	5	6
Duration (min)	2	2	2	2	2	2	2

Table 12.1
Comparison of various exercise protocols

of coronary artery disease to have asymptomatic ECG changes with ambulatory monitoring.[15]

Thallium perfusion imaging

When screening healthy populations aged more than 65 years, many will have ST-segment changes with exercise testing. As many as 15% of 80 year olds have asymptomatic changes.[16] In nearly 5 years of follow-up, a cardiac event occurred in 7% of patients with neither a positive electrocardiogram nor thallium perfusion study, 12% of patients with only a positive exercise electrocardiogram and 3% of subjects with only an ischemic thallium scan. In contrast, 48% of subjects with concordant exercise electrocardiogram and thallium scan positive for ischemia developed a cardiac event during follow-up. Also, 8–10% of subjects aged more than 70 years screened by Pollock[17] had asymptomatic ST changes. When Pollock's subjects were followed-up with thallium testing, only one had evidence for significant myocardial ischemia.[17] Thus, abnormal responses will occur and must be interpreted within the context of all of the factors mentioned previously. In the absence of other factors, especially symptoms of angina, a 1–2 mm ST-segment shift often represents a false-positive finding.

Dipyridamole thallium perfusion imaging and echocardiography (Table 12.2)

A limitation to exercise stress testing in the elderly is the frequent inability of older

High disease prevalence
Inability to exercise adequately
   Inactivity
   Weight gain
   Arthritis
   Peripheral vascular disease
Medications limiting heart rate response
Frequently abnormal baseline ECG
   ST-T wave abnormalities
   Atrial fibrillation
   Left ventricular hypertrophy
   Bundle branch block

Table 12.2
Limitations to exercise testing in the elderly

patients to perform vigorous exercise because of underlying medical conditions or physical deconditioning. Intravenous dipyridamole and adenosine are well tolerated in older subjects. In a series of 337 patients with suspected coronary artery disease who underwent dipyridamole thallium imaging, 101 subjects were older than 70 years of age.[18] The overall incidence of side-effects was 39% and was similar in younger and older patients. In those older patients who subsequently underwent coronary arteriography, the sensitivity of dipyridamole thallium scanning for the detection of coronary artery disease was 86% with a specificity of 75%, compared with respective values of 83% and 70% in younger patients. Therefore, dipyridamole thallium scanning has a similar side-effect profile in old and young patients and has a high sensitivity and specificity in older patients referred for evaluation for suspected coronary artery disease.

Dipyridamole thallium imaging also has excellent prognostic value in older populations. In 348 patients with known or suspected coronary artery disease aged 70 years or older who underwent this procedure, the presence of a fixed and/or reversible thallium defect was a powerful and independent predictor of cardiac death or nonfatal myocardial infarction during nearly 2 years of mean follow-up.[19] In a multicenter trial of 190 elderly (older than 65 years) survivors of myocardial infarction, a positive dipyridamole echocardiogram occurred in 45%.[20] During 14 months of follow-up, the relative risk of a cardiac event (angina, recurrent myocardial infarction or cardiac death) was three-fold and relative risk of death four-fold in those patients with a positive compared to a negative study.

Dobutamine stress testing

Dobutamine is also frequently used in conjunction with echocardiography or thallium scintigraphy as a pharmacological stress agent. Dobutamine is an attractive method to aid in the diagnosis of coronary artery disease in those patients who cannot exercise adequately, particularly those patients with obstructive lung disease in whom both dipyridamole and adenosine are contraindicated. Dobutamine is well tolerated and has a high sensitivity and specificity for detecting significant coronary artery disease, but its diagnostic and prognostic value specific to the elderly population is unknown.

Summary

Elderly patients constitute an increasing proportion of the patients evaluated and treated for coronary artery disease. Clinical and noninvasive evaluation are important in both the diagnosis and prognosis of coronary disease in the elderly, and stress testing is an important part of that evaluation. For older individuals capable of vigorous treadmill or cycle exercise, the exercise electrocardiogram, either alone or combined with radionuclide or echocardio-

	Advantages	Disadvantages
Exercise	Largest amount of diagnostic and prognostic information Allows for exercise prescription	Frequently nondiagnostic (see Table 12.1)
Dipyridamole/adenosine	Diagnostic and prognostic information available for the elderly	Expensive Contraindicated in COPD
Dobutamine	Inexpensive May use in COPD	Less data than with dipyridamole/adenosine

COPD, chronic obstructive pulmonary disease.

Table 12.3
Options for stress testing in the elderly

graphic imaging, remains an excellent diagnostic and prognostic tool. For the large percentage of elderly patients unable to perform adequate exercise, pharmacological stress testing with dipyridamole, adenosine or dobutamine is a valuable alternative (Table 12.3). The challenge is to choose the most appropriate cardiac stress test for the patient from among the many alternatives available. Future studies comparing the accuracy and cost–benefit ratio of various stress tests in the elderly will help achieve this goal.

Invasive testing (Table 12.4)

While coronary arteriography is used to define anatomy at any age, the specific indications may differ in the very elderly. By the time they are referred to the cardiac catheterization laboratory, these patients are more likely to be symptomatic from ischemia, and for such symptoms to be frequent and refractory to medical therapy. Such a selection bias might

Increasingly used
Patients more symptomatic
Greater extent of disease
Complications more frequent
Cost-effectiveness poorly tested

Table 12.4
Invasive testing in the very elderly

account for the findings of Cave and others[21] who reported that patients over the age of 70 years with positive adenosine SPECT thallium scans were one-third less likely to be referred for coronary arteriography.

The high incidence of coronary disease in the very elderly also puts them at a higher risk of being recommended for coronary revascularization prior to any noncardiac surgery. The cost–benefit ratio of such an approach has not been evaluated.

A recent study of Medicare patients documents a low, but growing, frequency of coronary arteriography following myocardial infarction.[22] Despite uniform Medicare coverage, there are up to three-fold variations between states in the use of coronary arteriography for the elderly patient postmyocardial infarction.[23] In GUSTO, the factor that most predicted whether the patient had coronary arteriography following myocardial infarction was age, with the rates being lowest in the very elderly.[24] This runs counter to the logic of selecting coronary arteriography for those patients at highest risk and more intensive evaluation of selected subgroups may also prove highly cost-effective.[25]

Simply quoting rates for coronary arteriography begs the question whether patients are being appropriately selected for study. When rates increase, is that due to more high-risk or more low-risk patients being studied? In an elegant comparison of US and Canadian rates, Tu and co-workers[26] found that US elderly patients had a 34.9% chance of having coronary arteriography following myocardial infarction in 1991 while in Ontario, the chance was 6.7%. Coronary angioplasty and coronary bypass surgery was performed 8 times more frequently in the US group despite lesser angina in US patients. However, 1-year mortality was no different.[26]

At coronary arteriography, the very elderly have a higher rate of coronary artery disease.[27] Indeed, age is a more powerful risk factor than any of the other classic risk factors. When disease is present, it is also more extensive in older patients.[28] Finally, the coronary anatomy found is less likely to be easily amenable to percutaneous transluminal coronary angioplasty (PTCA).[29]

The presence of coronary artery calcification increases with age. Recent studies combining electron beam computed-tomography and coronary arteriography reveal that while coronary calcification increases with age, it simply parallels the increased incidence of coronary atherosclerosis.[30] Indeed, the absence of coronary calcification on ultra-fast CT scan is a good predictor of angiographically normal coronary arteries in the elderly.[31]

The complications of coronary arteriography are increased in the elderly and the risk–benefit ratio must be adjusted accordingly. As early as age 65 years, coronary arteriography complications increase, as was found in the CASS study.[32] The complications of catheterization that are increased include death, nonfatal infarction and stroke.

Many very elderly patients have impaired renal function, an important predisposing factor for contrast-induced renal failure. This latter problem is not only an issue for coronary arteriography, but also applies to percutaneous catheter intervention.[33]

The vascular complications of catheterization include peripheral as well as coronary embolism, vascular dissection, hematoma, pseudoaneurysm and vessel perforation. All of these complications tend to occur more frequently at older age. The arteriographer should also be sensitive to identifying other areas of vascular disease when coronary disease is found in the very elderly. The association of carotid and renal artery stenoses with coronary disease is particularly common in this age group.

Finally, the very elderly are less tolerant of the discomfort and the immobilization associated with catheterization procedures. They are, therefore, more often exposed to high doses of sedatives and analgesics. To minimize immobilization some have recommended using the radial artery approach.[34] Clearly this may be useful in carefully selected patients, but aortic and subclavian tortuosity and calcification may make it more problematic.

An increased use of coronary arteriography in the elderly is being reported in many countries throughout the world.[35] With today's catheters and techniques, very low rates of complications are seen. However, evaluating elderly patients for revascularization brings with it a responsibility to provide a revascularization service promptly. Bengtson and co-workers[36] in Sweden found that old age was the most powerful risk factor for death or myocardial infarction while on the waiting list for surgery.

Future research (Table 12.5)

An informal review of the numbers of very elderly patients randomized in angiographic trials of new catheter technology reveals that very few have been included. Given that this subgroup of patients is rapidly growing in number, there are many issues that require future investigation.

It would be helpful to be able to identify the characteristics of patients who benefit most from intensive investigation for coronary disease. There is a difference between biological and chronological age, but putting a precise value on it is difficult.

Some technologies might have special application in the elderly. The use of hemostatic closure devices following coronary arteriography and angioplasty may be highly useful for the fragile femoral vessels of the old patient. They may allow more rapid mobilization and shorter hospital stay.

The sensitivity and specificity of various tests have been well defined in the overall pop-

Include in randomized controlled trials
Specific technologies helpful
Different tests, sensitivities and specificities
Normal values for aged
Age interaction with known risk factors
Patient and social expectations

Table 12.5
Future research

ulation, but these values may not be meaningful in the very elderly. Similarly, the normal values for an 85 year old are less certain than they are at younger age. For example, what is the normal intravenous dobutamine response of heart rate at age 85?

More data are needed on the cost effectiveness of tests in elderly age. This would include learning more about the patient's and society's expectations, and current levels of investigation and treatment. Paul and colleagues from the Massachusetts General Hospital found that the elderly had coronary thrombolysis, PTCA and coronary bypass surgery frequencies only one-third of that of younger patients and underwent catheterization following infarction less than half as frequently.[37]

Age needs to be considered in the interpretation of tests. A recent analysis of myocardial infarction performed at the Mayo Clinic demonstrated a powerful interaction between myocardial infarction size, age and mortality that had not been previously recognized.[38] It is likely that age significantly modifies the power of many risk factors and predictors.

References

1. Gehlbach SH, Adamche KW, Cromwell J. Changes in the user of diagnostic technologies among Medicare patients, 1985 and 1990. *Inquiry* (1996) **33**:363–72.

2. Manton KG, Vaupel JW. Survival after the age of 80 in the United States, Sweden, France, England and Japan. *N Engl J Med* (1995) **333**:1232–5.

3. Mihalick MJ, Fisch C. Electrocardiographic findings in the aged. *Am Heart J* (1974) **87**:117–28.

4. Samek L, Betz P, Schnellbacher K. Exercise testing in elderly patients with coronary artery disease. *Eur Heart J* (1984) **5**:(Supplement E): 69–73.

5. Hagberg JM. Effect of training on the decline of VO$_2$max with aging. *Federation Proceedings* (1987) **46**:1830–3.

6. Heath GW, Hagberg JM, Ehsani AA, Brown MM. A physiological comparison of young and older endurance athletes. *J Appl Physiol* (1981) **61**:634–40.

7. Bruce RA. Exercise testing of patients with coronary artery disease. *Ann Clin Res* (1971) **3**:323–30.

8. Naughton JB, Balke B, Nagle FJ. Refinements in methods of evaluation and physical conditioning before and after myocardial infarction. *Am J Cardiol* (1964) **14**:837–45.

9. Balke B, Ware RW. An experimental study of physical fitness of Air Force personnel. *US Armed Forces Med J* (1959) **10**:675–82.

10. Wilson PF, Winga ER, Edgett JW, Gushiken TT. *Policies and procedures of a Cardiac Rehabilitation Program.* (Lea & Febiger: Philadelphia, 1978).

11. Sheffield L, Haskell W, Heiss G et al. Safety of exercise-testing volunteer subjects: the Lipid Research Clinic's prevalence study experience. *J Cardiol Rehab* (1982) **2**:395–400.

12. Doan A, Peterson D, Blackman J et al. Myocardial ischemia after maximal exercise in healthy men. *Am Heart J* (1965) **69**:11–21.

13. Kasser I, Bruce R. Comparative effects of aging and coronary heart disease on submaximal and maximal exercise. *Circulation* (1969) **39**:759–74.

14. Vasilomanolakis E. Geriatric cardiology; when exercise stress testing is justified. *Geriatrics* (1985) **40**:41–57.

15. Kurita A, Takasa B, Uehata A et al. Painless myocardial ischemia in elderly patients compared with middle-aged patients and its relation to treadmill testing and coronary hemodynamics. *Clin Cardiol* (1991) **14**: 886–90.

16. Fleg JL, Gerstenblith G, Zonderman AB et al. Prevalence and prognostic significance of exercise-induced silent ischemia detected by thallium scintigraphy and electrocardiography in asymptomatic volunteers. *Circulation* (1990) **81**:428–36.

17. Pollock M. Geriatric stress testing and physical conditioning of the aged. In: *1991 Medical Section Proceedings, 16th Annual Meeting of the American Council of Life Insurance.* (ACLI: Washington DC, 1991) 99–110.

18. Lam JYT, Chaitman BR, Glaenzer M et al. Safety and diagnostic accuracy of dipyridamole thallium imaging in the elderly. *J Am Coll Cardiol* (1988) **11**:585–90.

19. Shaw L, Chaitman BR, Hilton TC et al. Prognostic value of dipyridamole thallium-201 imaging in elderly patients. *J Am Coll Cardiol* (1992) **19**:1390–8.

20. Camerieri A, Picano E, Landi P et al. Prognostic value of dipyridamole echocardiograph yearly after myocardial infarction in elderly patients. *J Am Coll Cardiol* (1993) **22**: 1809–15.

21. Cave V, Wasserleben V, Heo J, Iskandrian AS, Age- and sex-related differences in the use of coronary angiography in patients undergoing adenosine SPECT thallium imaging. *Coron Art Dis* (1993) **4**:1123–7.

22. Paschos CL, Newhouse JP, McNeil BJ. Temporal changes in the care and outcomes of elderly patients with acute myocardial infarction, 1987 through 1990. *JAMA* (1993) **270**: 1832–6.

23. Gatsonis CA, Epstein AM, Newhouse JP et al. Variations in the utilization of coronary angiography for elderly patients with an acute myocardial infarction. An analysis using hier-

archical logistic regression. *Med Care* (1995) **33**:625–42.

24. Pilote L, Miller DP, Califf RM et al. Determinations of the use of coronary angiography and revascularization after thrombolysis for acute myocardial infarction. *N Engl J Med* (1996) **335**:1198–205.

25. Kuntz KM, Tsevat J, Goldman L, Weinstein MC. Cost-effectiveness of routine coronary angiography after acute myocardial infarction. *Circulation* (1996) **94**:957–65.

26. Tu JV, Paschos CL, Naylor CD et al. Use of coronary procedures and outcomes in elderly patients with myocardial infarction in the United States and Canada. *N Engl J Med* (1997) **336**:1500–5.

27. Vlietstra RE, Frye RL, Kronmal RA et al. Risk factors and angiographic coronary artery disease: a report from the Coronary Artery Surgery Study (CASS). *Circulation* (1980) **62**:254–61.

28. Vlietstra RE, Kronmal RA, Frye RL et al. Factors affecting the extent and severity of coronary artery disease in patients enrolled in the Coronary Artery Surgery Study (CASS). *Arteriosclerosis* (1982) **2**:208–15.

29. Kowalchuk GJ, Siu SC, Lewis SM. Coronary artery disease in the octogenarian: angiographic spectrum and suitability for revascularization. *Am J Cardiol* (1990) **66**:1319–23.

30. Rumberger JA, Sheedy PF, Breen JF et al. Electron beam computed tomography and coronary artery disease: scanning for coronary artery calcification. *Mayo Clin Proc* (1996) **71**:369–77.

31. Shemesch J, Tenenbaum A, Fisman EZ et al. Absence of coronary calcification on double-helical CT scans: predictor of angiographically normal coronary arteries in elderly women? *Radiology* (1996) **199**:665–8.

32. Gersh BJ, Kronmal RA, Frye RL et al. Coronary arteriography and coronary artery bypass surgery: morbidity and mortality in patients ages 65 or older. A report from the Coronary Artery Surgery Study (CASS). *Circulation* (1983) **67**:483–90.

33. Vlietstra RE, Nunn CM, Narvarte J, Browne KF. Contrast nephropathy after coronary angioplasty in chronic renal insufficiency. *Am Heart J* (1996) **132**:1049–50.

34. Lotan C, Hasin Y, Mosseri M et al. Transradial approach for coronary angiography and angioplasty. *Am J Cardiol* (1995) **76**:164–7.

35. Ricou FJ, Suilen C, Rothmeier C et al. Coronary angiography in octogenarians: results and implications for revascularization. *Am J Med* (1995) **99**:16–21.

36. Bengtson A, Karlsson T, Hjalmarson A, Herlitz J. Complications prior to revascularization among patients waiting for coronary artery bypass grafting and percutaneous transluminal coronary angioplasty. *Eur Heart J* (1996) **17**:1846–51.

37. Paul SD, O'Gara PT, Mahjoul ZA et al. Geriatric patients with acute myocardial infarction: cardiac risk factor profiles, presentation, thrombolysis, coronary interventions, and prognosis. *Am Heart J* (1996) **131**:710–15.

38. Miller TD, Christian TF, Hopfenspirger MR et al. Does larger infarct size explain the higher mortality in the elderly with myocardial infarction? *Circulation* (1997) **96**:1–28 (abst).

13

Angina and myocardial infarction in the elderly

Joseph A Guzzo and Sidney C Smith Jr

Introduction

Cardiovascular disease is the most common disabling and lethal medical problem in the elderly population. It accounts for approximately two-thirds of all deaths in the age group greater than 65 years and over half of the patients hospitalized with an acute myocardial infarction (AMI) belong to this age group.[1] The fastest growing segment of the population is the group over 85 years of age. This portion of the population will probably continue to increase, so it is essential to understand better the nature of cardiovascular disease among the elderly. This is a difficult task for many reasons. Many previous studies in cardiology excluded patients from enrolment based solely on age criteria. This has resulted in a relative lack of evidence-based medicine for the treatment of cardiovascular disease in the elderly. The presentations of acute coronary syndromes are significantly different in the elderly compared with the younger population. This makes the diagnosis and treatment of unstable coronary syndromes more difficult. This continuously expanding age group should be considered a separate entity when considering all facets of cardiovascular management. Symptomatology, prognosis and relative risk factors take on separate meanings when dealing with the elderly patient.

There has been an age-adjusted decrease in mortality rates for AMI of approximately 3.5% per year over the past three decades. The decline in mortality in the elderly has been less impressive.[2] Evidence suggests that the reduction in mortality among elderly patients is largely due to decreased in-hospital mortality.[3] Further improvements in the diagnosis and management of elderly patients are indicated and should significantly improve outcomes.

Baseline characteristics

It is likely that improvements in the acute management and chronic stabilization of middle-aged patients with coronary heart disease (CHD) will result in a large increase in the elderly population. Pepine et al,[4] recently published an observational study of approximately 5000 outpatients with angina and known CHD. Their study sample was composed of 53% women with an average age of 71 years. The average age for men was 67 years. They found significantly more women with hypertension, diabetes and heart failure, while men had more myocardial infarctions and revascularization procedures. 62% of patients perceived their health to be either fair or poor, with the worst perception being in the 80+ years age group. The majority of patients also had more than one cardiovascular-associated illness other than angina, such as hypertension, congestive heart failure (CHF) and conduction disturbances. 25%

of the group noted angina that awakened them at night; over half of this group were women. 37% had mental-stress-related angina, again with over half being women. Rest pain occurred in 47% of subjects, again with a similar trend of a 17% excess of women in this group. Interestingly, although perception of health was associated with all types of angina (exertional, rest and mental-stress), there was a trend toward decreased prevalence of mental-stress angina as age increased. These data suggest that the current demographic profile of patients with angina frequently includes women, the elderly, patients with high rates of associated illness, and exertional, rest, and mental-stress-associated angina. This type of profile may partly contribute to the variability in determining prognosis in the elderly patient.

This variability was recently demonstrated in a study by Normand et al.[5] in which they attempted to develop a predictive model for mortality in a cohort of 14 501 elderly patients admitted with AMI, based on admission variables. Demographic data, comorbid conditions and severity variables related to the AMI were used as independent predictor variables. The most predictive model developed could only account for 27% of the total variability in predicting 30-day mortality. The authors proposed several reasons for the inability of their models to predict outcome. Part of the variability could be accounted for by differences in the types and frequencies of acute interventions among the various states analyzed. Hospital interventions accounted for only a small portion of the unexplained variability. Differences in quality of care, systematic differences in unobserved patient characteristics (unlikely as many variables were examined) or random error were cited as possible reasons for the persistent large unexplained variability. The 30-day mortality rate

for AMI in the elderly is approximately 20%.[6] Prediction of mortality is poorly understood, however. This inability to predict which elderly patients are most at risk for death compromises our ability to fully predict who will benefit most from treatment.

In a prospective study from the Myocardial Infarction Registry at the Massachusetts General Hospital, Paul et al[7] showed that hypertension, diabetes, congestive heart failure and non-Q-wave MI were more frequent in the elderly. Evidence has shown that these risk factors, along with age itself, contribute to increased mortality.[1,7] Elevated lipids have also been linked to mortality in the elderly.[8,9] Given the increase in comorbidities in the elderly, it is likely that the attributable risks of these factors for coronary disease are different from those in younger people. These differences further contribute to the dilemma of identifying which elderly patients are at increased risk of having an ischemic event. Furthermore, they demonstrate the problems of using classical risk factors to develop preventive guidelines for unstable coronary syndromes in the elderly.

Presentation

Typical angina is very common in the elderly population as a presenting symptom of myocardial ischemia. However, the proportion of patients with atypical symptoms increases with age. As many as 90% of elderly patients may present with symptoms other than classic angina.[10]

Many elderly people have limited physical activity which may mask exertional angina. Furthermore, ischemic pain may be misdiagnosed as esophageal reflux, joint pains, nonspecific weakness or vague neurological or abdominal symptoms. One major difference in the presentation of ischemia in the elderly is that dyspnea and worsening heart failure are more frequent manifestations than in younger patients. Seigel et al[11] reported on a group of elderly patients who had worsening congestive heart failure as their initial manifestation of CHD: 90% had a history of hypertension and the majority were diagnosed with multivessel coronary disease but with only moderately depressed left ventricular systolic function. The increased prevalence of left ventricular hypertrophy and diastolic dysfunction in this age group probably contributes to these findings. A study by Paul et al[7] examined symptom characteristics in 561 patients with AMI. The subset of patients over 75 years old had 20% more CHF and 23% less chest pain than the younger subset.

Another major difference in the presentation of CHD in the elderly is the increased prevalence of silent ischemia. Bruyne et al.[12] reported on 3272 patients with a documented MI. The prevalence of silent ischemia increased by 50% in men and by 300% in women as age increased from 65 years to 85 years and over. Theories of possible mechanisms for silent ischemia in the elderly include decreased pain perception, increased endorphins, autonomic dysfunction and increased collateral flow reducing the severity of angina. However, increased mortality in patients with silent ischemia has not been documented conclusively. Studies involving patients with stable angina and known CHD have shown mixed results for the predictive power of silent ischemia on both cardiovascular mortality and the composite endpoints of mortality and cardiovascular events.[12–14] Most studies have not included the very elderly; thus extension of results to this age group is not possible. Based on the available studies it can be concluded that silent ischemia increases with age but its effect on mortality is not conclusive.

The electrocardiogram can be very helpful in confirming AMI or a previous infarction in younger patients, yet analysis of its contribution in the elderly has provided interesting findings. Typical ECG changes of a previous MI may not be present. Reasons for this discrepancy are that ECG changes may resolve, the patient may never have had an MI, or an apparent MI occurred, possibly with atypical features, without coming to medical attention. The Rotterdam Study[12] examined ECG criteria for a previous MI and the degree of discrepancy between past history and ECG findings in 3272 elderly patients. They found that the prevalence of silent MI increased with age, being most common in the group over 85 (7.5% for men and 9.8% for women). For all age groups, silent MI was 2.45 times more common in women. Furthermore, the incidence of self-reported MI without ECG or other confirmatory evidence increased with age, and was maximum in the oldest subgroup (5.0% for men and 1.2% for women). These findings indicate that the elderly not only have an increased incidence of silent ischemia (infarct or angina) but that the incidence of a falsely reported MI also increases with age.

Preconditioning

An interesting topic related to silent ischemia, angina and myocardial infarction is that of preconditioning, and how it may influence mortality from a cardiac event. Preconditioning is a phenomenon whereby repeated brief periods of coronary artery occlusion are thought to protect the heart from ischemia and lead to less damage during an acute infarction. Preconditioning is thought to result in both smaller infarctions and less severe postinfarction complications. Murry et al,[15] in a canine model, showed that brief (5 minute) sequential coronary artery occlusions followed by a sustained 40-minute occlusion caused less myocardial necrosis on histological examination than a single 40-minute sustained occlusion. Although the exact mechanism of preconditioning is speculative, it appears to be related to activation of protein kinase C through a variety of stimuli. These include the opening of potassium-dependent channels[16,17] and activation of alpha-adrenergic receptors by norepinephrine.[18] Although studied extensively in the adult population (<65 years), preconditioning has only recently begun to be evaluated in the elderly, who may have decreased benefit from preconditioning. It is possible that the absence of anginal symptoms in this age group reflects a lack of preconditioning, thus explaining the higher mortality from an ischemic event.

Clinical studies have since shown that similar preconditioning may occur in humans. In a study of balloon angioplasty, Deutsch et al[19] reported that repetitive balloon inflations during percutaneous coronary angioplasty resulted in progressively less ST segment elevation and less angina during the procedure. Matsuda et al[20] reported that patients with an AMI due to an occluded proximal LAD artery who had pre-infarction angina had a higher postevent ejection fraction than those patients without angina. Kloner et al,[21] in a subanalysis of patients enrolled in the TIMI-4 trial (a randomized trial to compare the effectiveness of two thrombolytic agents), evaluated the influence of pre-infarction angina on hospital mortality. The average age of this patient sample was 58 years. In their logistic regression analysis, subjects with a history of angina within 48 hours of their AMI were less likely to suffer in-hospital mortality, congestive heart failure or cardiogenic shock after adjusting for thrombolytic therapy and demographic variables.[21]

There has been only one study to date that specifically addressed the existence of preconditioning in the elderly. Abete et al[22] recently reported results on 210 elderly (65 years or older) patients admitted with myocardial infarction. They also evaluated multiple outcomes of younger patients with an AMI, one of which was in-hospital mortality. It was shown that pre-infarction angina was an independent protective factor for in-hospital mortality in the younger but not in the older age group. In a logistic regression analysis adjusting for use of thrombolytic therapy, demographic variables and anti-anginal medications, age was the only factor significantly associated with death in the elderly. The authors concluded that the lack of a protective effect of previous angina in the elderly suggested a lack of preconditioning, and may in part account for the higher mortality of elderly patients with AMI. One difficulty in evaluating the role of preconditioning among the elderly is that they are known to have increased silent ischemia. Strictly speaking, if silent ischemia occurred just prior to an AMI, it should constitute preconditioning, thus making the lack of angina an inaccurate surrogate marker for lack of preconditioning. Further studies are needed to determine how these two entities may interact to possibly influence mortality in the elderly.

Therapy

Overall, thrombolytic therapy given within 6–12 hours (and in some cases longer) of infarct onset reduces myocardial infarction size and improves survival. Rich[23] pooled the results of five major thrombolytic trials and showed an absolute reduction in mortality of 3.5% in the elderly (age over 65) compared with 2.2% in the younger population. Furthermore, after adjusting for age, there is an absolute excess of stroke and other bleeding complications of less than 1%.[23] However, elderly patients are less likely to receive thrombolytics for AMI. Depending on the study, between 10 and 50%[24,25] of elderly are excluded from the therapy solely on the basis of age. A partial explanation is that age alone may be considered an absolute contraindication to such therapy by some investigators, but one must also consider the contribution of atypical presentation. Lack of anginal symptoms and atypical presentation of ischemia among the elderly have important therapeutic ramifications. The lack of recognition of angina or anginal equivalents among the elderly can influence post-event treatment.

The ISIS-2 trial showed that aspirin at the time of infarct reduced vascular death by 2.1% in 3411 patients over the age of 70 years.[26] Results of meta-analyses have shown a substantial mortality reduction in patients greater than 65 years old given early intravenous beta-blockade during AMI. The proportionate reduction in mortality was greatest in elderly patients in whom absolute contraindications to beta-blockers and aspirin were absent.[27] Despite the proven efficacy of aspirin and beta-blockers in the treatment of AMI in the elderly population, many do not receive either in a timely manner or at all. Support for this notion was provided in a recent retrospective study by the Cooperative Cardiovascular Project, which analyzed 10 018 elderly Medicaid patients admitted with AMI with no absolute contraindication to aspirin therapy.[28] They found that only 61% of these patients received the medication at the time of hospitalization. Furthermore, the use of aspirin was associated with a 22% reduction in 30-day mortality.[28] Importantly, those patients who presented with either no anginal symptoms or atypical angina, both of which are frequently encountered in the elderly, or those who were critically ill were much less likely to receive aspirin. Using the same cohort, the authors

further showed that of the 5490 patients discharged who were candidates for aspirin therapy, only 48% were eventually instructed to use aspirin. Patients who were older, had more comorbid conditions, or who were not given aspirin on admission were less likely to receive it upon discharge. Atypical presentation of ischemia in this age group has been shown to cause similar undesirable treatment trends for thrombolytic therapy and use of beta-blockers both during acute infarction and post-hospitalization.[25,29]

ACE inhibitors have also been shown to be beneficial after AMI in reducing both cardiovascular mortality and total mortality.[30,31] The Trandolapril Cardiac Evaluation study was performed in a group of post-MI patients with a mean age of 68. There was no age limitation in this study. Results revealed a 22% reduction in total mortality for those receiving ACE inhibitor therapy.[31] In another recently published observational study of heart failure patients in a community setting, age was found to be independently associated with lack of ACE inhibitor use, even in those with no absolute contraindications to their use.[32] This association was only partially explained by the increased prevalence of congestive heart failure caused by diastolic dysfunction and renal impairment in the older age group. Also, those without a documented ejection fraction or without cardiomegaly on chest X-ray were also less likely to receive ACE inhibitors for heart failure. It is possible that lack of awareness due to atypical presentations, as described earlier, may also contribute to lack of treatment in this situation. Atypical features in the elderly not only present a diagnostic challenge, but also greatly influence subsequent treatment and outcomes.

One very interesting study evaluated the treatment of AMI in two comparable population samples from Canada and the United

States, followed for 1 year post-MI.[33] The influence of cardiac interventions, both acute and post-MI, on 1-year mortality was evaluated. Coronary angiography was performed 5.2 times more frequently in the US compared with Canada, and revascularization procedures were 7.9 times more frequent in the US. Additionally, twice as many patients in the United States underwent the revascularization procedures within 30 days of infarct. Six months after the index AMI, the rate of revascularization in the US cohort was quadruple that in the Canadian cohort. There was a very small 30-day difference in mortality between the two cohorts, favoring the US (21.4% versus 22.3%). However, at 1 year the mortality rates were virtually identical at 34%. These results support those reported in the TIMI-3B elderly subgroup, showing that an early invasive strategy in the elderly is effective in improving short-term mortality.[34] The authors speculate that the lack of benefit in the United States cohort at 1 year is possibly due to less access to primary care, less use of prescription and non-prescription medications (such as beta-blockers and aspirin), and less access to long-term care which is universally provided to the elderly with minimal co-payments under the Canadian health-care system. These observations also underscore the need for broad and prolonged application of secondary prevention strategies among the elderly after acute myocardial infarction and the continued effort to identify patients with possibly atypical features who are at increased risk for subsequent cardiac events.

Evaluation of elderly patients

The evaluation of elderly patients thought to have angina is difficult. Atypical features and silent ischemia account for some of this difficulty. Also, the elderly are more likely to have left ventricular hypertrophy, conduction abnormalities and comorbidities[4] that may make the feasibility, interpretation, and clinical correlation of noninvasive testing difficult. An example is the use of exercise testing. According to the ACC/AHA guidelines for exercise testing, older age is not a contraindication to performing the test.[35] Pretest probability data for ischemic coronary artery disease is provided in the guidelines only to age 69 years. However, the prevalence of CHD is known to increase with age. The guidelines note that men and women 69 years of age with atypical/probable angina pectoris have an intermediate probability (10% to 90%) of CAD. The same intermediate probability is reported for those with nonanginal chest pain in this age group. The probability for those with classic angina in this elderly age group is higher (>90%). Thus, elderly patients with either atypical angina or symptoms thought not to be angina have the same pre-test probability of receiving a diagnosis of CHD by exercise testing. This adds to the difficulty of noninvasive testing in the elderly population. Diagnosis of those patients with classic angina is likely not to be influenced by noninvasive testing. However, testing is more helpful in those with unusual features of angina who are at intermediate risk of having CAD. Both atypical angina and symptoms regarded as nonanginal in nature increase with age and these two categories of patients have identical pretest probabilities for diagnosing CHD by exercise testing.

Non-Q-wave MI and angina

The occurrence of non-Q-wave MI increases with age, and hospital admissions for both non-Q-wave MI and unstable angina may be increasing at a faster rate than Q-wave MI.[4] Early mortality is greater for Q-wave MI but 1-year mortality rates for both Q-wave and non Q-wave MI are comparable. Smith et al[1] compared the outcome of AMI in patients over 75 years old to that of patients age 65–75 years. After discharge, cardiac mortality at 1 year was 17.6% for patients over 75 years and 12% for those aged 65–75% years. Although cardiac mortality was not statistically different between those with Q-wave and non-Q-wave MI, there was a trend towards higher mortality in the non-Q-wave elderly group compared to the younger group (15.7% versus 12.1%). Chung et al[36] followed two cohorts of patients under and over 70 years old admitted with a non-Q-wave MI. Mortality rate at 1 year was 29% in the elderly cohort compared with 14% in the younger group. Total mortality was also higher in the elderly group (36% versus 16%). Interestingly, the authors also found that the younger patients were more likely to receive beta-blockers, intravenous heparin and coronary intervention for non-Q-wave MI. This is further evidence that despite treatment advances for MI and angina, the elderly population may not be receiving the maximal treatment possible.

Current data suggest that an invasive strategy can be used in the elderly for the treatment of unstable angina and non-Q-wave MI. For a 6-month period the TIMI-3B investigators included 48 patients between the ages of 76 and 79 into their total population of 471 patients in a study of early invasive versus early conservative approaches for the treatment of unstable angina and non-Q-wave MI.[34] Results showed a higher composite end-point of death and AMI among elderly patients. However, there was a statistically significant difference in the composite endpoint of death and AMI between the early invasive and early conservative approaches (7.9% versus 14.8%). There was no such statistical difference in the younger group. Reports have shown that elderly patients, compared with younger patients, have a higher incidence of procedure-related complications during invasive cardiac procedures. Thompson et al studied 1750 elderly patients undergoing angioplasty at the Mayo Clinic between the years 1980 and 1990, and compared procedural success rates with a similar sample of subjects who had the procedure between 1990 and 1992. Success rate, when attempted angioplasty of total coronary occlusions was excluded, increased from 88% to 93%. Emergent bypass surgery decreased from 5.5% to 0.5% and procedure-related mortality decreased from 3.3% to 1.4%.[37] Coronary artery stenting was introduced in 1989 and only the later group had the opportunity to receive this therapy in a rescue fashion. This probably contributed to the difference in outcomes. There is also evidence that if the elderly can achieve complete revascularization, their age-adjusted cardiac mortality and angina-free period approaches that of younger patients.[38]

Conclusion

Coronary artery disease is prevalent in our aging population. It is safe to say that as age increases, the characteristics of unstable coronary syndromes become less typical. The diagnosis of an acute myocardial infarction in a middle-aged patient with classic symptoms and ECG changes is relatively straightforward. A heightened level of suspicion is needed for the elderly population because of the atypical presentation of coronary artery syndromes. Increased awareness and understanding of these characteristics will hopefully bring about increases in diagnosis and therapeutic interventions. The art of medicine implies that we be creative, inquisitive and persistent in our instincts above and beyond that dictated by facts and figures. This truly applies to the elderly population with regard to our efforts in recognizing and treating coronary heart disease.

References

1. Smith SC, Gilpin E, Ahnve S et al. Outlook after acute myocardial infarction in the very elderly compared with that in patients age 65 to 75 years. *J Am Coll Cardiol* (1990) **16**: 784–92.
2. Pepine CJ. Changing myocardial infarction population characteristics: reasons and implications. *Am Heart J* (1997) **134**:S1–4.
3. McGowan PG, Pankow JS, Shakar E et al. Minnesota Heart Survey. *N Engl J Med* (1996) **334**:884–90.
4. Pepine CJ, Abrams J, Marks RG et al. Characteristics of contemporary population with angina pectoris. *Am J Cardiol* (1994) **74**: 226–31.
5. Normand ST, Glickman ME, Sharma RG et al. Using admission criteria to predict short-term mortality from myocardial infarction in elderly patients: results from the Cooperative Cardiovascular Project. *JAMA* (1996) **275**:1322–8.
6. Udvarhelyi IS, Gatsonis C, Epstein AM et al. Acute myocardial infarction in the Medicare population. *JAMA* (1992) **268**:2530–6.
7. Paul SD, O'Gara PT, Mahjoub ZA et al. Geriatric patients with acute myocardial infarction: cardiac risk factor profiles, presentation, thrombolysis, coronary interventions, and prognosis. *Am Heart J* (1996) **131**:710–15.
8. Scandinavian Simvistatin Survival Study Writing Group. Randomized trial of cholesterol lowering in 4444 patients with coronary heart disease: The Scandinavian Simvistatin Survival Study (4S). *Lancet* (1994) **344**:1383–9.
9. Sacks FM, Pfeffer MA, Moye LA et al and the Cholesterol and Recurrent Events Trial Investigators. The effects of pravistatin on coronary events after myocardial infarction in patients with average cholesterol levels. *N Engl J Med* (1996) **335**:1001–9.
10. Gregoratos G. Clinical presentation of coronary artery disease in the elderly: how much does it differ from the younger population. *Am J Geriatr Cardiol* (1998) **7**:35–40.
11. Siegel R, Clemens T, Wingo M. Acute heart failure in the elderly: another manifestation of unstable angina. *J Am Coll Cardiol* (1991) **17**:149A.
12. Bruyne MC, Mosterd A, Hoes AW et al. Prevalence, determinants, and misclassification of myocardial infarction in the elderly. *Epidemiology* (1997) **8**:495–500.
13. Gandhi MM, Wood DA, Lampe FC. Characteristics and clinical significance of ambulatory myocardial ischemia in men and women in the general population presenting with angina pectoris. *J Am Coll Cardiol* (1994) **23**:74–80.
14. Quyyumi AA, Panza JA, Diodati JG et al. Prognostic implications of myocardial ischemia during daily life in low risk patients with coronary artery disease. *J Am Coll Cardiol* (1993) **21**:700–8.
15. Murry CE, Jennings RB, Reimer KA. Preconditioning with ischemia: a delay of lethal cell injury in ischemic myocardium. *Circulation* (1986) **74**:1124–36.
16. Hearse DJ. Activation of ATP-sensitive potassium channels; a novel pharmacological approach to myocardial protection. *Cardiovasc Res* (1995) **30**:1–17.
17. Cole WC, McPherson CD, Sontag D. ATP regulated K channels protect the myocardium against ischemic/reperfusion damage. *Circ Res* (1991) **69**:571–81.
18. Banerjee A, Lock-Winter C, Rogers KB et al. Preconditioning against myocardial dysfunction after ischemia and reperfusion by alpha-1 adrenergic mechanism. *Circ Res* (1993) **73**:656–70.
19. Deutsch E, Berger M, Kussmal WG et al. Adaptation to ischemia during percutaneous transluminal coronary angioplasty, clinical, hemodynamic, and metabolic features. *Circulation* (1990) **82**:2044–51.
20. Matsuda Y, Ogawa H, Moritani K et al. Effects of the presence or absence of preceding angina pectoris on left ventricular function after acute myocardial infarction. *Am Heart J* (1984) **108**:955–8.

21. Kloner RA, Shook T, Przyklen K et al. Previous angina alters in-hospital outcome in TIMI 4. A clinical correlate to preconditioning. *Circulation* (1995) **91**:37–47.

22. Abete P, Ferrara N, Cacciatore F et al. Angina-induced protection against myocardial infarction in adult and elderly patients: a loss of preconditioning mechanism in the aging heart? *J Am Coll Cardiol* (1997) **30**:947–54.

23. Rich MW. Acute myocardial infarction in the elderly. *Cardio* (1990) **7**:81.

24. Gottlieb S, Goldbourt U, Boyko V et al. Improved outcome of elderly patients (greater than or equal to 75 years of age) with acute myocardial infarction from 1981–1983 to 1992–1994 in Israel. *Circulation* (1997) **95**: 342–50.

25. Krumholz HM, Murillo JE, Chen J et al. Thrombolytic therapy for elderly patients with acute myocardial infarction. *JAMA* (1997) **277**:1683–8.

26. ISIS-2 Collaborative Group. Randomized trial of intravenous streptokinase, oral aspirin, both, or neither among 17 187 cases of suspected acute myocardial infarction: ISIS-2. *Lancet* (1988) **ii**:349–60.

27. Antman EM, Lay J, Kupelnick B et al. A comparison of results of meta-analyses of randomized control trials and recommendations of clinical experts: treatments for myocardial infarction. *JAMA* (1992) **268**:240–8.

28. Krumholz HM, Radford MJ, Ellerbeck EF et al. Aspirin in the treatment of acute myocardial infarction in elderly Medicare beneficiaries: patterns of use and outcomes. *Circulation* (1995) **92**:2841–7.

29. Soumerai SB, McLaughlin TJ, Spiegelman D et al. Adverse outcomes of under use of beta-blockers in elderly survivors of acute myocardial infarction. *JAMA* (1997) **277**:115–21.

30. Pfeffer MA, Braunwald E, Moye LA et al, on behalf of the SAVE Investigators. Effect of captopril on mortality and morbidity in patients with left ventricular dysfunction after myocardial infarction: results of Survival and Ventricular enlargement. *N Engl J Med* (1992) **327**:669–77.

31. Kober L, Torp-Pederson C, Carlsen JE et al. A clinical trial of the angiotensin-converting enzyme inhibitor trandolapril in patients with left ventricular dysfunction after myocardial infarction. *N Engl J Med* (1995) **333**:1670–6.

32. Tu JV, Pashos CL, Naylor CD et al. Use of cardiac procedures and outcomes in elderly patients with myocardial infarction in the United States. *N Engl J Med* (1997) **336**: 1500–5.

33. Philbin EF. Factors determining angiotensin-converting enzyme inhibitor under utilization in heart failure in a community setting. *Clin Cardiol* (1998) **21**:103–8.

34. The TIMI IIIB Investigators. Effects of tissue plasminogen activator and a comparison of early invasive and conservative strategies in unstable angina and non-Q-wave infarction. *Circulation* (1994) **89**:1545–56.

35. American College of Cardiology/American Heart Association. Guidelines for exercise testing. *J Am Coll Cardiol* (1997) **3**:260–315.

36. Chung MK, Bosner MS, McKenzie JP et al. Prognosis of patients ≥70 years of age with non-Q-wave infarction compared with younger patients with similar infarcts and with patients ≥70 years of age with Q-wave acute myocardial infarction. *Am J Cardiol* (1995) **75**: 18–22.

37. Thompson RC, Holmes DR, Grill DE et al. Changing outcomes of angioplasty in the elderly. *J Am Coll Cardiol* (1996) **27**:8–14.

38. tenBerg JM, Voors AA, Suttorp MJ et al. Long-term results after successful percutaneous transluminal coronary angioplasty in patients over 75 years of age. *Am J Cardiol* (1996) **77**:690–5.

14

Coronary angioplasty and other transcatheter revascularization procedures

Claudia F Gravina Taddei, William S Weintraub, Leslee Shaw and Andrzej S Kosinski

Introduction

The world population is aging. In the United States, in 1995, the population was 262 million, with 14 million over age 75 years. By the year 2000, this age group will have grown to 16 million, of which one-quarter will be older than 85 years.[1] The size of this oldest subset of the world population is increasing rapidly in industrialized nations and the fastest increasing group of older people is that aged 85 years and above.[2–5]

The leading disease in octogenarians is coronary heart disease, responsible for half of the deaths and one-quarter of the disabilities in this age group.[6,7] This disability leads to a decrease in the active life expectancy, that is the period of life in which one is able to take care of oneself and lead a relatively independent life.[8–10] The average life expectancy of a non-institutionalized elderly American aged 80–84 years is 7.5 years, and the active life expectancy is 5 years. For those aged 85 years and over, the life expectancy is 6 years, and the active life expectancy is 3 years.[11] A recent report shows that, for a 90 year old, the life expectancy for women is 5 years, and for men is 3 years, but the active life expectancy for both is 2 years.[8]

The ideal treatment in the octogenarian is the one that not only prolongs life expectancy, but one that, as a priority, prolongs active life expectancy. Several strategies can be used to control disability due to coronary artery disease in octogenarians, and one of these is percutaneous transluminal coronary angioplasty (PTCA).

PTCA was introduced by Andreas Gruentzig in 1977.[12] Initially, it was used for non-calcific lesions and single vessel disease in younger, symptomatic patients. Increased operator and institutional experience and improvements in technical equipment resulted in progressively increased use in more complex lesions and in elderly patients.[13,14] Several studies showed that it could be used in patients 65 years of age and older with similar results to those in the younger population.[15–17] In fact, most individuals aged 65–74 years have results that are more similar to the younger population than to those who are older than 75.[18]

Compared with younger patients, there are few data regarding the use of angioplasty in the oldest subset, the octogenarian and beyond, for several reasons. First, there is a systematic exclusion of aged patients, particularly octogenarians, from clinical trials of all types.[19] Second, the first choice for treatment of coronary disease at this age is often medical therapy.[15] Nevertheless, medical therapy is not always able to control anginal symptoms in a severely symptomatic older patient, as shown in a report of 1-year survival of octogenarians with unstable angina treated conservatively.[20] The 1-year overall survival for medical treatment was 82%, the cardiac survival was 89%, but the event free survival decreased to 55%, with many patients remaining symptomatic, and a high rate of repeated hospitalizations. An analysis of mortality of coronary heart disease in Medicare patients treated medically, interventionally and surgically revealed a 30-day mortality expressed as death/1000 discharges, of 245.1 (24.5%) in the patients aged 85 years and over treated medically.[21]

Moreover, it can be difficult to manage an aged patient who cannot easily tolerate several antianginal medications. Therefore, the difficulty in controlling symptoms, associated with the consideration of the impact of coronary bypass surgery in the octogenarian, coupled with the generally successful outcome of PTCA in younger patients, has resulted in physicians becoming more aggressive in the use of PTCA in the octogenarian and older with severe angina, when the coronary lesions are suitable for PTCA.

In recent years, the use of angioplasty has expanded in very old patients. Data on PTCA use in 20 006 Medicare patients over the age of 80 in the United States showed that between 1987 and 1990 the number of angioplasties in this age group more than doubled.[22]

PTCA in symptomatic coronary artery disease

Fourteen studies concerning coronary angioplasty in a total of 1427 patients with a mean age of 75–92 years, published since 1989, are reviewed.[23–25] Ten studies were carried out in the United States, and one each in Brazil,[27] Italy,[30] Holland,[32] and Israel.[34]

The number and clinical characteristics of the patients are summarized in Table 14.1,

and show the severity of coronary heart disease in this population. There was a high prevalence of class III-IV angina, reaching 100% in some studies.[24,33] Unstable angina varied from 33 to 80%[27,28] and previous myocardial infarction from 21 to 72%[27,30] among the patients who underwent PTCA. Congestive heart failure was present in 19 to 43%[27,28] and previous coronary artery bypass grafting in 8 to 28% of the patients in different series.[31,25]

Table 14.2 shows the angiographic success rates and major in-hospital complications: death, myocardial infarction (MI), and coronary artery bypass graft surgery (CABG). The procedural success rate in aged patients has increased significantly since the initial reports, showing an angiographic success rate of about 90%, comparable to the rates in younger patients.[36] One study in patients aged 90–95 years showed an angiographic success rate of 92%.[35] There was great variation of the percentage of major complications, probably related to differences in patient selection, severity of the disease, and the relatively small numbers of patients in 10 of 14 studies. The procedure-related deaths ranged from zero to 23%.[24,35] The myocardial infarction rate (MI) varied from zero to 19%,[30,35] and the need for emergency coronary artery bypass surgery (CABG), from zero to 10%.[24,29] The patients who consistently showed high mortality and major myocardial infarction were the group over 90 years. This suggests that, despite the high angiographic success rate, the nonagenarians have higher complication rates.

Table 14.3 shows the mean follow-up of patients in the various series, which ranged from 6 to 36 months. One-year survival varied from 76 to 98%,[6,34] except in the group of 90 years and older, which had a 1-year survival of 59%.[35] The freedom from death, myocardial infarction, and coronary bypass surgery

Table 14.1
Characteristics of aged patients who underwent PTCA

Author	Number	Mean Age (years)	Male (%)	Angina III–IV (%)	Unstable angina (%)	Previous MI (%)	CHF (%)	Previous CABG (%)	Previous PTCA (%)	Three-vessel disease (%)
Imburgia et al[23]	43	79	42	86						
Rich et al[24]	22	82		100		56				
Jeroudi et al[25]	54	82	54	91	59	48		28		
Rizo-Patron et al[26]	53	83	58	19	64	26		25		
Sousa et al[27]	452	75	70		33	21	19			
*Thompson et al[28]	193	79	56	65	80	52	43	12		
Jackman et al[29]	31	82	42		55	68				10
Maiello et al[30]	47	77	60	98		72				44
†Forman et al[31]	67	≥80	39		73	59	42	8		
ten Berg et al[32]	212	78	59	88		45		13	15	
Santana et al[33]	53	84	36	100		55	21	6	6	51
Little et al[6]	118	83	43	87		25				
Shapira et al[34]	56	77	84	93		63				34
Weyrens et al[35]	26	92	50		77	46	23			

* Group ≥75 years.
† Group ≥80 years.

Author	Angiographic success (%)	Major complications (%)		
		Death	MI	CABG
Imburgia et al[23]	68	6	14	8
Rich et al[24]	89	0	14	0
Jeroudi et al[25]	93	4	4	0
Rizo-Patron et al[26]	83	2	5.5	7.5
Sousa et al[27]	90	1	2	1
*Thompson et al[28]	93	6	7	3
**Jackman et al[29]	90	6.5	7	10
Maiello et al[30]	93	8.5	0	2
†Forman et al[31]	84	6	5	2
ten Berg et al[32]	91	2	3	1
Santana et al[33]	83	15	4	0
Little et al[6]	89	2	1	1
Shapira et al[34]	91	2	2	0
Weyrens et al[35]	92	23	19	0

* Group ≥75 years.
**One patient died after MI, and the other after CABG
 † Group ≥80 years.

Table 14.2
Procedural results of PTCA in the aged

ranged from 63 to 87%.[6,26] In addition recurrent angina was noted in some series. In one study freedom from death, MI, CABG and angina was 58% in the first year, decreasing to 36% in the third year.[28] Differences in patient characteristics and in the use of repeated procedures may be responsible for much of the variation in outcome.

A meta-analysis of univariable outcome assessment in the 14 published reports is detailed in Figures 14.1–14.4. This analysis includes the use of averaged outcomes rates, weighted by the proportional sample size. The summary odds ratio is an empirical Bayes random-effects model that incorporates a wider range of uncertainty about the outcome of interest. This analysis assumes that other factors are affecting outcomes that are uncontrolled in this analysis. A chi-square test for heterogeneity was calculated for each of the individual outcomes. A statistically significant chi-square statistic indicates that the included reports are not homogeneous. Annual rates include events occurring from hospital discharge to an annualized event rate.

For Figure 14.1, the procedural and annual cardiac death rates (±95% confidence intervals) are reported. The reports are ordered by

Author	Number	Mean follow-up (months)	Survival (%)	MI (%)	CABG (%)	Angina (%)	Repeat PTCA (%)	Restenosis (%)	Event free from death, MI, CABG
Imburgia et al[23]	26	15	88		7.7		15		26% (Death/CABG/repeat PTCA)
Rich et al[24]	22	11	91 1 year 87%	0	4.5	4.5			86% 1 year: 81%
Jeroudi et al[25]	55	19	3 year: 80%				34.5	20	3 years: 78% 1 year: 87%
Rizo-Patron et al[26]	40	14	97.5						subsequent 2 years: 75%
Sousa et al[27]	349	24	92	0.6	9	29	11	19	70,5% (Death/MI/CABG/angina) Free of MI/CABG 1 year: 83%
*Thompson et al[28]		24	5 years > 75					17	Free of angina/CABG/MI 1 year: 58%
Jackman et al[29]	31	16	1 year 90%					31	1 year: 84% Free of death/MI/CABG/re-PTCA
Maiello et al[30]	35	14	94	3	6		6		94%
†Forman et al[31]	34	36	82	3	6				
ten Berg et al[32]	181	6	7 years 69 1 year 76	2	3		5.5		Freedom of angina 7 years: 26% 1 year: 63%
Little et al[6]	110	18	3 years 61						3 years: 52%
Shapira et al[34]	51	21	98		4		18		Asymptomatic 43% Freedom from further intervention
Weyrens et al[35]	17	12	59		6		12	18	with mild or moderate symptoms: 41%

* Group ≥75 years.
† Group ≥80 years.

Table 14.3
Late results of PTCA in the aged

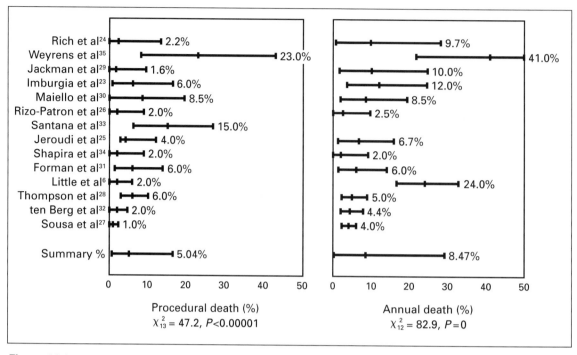

Figure 14.1
Procedural and late cardiac death rates in patients with mean age of 75–92 years undergoing PTCA. Authors are listed incrementally by sample size. Weighted average (by the sample size) death rate. The summary % death is the empirical Bayes random-effects model.

the sample sizes ranging from 22 to 452 patients. In general, the outcome rates decrease and the 95% confidence intervals become more precise and narrow with increasing sample size. The summary procedural and annual rates of death are 5.0 and 8.5%. The procedural and annual rates of myocardial infarction (±95% confidence intervals) are reported in Figure 14.2. Procedural rates of myocardial infarction range from 2–19% (summary rate = 5.6%) with lower rates occurring more often in larger patient populations (i.e. >175 patients, rates ranged from 2 to 3%). Annual rates (from discharge for-

ward) of myocardial infarction ranged from 0.3 to 2.3% with an average of 1.2%. For procedural and annual rates of CABG in the PTCA population (Figure 14.3), the summary rates are 2.8% (range = 1–10%) and 4.3% (range = 2.0–7.6%). Finally, Figure 14.4 details the summary procedural and annual outcomes rates for patients with mean age varying from 75 to 92 years. Annual rates of recurrent angina, repeat PTCA and restenosis were 4.3%, 14.2%, and 11.7%, respectively.

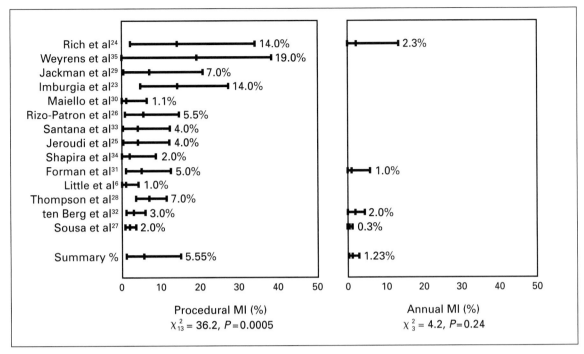

Figure 14.2
Procedural and late myocardial infarction rates in patients with mean age of 75–92 years undergoing PTCA. Authors are listed incrementally by sample size. Late MI reflects past-discharge rates. Weighted average (by the sample size) death rate. The summary % death is the empirical Bayes random-effects model.

Emory University experience with elective PTCA in octogenarians

At the Emory University Hospital, 15 360 coronary angioplasty were performed in 11 846 patients between January 1990 and December 1996. Octogenarians and older patients represented 4% of this total (478 patients and 625 procedures). The great majority of the PCTAs performed in these patients was with balloon angioplasty (80.3% of the procedures). New devices including stent, atherectomy and laser were responsible for the interventional treatment of coronary heart disease in a small proportion of very aged patients (19.7% of the procedures).

The proportion of procedures in octogenarians gradually increased from 2.1% of all angioplasties performed in 1990, to 5.7% in 1996 (Figure 14.5). The mean age of these elderly patients was 82.6 ± 2.7 years, and 48% were male. Hypertension was the most frequent risk factor, occurring in 55%, followed by hyperlipidemia in 35% of the patients. Diabetes was noted in 19%, obesity in 4% and smoking in 3% (past smoking in 33%). Ejection fraction no more than 40% was present in 20%.

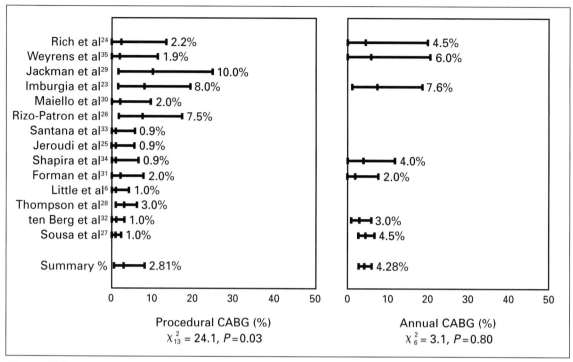

Figure 14.3
Procedural and late coronary artery bypass graft surgery rates in patients with mean age of 75–92 years undergoing PTCA. Authors are listed incrementally by sample size. Late CABG reflects past-discharge rates. Weighted average (by the sample size) death rate. The summary % death is the empirical Bayes random-effects model.

Angina class 0 was present in 7%, angina class I–II in 9%, and class III–IV in the great majority of the patients (84%). Congestive heart failure class III–IV occurred in 8%. Single-vessel disease was noted in 36%, two-vessel disease in 31% and three-vessel disease in 33%. Previous myocardial infarction was noted in half of the patients (52.4%), previous PTCA in 33% of the procedures, and previous coronary bypass surgery in 23% of the patients. PTCA was performed in one vessel in 89% of the aged patients, in two vessels in 10%, and in three vessels in just 0.5% (three patients). It was per-

formed in the left main coronary artery in 0.5% (three patients).

The procedural success rate between 1990 and 1996 for all angioplasties performed at Emory University Hospitals, and specifically in the angioplasties performed in octogenarians, is shown in Figure 14.6. The mean procedural success rate for all angioplasties was 93.5%, and the mean procedural success rate in the procedures performed in the octogenarians was quite similar at 91.9%. These results corroborate the results of the studies mentioned above, with a high angiographic success rate in the procedures in the aged.

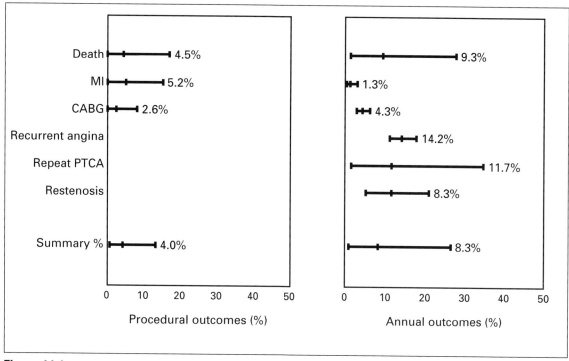

Figure 14.4
Procedural and late complications in patients with mean age of 75–92 years undergoing PTCA. Authors are listed incrementally (by sample size) death rate. The summary % death is the empirical Bayes random-effects model.

The major in-hospital complications that occurred among the octogenarians in the period analyzed were death in 2.7%, myocardial infarction in 1.5% and emergency coronary bypass surgery in 2.1%. These results are also similar to those found in other studies,[6,27,32,34] and to those of the 1985–1986 NHLBI PTCA Registry: death, 1.6%, myocardial infarction, 5.5%, CABG, 4.4%.[37] Dissection during the procedure occurred in 8% of the patients corresponding to 6.4% of the procedures.

The mean time to follow-up was 2.4 ± 1.9 years. Figure 14.7 shows the Kaplan–Meier survival curve, the event-free from death, MI, CABG curve, and the event-free from death, MI, CABG and angina curve in the period analyzed. Figure 14.8 displays survival percentages. For the first year, the survival rate was 89.3%, the event-free rate from death, MI and CABG was 86%, and the event-free rate from death, MI, CABG, and PTCA was 73.7%. At the end of the second year, the survival rate was 82.0%, the survival rate free from death, MI and CABG was 74.8%, and the event-free rate from death, MI, CABG and PTCA was 62.6%. During third, fourth, fifth

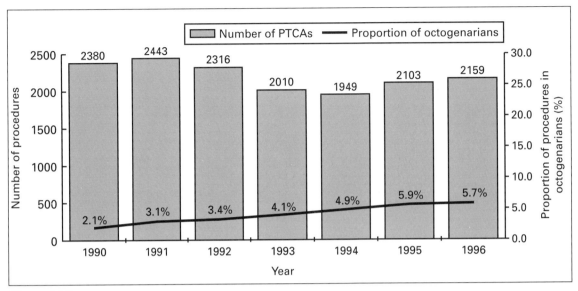

Figure 14.5
Number of angioplasties at Emory University and proportion of procedures in octogenarians for 1990–96.

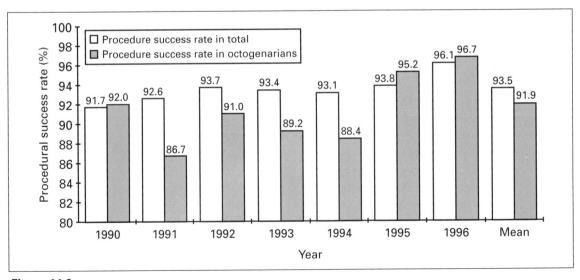

Figure 14.6
Percentage of procedural success rate of all angioplasties compared with angioplasties in octogenarians from 1990–96.

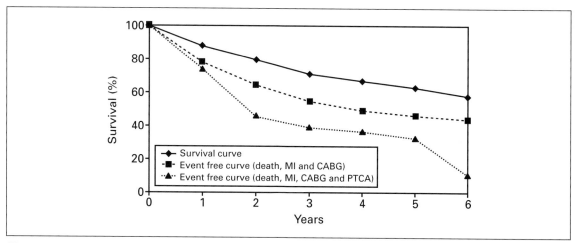

Figure 14.7
Kaplan–Meier survival curves in octogenarians post-PTCA.

and sixth years, there were continuing events.

The results of the last 7 years of Emory experience with PTCA in symptomatic octogenarians show a high angiographic success rate, a low in-hospital complication rate and a reasonable survival. It is important to mention that the 5-year survival in the United States in 1987 for all persons aged 80–85 years was

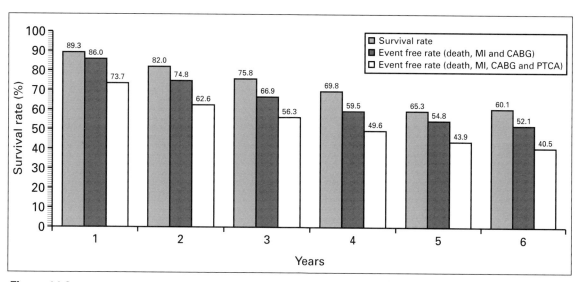

Figure 14.8
Percentage of survival rate, event free rate from death, MI, CABG, and event free rate from death, MI, CABG, PTCA in octogenarians who underwent angioplasty from 1990–96.

66%,[38,39] close to the 65% found in the Emory experience in cardiac octogenarians undergoing angioplasty. When, in addition to the evaluation of death, MI and CABG, the evaluation of repeat PTCA was included, the event-free survival was not so favorable after the first year, probably reflecting recurrent angina. Angina can be related to restenosis, to progression of the disease, or to incomplete revascularization. Restenosis occurs most frequently in the first 6 months after angioplasty. The rate of restenosis in the aged may not be precisely known, as angiographic restudy is generally performed only in symptomatic patients. In the series analyzed, it ranged from 17 to 31%, in the symptomatic patients undergoing restudy.[28,29] Several strategies, such as intracoronary stents, may decrease late stenosis, and the experience with their use in octogenarians is beginning. In any case, repeat angioplasty should not be excluded in the elderly because of age alone, and some authors recommend its use up to three times if necessary, before abandoning further attempts at PTCA.[40]

Completeness of revascularization has been associated with improved long-term survival and event-free survival in the surgical series.[41] In relation to angioplasty, recent studies show that late outcome is more influenced by the patient characteristics than the degree of revascularization.[42–44] Nevertheless, these results have to be confirmed by long-term prospective studies.

These data about survival and event-free survival must be analyzed with consideration of the patient's perceptions about his/her disease. In a study of late outcomes and quality of life, Little and colleagues[6] found an overall survival of 76% at 1 year, 73% at 2 years and 61% at three years. Event-free survival was 63% at 1 year, 58% at 2 years and 52% at 3 years. Outcomes were similar for men and women. Prior to the PTCA, 87% of the octogenarians had unstable angina. Among the survivors, 88% indicated they would be willing to undergo PTCA again if needed, 90% appreciated the benefits of PTCA, 66% continued to live independently, 55% could drive an automobile, and 38% were capable of taking care of a spouse.

The results of the Emory experience with PTCA in octogenarians and older are complemented by information from the EAST trial (Emory Angioplasty versus Surgery Trial), which included a small subset of aged patients, presented next.

PTCA versus CABG in octogenarians: East Trial

There are few studies comparing CABG with PTCA in octogenarians,[45–47] and they are retrospective. In one prospective, randomized trial, with 3 years of follow-up, that compared the clinical outcomes of coronary angioplasty and coronary bypass surgery in patients with multivessel disease,[48,49] there is a small subset of patients aged 75–81 years old, the Emory Angioplasty versus Surgery Trial (EAST). The final results in a population with mean age of 62 years showed that the two procedures had equivalent 3-year outcomes with respect to survival, myocardial infarction and major myocardial ischemia.[50] The study also revealed that revascularization was more complete with surgery than angioplasty at 1 and 3 years, but this fact became less significant when the severity of the residual stenosis and the physiological priority of the lesion were analyzed.[51] The initial advantage of lower costs for PTCA lost its importance, because costs with repeated procedures are similar to CABG costs. Finally, in relation to quality of life, more patients who underwent angioplasty had angina, but they were also more optimistic about their health

Clinical characteristics	CABG group	PTCA group
Number	18	18
Mean age ± SD	77.1 ± 1.8	76.8 ± 1.6
Male (%)	38.9	55.6
Number of vessels (%)		
Two	55.6	61.1
Three	44.4	38.9
Number of lesions per patient	3.3 ± 1.2	3.6 ± 1.1
Ejection fraction	60.6 ± 9.8	60.1 ± 12.4
Prior MI (%)	44.4	33.3
Congestive heart failure (%)	5.6	0
Angina (%)		
CCS class I–II	11.2	0
CCS class III–IV	88.8	100
Diabetes mellitus (%)	11.1	50.0
Hypertension (%)	55.6	77.8

Table 14.4
Clinical characteristics of the oldest subset of EAST trial

than the patients who underwent CABG surgery.[52]

The elderly subset of the EAST trial represented 9.2% of the total, comprising 36 patients.[49] The clinical characteristics of the patients randomized to CABG and PTCA are summarized in Table 14.4. They are quite similar, except for diabetes, hypertension and male gender being more prevalent in the PTCA group. Table 14.5 shows the angiographic success rates and in-hospital complications of the two groups. One CABG patient who received PTCA instead of CABG was excluded. Table 14.6 shows the 3-year outcomes. The survival after a follow-up of 3-years in the CABG group was 100%. The survival in the PTCA group was 77.8%. Death in the PTCA group occurred in four patients: the first patient who died had an MI after the PTCA, had CABG surgery and died on the sixth day, during the in-hospital period. The second patient died at 23.9 months, because of a noncardiac cause (urosepsis). The third patient died at 33.9 months of a cerebrovascular accident. The fourth died at 34.8 months of a probable MI.

Quality of life was measured by the patient's subjective responses concerning daily activity level, and was available in 14 patients in the PTCA group, and in 17 patients in the CABG group. In the PTCA group, 10 patients (71%) had a sedentary/mild activity level, and four (29%) had a moderate/strenuous activity level. In the CABG group, 16 patients (94%) had a sedentary/mild activity level, and one patient (6%) had a moderate/strenuous activity level ($P = 0.148$).

Although the small size of the sample limits comparison between these two procedures, the fact that it was a prospective, randomized

	CABG group	PTCA group
Angiographic success	94.1	In all segments attempted: 83.3%
		At least one segment attempted: 94.4%
In-hospital complications (%)		
Death	0.0	*5.6
Q wave MI	11.1	*5.6
CABG	—	*5.6
Thoracotomy for bleeding	5.6	—
Stroke	5.6	0

* Same patient

Table 14.5
Angiographic success and in-hospital complication of the oldest subset of the EAST trial

	CABG group	PTCA group
Survival (%)	100	78
Events (%)		
Q-wave MI	25.0	15.4
Subsequent PTCA	16.7	38.9
Subsequent CABG	0.0	11.1
Angina class II, III, IV	12	29

Table 14.6
Three-year outcome of the oldest subset of the EAST trial

study offers insight into this growing segment of the population. Two patterns can be identified. The CABG group had more serious in-hospital events (two myocardial infarctions, one stroke, and one thoracotomy for bleeding), and a better subsequent course with a high survival rate, and fewer events at follow-up (four myocardial infarctions and three angioplasties). The PTCA group had fewer in-hospital events (one patient had a myocardial infarction, went to CABG, and died), and more subsequent events at follow-up (two myocardial infarctions, seven angioplasties and two CABGs).

The decision to take an octogenarian or older to coronary bypass surgery must be preceded by a careful evaluation of the general physical and cognitive status and severity of the comorbid illness. The perceptions of the aged patient about surgery and hospitalization are crucial, and responsibility for the final decision must lie with the patient. The in-hospital mortality is high, ranging from 9 to 16%.[38,53–58] The postoperative complications are frequent, the length of hospitalization is increased compared with younger patients, and stroke and neurophysiological disturbance are more prevalent in the aged.[59] It can be emotionally difficult for a very old patient to cope with the pain and discomfort of a thoracotomy, the isolation and the noise of equipment in an intensive care unit, the fear of being separated from family for several days, and prolonged dependence during the period of recuperation. But, for the aged patient who decides to undergo surgery and who has success, the quality of life is excellent, with an absence of angina in 82% of the octogenarians at an average of 35 ± 22 months after surgery,[38] and a 5-year survival of 62%,[38] comparable to the survival of the 80–85 year old population of the United States already mentioned (66%). It is also comparable with the 5-year survival of 65%, found in Emory experience with PTCA in octogenarians.

Emergency PTCA post acute myocardial infarction

Acute myocardial infarction in the aged is associated with an increased risk of in-hospital death and a shorter life expectancy after survival estimated at 2.7 years for an 80 year old patient.[60] In the Worcester Heart Attack Study, the in-hospital mortality increased from 16.1% in patients of 65–74 years, to 32.1% in those of 75 years or older.[61] Smith and colleagues found in-hospital cardiac death for patients over 75 years old of 19.9%, compared with 12.2% for patients between 65–75 years.[62] Naylor and colleagues, in a study carried out in Ontario to determine population-based trends in hospital patient fatality from acute myocardial infarction, found mortality rates in the octogenarian of 43.0% in 1981, and 35.9% in 1991.[63]

Although the mortality associated with medical treatment in the aged with acute myocardial infarction is high, there are few reports about more aggressive approaches to attempt to change this situation. Laster and colleagues analyzed retrospectively the acute and long-term results of emergency PTCA in 55 consecutive postmyocardial infarction patients, aged 80–89 years.[64] Ejection fraction less than 40% was noted in 40%, and cardiogenic shock in 11%. The myocardial infarction was anterior in 49% and inferior in 51%. PTCA was successful in 96%. Urgent repeat PTCA of the infarct-related vessel was needed in 11%. While no urgent coronary bypass surgery was necessary, one elective coronary bypass surgery occurred during the hospitalization. The in-hospital mortality was 16%, including 4 of 6 (67%) in patients with cardiogenic shock and 5 of 49 (10%) in patients without cardiogenic shock. Cardiogenic shock was an independent predictor of in-hospital mortality. One-year survival was 67%, and freedom from death and myocardial infarction was 65%. At a follow-up of 25 ± 4 months, 64% were alive, with angina class I–II in 77% (27 patients) and III–IV in 23% (8 patients).

During the period from 1990 to 1996, emergency PTCA was performed in 15 octogenarians post-acute MI at the Emory University

Hospital corresponding to 20 procedures. The mean age was 83.2 ± 3.9, ranging from 80 to 95 years. The gender distribution was 53% male. Prior PTCA had been performed in 20% of the procedures, and prior CABG in 27% of the patients. Ejection fraction was available in 11 patients, and was less than or equal to 40% in 36%. Angiographic success was achieved in 85% of the procedures corresponding to 87% of the patients. The in-hospital mortality was 20% (three patients). No patient underwent in-hospital CABG and two patients (13%) underwent repeated PTCA. The Kaplan–Meier survival rate after 1 year was 76.9%. Freedom from death, MI or CABG was 66.7% after 1 year. Freedom from death, MI, CABG and PTCA was 58.3% after one year.

These two analyses, although not randomized, suggest a reduction in the high in-hospital mortality rate with more aggressive treatment. The high in-hospital mortality rate is probably related to severe comorbidity, multivessel coronary disease, and perhaps less aggressive treatment in this population.[65] The procedural success rate varied from 85 to 96% and the in-hospital mortality ranged from 16 to 20% in severely compromised patients. The 1-year survival free of death and MI was 65% in one series, and the survival free of death, MI, CABG was 66.7% in the other.

Intracoronary stents

Of the new devices used to perform PTCA in the octogenarian and above in the Emory University Hospitals during the period 1990–1996, the most commonly used was an intracoronary stent, placed in 11% of the total procedures. Rotational atherectomy (rotoblator) was used in 3.8% of the procedures, directional atherectomy in 2.7%, laser in 1.8%, and extraction atherectomy in 0.3% of the procedures.

Stents were placed during this period in 43 elderly patients, ranging from 80 years old to a centenarian and corresponding to 69 procedures in this age group. The mean age was 82.8 ± 3.6, and 56% were male. Prior PTCA had been performed in 42% of the procedures, and prior CABG in 35% of the patients. The procedure was angiographically successful in almost all patients, failing in just one patient (98%) and corresponding to 98.5% of success at the procedures. In-hospital death occurred in 4.8% (two patients), and in-hospital CABG in 2.3% (one patient). No one had in-hospital MI or stroke.

The Kaplan–Meier survival rate curve was 90.2% in the first year, decreasing to 72.4% in the second year. Freedom from death, MI and CABG was 81.1% in the first year, 62.0% in the second year. Freedom from death, MI, CABG, and PTCA was 62.9% at 1 year, 44.4% at 2 years.

It is interesting that the 100 year old patient had a successful combined procedure, with the use of rotablator and stent, and a reduction of a 71% stenosis of the proximal right coronary artery to 2% stenosis after the procedures. After almost 4 months, in 1997, he underwent another interventional procedure and died.

The New Approaches to Coronary Interventions (NACI) Registry, in a comparison between patients aged less than 70 years and a small group older than 70, showed that the use of a Palmaz–Schatz stent had a deployment success rate comparable in both groups, but the frequency of complications was higher in the elderly, particularly vascular complications.[66] Fishman studied the acute and long-term results of coronary stents and atherectomy in women and elderly of less than and older than 70 years. He concluded that both can be performed successfully, and that, although they have no risk of major complications, the risk of other complications (in particular non-Q-wave myocardial infarction and vascular complications), was increased.[67] Suilen and colleagues recently reported coronary stenting following failed balloon angioplasty in a small group (18 patients) of selected octogenarians, and reported successful results, with complication rates similar to the younger patients.[68]

The experience with stents in the octogenarian is just beginning. As it increases, the benefits and complications will be more precise. For now, it offers an excellent option of a procedure other than emergency coronary bypass surgery for the octogenarian who has an abrupt vessel closure after PTCA.

Conclusions

Octogenarians and older patients make up a heterogeneous group, where more than in any other group, the chronological age does not necessarily reflect the biological age. The medical care must be highly individualized, and should consider the biological age, the functional capacity, comorbidity, way of living and expectations of the patient about his/her life. This demands close physician–patient relationship, up-to-date scientific knowledge and mature clinical judgement.

Percutaneous transluminal coronary angioplasty provides an effective way to handle some of the disabilities caused by coronary heart disease, and perhaps to improve survival and quality of life, without submitting the very elderly patient to the stress of coronary bypass surgery, followed by a long convalescence. In no other age group is quality of life so relatively valued compared to survival, probably because, after a long life, the worst fear is not of death, but of dependence, of pain and apprehension over becoming a burden to others. High-quality medical care of the octogenarian and older patient must have as a main goal the preservation of an autonomous life, with dignity and self-respect.

References

1. US Bureau of the Census. Statistical Abstract of the United States: 1996 (116th edn). Washington, DC, 1996.
2. Wenger NK. Cardiovascular disease in the elderly. *Curr Probl Cardiol* (1992) **17**:615–90.
3. Williams T. Demographics of aging. *Cardiovasc Clin* (1992) **22**:3–7.
4. Stason W, Sanders C, Smith H. Cardiovascular care of the elderly: economic considerations. *J Am Coll Cardiol* (1987) **10**:18–21A.
5. Shapira I, Pines A, Fisman E, Drory Y. Percutaneous transluminal coronary angioplasty in the elderly. *Cardiol Elder* (1996) **4**:119–24.
6. Little T, Milner M, Lee K et al. Late outcome and quality of life following percutaneous transluminal coronary angioplasty in octogenarians. *Cathet Cardiovasc Diagn* (1993) **29**:261–6.
7. Little T, Lindsay J. Percutaneous transluminal coronary angioplasty and coronary artery bypass graft surgery in octogenarians: indications and outcome. *Heart Dis Stroke* (1994) **3**:261–5.
8. Crimmins E, Hayward M, Saito Y. Differentials in active life expectancy in the older population of the United States. *J Gerontol* (1996) **51**(Suppl B):S111–20.
9. Branch L, Guralnik J, Foley D et al. Active life expectancy for 10 000 caucasian men and women in three communities. *J Gerontol* (1991) **46**(Suppl A):M145–50.
10. Tsuji I, Minami Y, Fukao A, et al. Active life expectancy among elderly Japanese. *J Gerontol* (1995) **50**:M173–6
11. Katz S, Branch L, Branson M et al. Active life expectancy. *N Engl J Med* (1983) **309**:1218–24.
12. Grüntzig A. Transluminal dilatation of coronary-artery stenosis. *Lancet* (1978) **i**:263.
13. Sousa JE, Sousa AG, Feres F. Percutaneous transluminal coronary angioplasty: indications and results. *Arq Bras Cardiol* (1988) **51**:69–76.
14. Sousa AG, Sousa JE. Percutaneous transluminal coronary angioplasty and coronary artery bypass graft surgery: partners or opponents? *Rev Assoc Med Bras* (1993) **39**:63–4.
15. Mills T, Smith H, Vlietstra R. PTCA in the elderly: results and expectations. *Geriatrics* (1989) **44**:71–9.
16. Voudris V, Antonellis G, Salachas A et al. Coronary angioplasty in the elderly: immediate and long-term results. *Angiology* (1993) **44**:933–7.
17. Le Feuvre C, Bonan R, de Guise P et al. Long-term medical care after multivessel percutaneous transluminal coronary angioplasty in older patients: comparison with younger subjects. *Cardiol Elder* (1996) **4**:45–9.
18. Wenger N. Aging in the Americas: its impact on cardiovascular health. *Clin Cardiol* (1992) **15**:627–9.
19. Gurwitz J, Col N, Avorn J. The exclusion of the elderly and women from clinical trials in acute myocardial infarction. *JAMA* (1992) **268**:1417–22.
20. Meadaa R, John B, Little T. One year survival of octogenarians with unstable angina treated conservatively. *Clin Res* (1992) **40**:254A.
21. Little T. Mortality of ischemic heart disease in Medicare patients treated medically, interventionally and surgically after cardiac catheterization. *Clin Res* (1992) **40**:254A.
22. Jollis J, Peterson E, Bebchuk J et al. Coronary angioplasty in 20 006 patients over age 80 in the United States. *J Am Coll Cardiol* (1995) **26**(Suppl 1):47A.
23. Imburgia M, King T, Soffer A et al. Early results and long-term outcome of percutaneous transluminal coronary angioplasty in patients aged 75 years or older. *Am J Cardiol* (1989) **63**:1127–9.
24. Rich J, Crispino C, Saporito J et al. Percutaneous transluminal coronary angioplasty in patients 80 years of age and older. *Am J Cardiol* (1990) **65**:675–6.
25. Jeroudi M, Kleiman N, Minor S et al. Percutaneous transluminal coronary angioplasty in octogenarians. *Ann Intern Med* (1990) **113**:423–8.

26. Rizo-Patron C, Hamad N, Paulus R et al. Percutaneous transluminal coronary angioplasty in octogenarians with unstable coronary syndromes. *Am J Cardiol* (1990) **66**:857–8.

27. Sousa AG, Feres F, Pinto I, Tanajura L et al. Transluminal coronary angioplasty in patients 70 years of age and older: an effective technique for myocardial revascularization? *Arq Bras Cardiol* (1991) **57**:197–202.

28. Thompson R, Holmes D, Gersh B et al. Percutaneous transluminal coronary angioplasty in the elderly: early and long-term results. *J Am Coll Cardiol* (1991) **17**:1245–50.

29. Jackman J, Navetta F, Smith J et al. Percutaneous transluminal coronary angioplasty in octogenarians as an effective therapy for angina pectoris. *Am J Cardiol* (1991) **68**: 116–19.

30. Maiello L, Colombo A, Gianrossi R et al. Results of coronary angioplasty in patients aged 75 years and older. *Chest* (1992) **102**: 375–9.

31. Forman D, Berman A, McCabe C et al. PTCA in the elderly: the 'young-old' versus the 'old-old'. *J Am Geriatr Soc* (1992) **40**:19–22.

32. ten Berg J, Bal E, Tjon R et al. Initial and long-term results of percutaneous transluminal coronary angioplasty in patients 75 years of age and older. *Cathet Cardiovasc Diagn* (1992) **26**:165–70.

33. Santana J, Haft J, LaMarche N et al. Coronary angioplasty in patients 80 years of age and older. *Am Heart J* (1992) **124**:13–18.

34. Shapira I, Frimerman A, Rosenschein U et al. Percutaneous transluminal coronary angioplasty in elderly patients. *Cardiology* (1994) **85**:88–93.

35. Weyrens F, Goldenberg I, Mooney J et al. Percutaneous transluminal coronary angioplasty in patients aged ≥90 years. *Am J Cardiol* (1994) **75**:397–8.

36. Thompson R. Coronary angioplasty in the elderly. In: Aronow WS, Stemmer EA, Wilson SE, eds, *Vascular Disease in the Elderly.* (Futura: Armonk, NY, 1997) 317–37.

37. Bourassa M. Complete versus incomplete revascularization. In: Ellis S, Holmes D, eds, *Strategic Approaches in Coronary Intervention.* (Williams & Wilkins: Baltimore, 1996) 440–54.

38. Weintraub W, Clements S, Ware J et al. Coronary artery surgery in octogenarians. *Am J Cardiol* (1991) **68**:1530–4.

39. National Center for Health Statistics Mortality. Public Health Service, 1990 (Vital Statistics of the United States), 1987 vol II, Section 6, p. 6. Washington, DC.

40. Shimshak T, McCallister B. Coronary artery bypass surgery and percutaneous transluminal coronary angioplasty in the elderly patients with ischemic heart disease. In: Tresch D, Aronow W, eds, *Cardiovascular Disease in the Elderly Patient.* (Marcel Dekker: New York, 1994) 323–44.

41. Jones EL, Weintraub WS. The importance of completeness of revascularization during long-term follow-up after coronary artery bypass surgery. *Circulation* (1991) **84**(Supplement II): II-463.

42. Cowley M, Vandermael M, Topol E et al. Is traditionally defined complete revascularization needed for patients with multivessel disease treated by elective coronary angioplasty? *J Am Coll Cardiol* (1993) **22**:1289–97.

43. Weintraub W, King III S, Jones E et al. Completeness of revascularization after coronary angioplasty and coronary surgery: different strategies, different results. *J Am Coll Cardiol* (1993) **21**:73A.

44. Bell M, Bailey K, Reeder G et al. Percutaneous transluminal coronary angioplasty in patients with multivessel coronary disease: how important is complete revascularization for cardiac event-free survival? *J Am Coll Cardiol* (1990) **16**:553–62.

45. Kaul T, Fields B, Wyatt D et al. Angioplasty versus coronary artery bypass in octogenarians. *Ann Thorac Surg* (1994) **58**:1419–26.

46. Mick M, Simpfendorfer C, Arnold A et al. Early and late results of coronary angioplasty and bypass in octogenarians. *Am J Cardiol* (1991) **68**:1316–20.

47. Myler R, Webb J, Nguyen K et al. Coronary angioplasty in octogenarians: comparisons to coronary bypass surgery. *Cathet Cardiovasc Diagn* (1991) **23**:3–9.

48. King III S, Lembo N, Weintraub W et al. A randomized trial comparing coronary angioplasty with coronary bypass surgery. *N Engl J Med* (1994) **331**:1044–50.

49. King III S, Lembo N, Weintraub W et al. Emory Angioplasty versus Surgery Trial

(EAST): design, recruitment, and baseline description of patients. *Am J Cardiol* (1995) **75**:42–59C.

50. King III S, Barnhart H, Kosinki A et al. Angioplasty or surgery for multivessel coronary artery disease: comparison of eligible registry and randomized patients in the EAST trial and influence of treatment selection on outcomes. *Am J Cardiol* (1997) **79**:1453–9.

51. Zhao X, Brown B, Stewart D et al. Effectiveness of revascularization in the Emory Angioplasty versus Surgery Trial. *Circulation* (1996) **93**:1954–62.

52. Weintraub W, Mauldin P, Becker E et al. A comparison of the costs and quality of life after coronary angioplasty or coronary surgery for multivessel coronary disease. *Circulation* (1995) **92**:2831–40.

53. Peterson E, Cowper P, Jollis J et al. Outcomes of coronary artery bypass graft surgery in 24 461 patients aged 80 years or older. *Circulation* (1995) **92**(Supplement II):II-85–91.

54. Ko W, Krieger K, Lazenby D et al. Isolated coronary artery bypass grafting in 100 consecutive octogenarian patients. *J Thorac Cardiovasc Surg* (1991) **102**:532–8.

55. Kowalchuk G, Siu S, Lewis S. Coronary artery disease in the octogenarian: angiographic spectrum and suitability for revascularization. *Am J Cardiol* (1990) **66**:1319–23.

56. Glower D, Christopher T, Milano C et al. Performance status and outcome after coronary artery bypass grafting in persons aged 80–93 years. *Am J Cardiol* (1992) **70**:567–71.

57. Cane M, Chen C, Bailey B et al. CABG in octogenarians: early and late events and actuarial survival in comparison with a matched population. *Ann Thorac Surg* (1995) **60**:1033–7.

58. Williams T, Carrillo R, Traad E et al. Determinants of operative mortality in octogenarians undergoing coronary bypass. *Ann Thorac Surg* (1995) **60**:1038–43.

59. Weintraub W, Craver J, Cohen C et al. Influence of age on results of coronary artery surgery. *Circulation* (1991) **84**(Supplement III): III-226–35.

60. Goodman S, Armstrong P. Invasive strategies in acute myocardial infarction in the elderly. *Cardiol Elder* (1994) **2**:43–9.

61. Goldberg R, Gore J, Gurwitz J et al. The impact of age on the incidence and prognosis of initial acute myocardial infarction: the Worcester Heart Attack Study. *Am Heart J* (1989) **117**:543–9.

62. Smith S, Gilpin E, Ahnve S et al. Outlook after acute myocardial infarction in the very elderly compared with that in patients aged 65–75 years. *J Am Coll Cardiol* (1990) **16**:784–92.

63. Naylor C, Chen E. Population-wide mortality trends among patients hospitalized for acute myocardial infarction: the Ontario experience, 1981–1991. *J Am Coll Cardiol* (1994) **24**: 1431–8.

64. Laster S, Rutherford D, Giorgi L et al. Results of direct percutaneous transluminal coronary angioplasty in octogenarians. *Am J Cardiol* (1996) **77**:10–13.

65. Wenger N. Coronary disease in elderly patients: myocardial infarction and myocardial revascularization. *Heart Dis Stroke* (1994) **3**: 401–6.

66. Saenz C, Killinger G, Baim D et al. Palmaz–Schatz intracoronary stent in the elderly: NACI experience. *J Am Coll Cardiol* (1992) **19**:109A.

67. Fishman R, Kuntz R, Carrozza Jr J et al. Acute and long-term results of coronary stents and atherectomy in women and the elderly. *Coron Art Dis* (1995) **6**:159–68.

68. Suilen C, Urban P, Chatelain P et al. Coronary stenting in octogenarians following failed balloon angioplasty. *Cardiol Elder* (1996) **4**: 157–60.

15

Dilatation versus thrombolytic therapy in elderly patients

David R Holmes Jr

Introduction

The treatment of elderly patients with acute myocardial infarction remains difficult. The number of elderly patients with symptomatic coronary artery disease continues to increase steadily. By the middle of the next century, 20–25% of most Western populations will be elderly.[1] When these patients present with acute myocardial infarction, the risk of mortality is markedly increased. Up to 30–50% of all deaths in patients hospitalized for acute infarction occur in patients older than 75 years.[2-4] Advanced age has been found to be the most important predictor of short- and longer-term mortality after infarction.[5,6] Some of the effect of age on outcome relates to a higher incidence of comorbid conditions while some relates to more extensive coronary artery disease with more prior infarction and more multivessel coronary disease.

Daida et al[7] reviewed the outcome in a population-based study of 309 elderly patients with acute myocardial infarction in Olmsted County, Minnesota from 1976 to 1991. During that time, there were marked changes in the care given to these patients. These changes included the introduction of aspirin, heparin, beta-blockers, thrombolytic therapy and mechanical reperfusion. The patients were divided by age into two groups: those aged 70–79 years and those 80 years and over. During this study time, 30-day survival improved

for patients 80 years of age or older. From 1976 to 1978, 30-day survival was 45%; from 1987 to 1989, it was 69%; and for 1991 it was 78% ($P = 0.01$) (Figure 15.1). However, there were only minimal changes in 30-day survival rates over time for patients from 70 to 79 years of age during the same three time periods 77%, 76%, 81% ($P = 0.65$). In a model adjusted for comorbidity and severity of myocardial infarction, the hazard in this group declined only 10% from 1.15 to 1.045. For the older group (>80 years), the hazard during the first 30 days in an adjusted model has declined by 72% from 3.176 to 0.883. When followed beyond 30 days, however, there was no improvement in survival from 1976 to 1991 in patients over the age of 80 (Figure 15.2). Although initial outcome was improved, longer-term outcome remains problematic.

The mainstay for therapy for acute myocardial infarction is reperfusion; this can be accomplished with thrombolytic therapy or by mechanical means with a catheter-based approach, usually percutaneous transluminal coronary angioplasty (PTCA). Surgical revascularization is also a potential approach; but in actual fact is limited by obvious practical considerations. Comparing the two approaches has been the subject of intense study with multiple randomized trials. In the most recent meta-analysis of these randomized

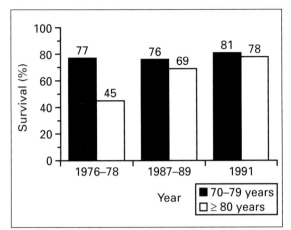

Figure 15.1
Thirty-day survival in three patients from 1976 to 1991. During this time, survival in patients 80 years of age or older has increased from 45 to 78%. (From Daida et al[7])

trials, Weaver et al[8] evaluated the outcome of 10 trials enrolling 2606 patients. The mortality at 30 days was 4.4% for primary PTCA compared to 6.5% for thrombolytic therapy. This represents a 34% reduction (odds ratio (OR): 0.66; 95% confidence interval (CI): 0.46–0.94; $P = 0.02$). The incidence of death or nonfatal reinfarction was 7.2% and 11.9% respectively (OR: 0.58; 95% CI: 0.44–0.76; $P < 0.001$). There was also a marked reduction in both total and hemorrhagic stroke with PTCA. Based on this meta-analysis, primary PTCA appears to be superior to thrombolytic therapy. This conclusion is based upon the essential assumption that angioplasty is carried out expeditiously by trained interventional cardiologists in an experienced laboratory setting.

None of these trials has focused specifically on the elderly. In this population of patients with acute myocardial infarction, there are some unique aspects including the following.

The potential risk of stroke

This is one of the most feared complications; in many patients the most feared adverse outcome is not death but nonfatal disabling stroke.

The potential for application of the selected reperfusion strategy

Thrombolytic therapy, although widely available, is administered in only approximately 40% of patients with acute myocardial infarction often because of relative or absolute contraindications.[9–12,13] The elderly may have more of these relative or absolute contraindications because of the presence of comorbid conditions. This is particularly true in estimating potential risk of stroke. In older patients, thrombolytic therapy may not be administered because of concern about these increased stroke rates.

Krumholz et al[10] evaluated the administration of thrombolytic therapy in a cohort of 3093 patients 65 years of age and over, treated in all acute nongovernmental hospitals in Connecticut from 1992 to 1993. In this cohort, there were 753 patients who were candidates for thrombolytic therapy defined as patients with ST segment elevation of at least 1 mm, left bundle branch block if it was not chronic and who had no contraindication to thrombolytic therapy. In this subset, 56% did not receive thrombolytic therapy. The specific reasons for not administering thrombolysis were documented in only 19% of these patients; the two most common reasons were either a delay in presentation or 'advanced age'. Increasing age was strongly associated with not administering thrombolytic therapy.

The application of thrombolytic therapy in the elderly has been increasing. This was

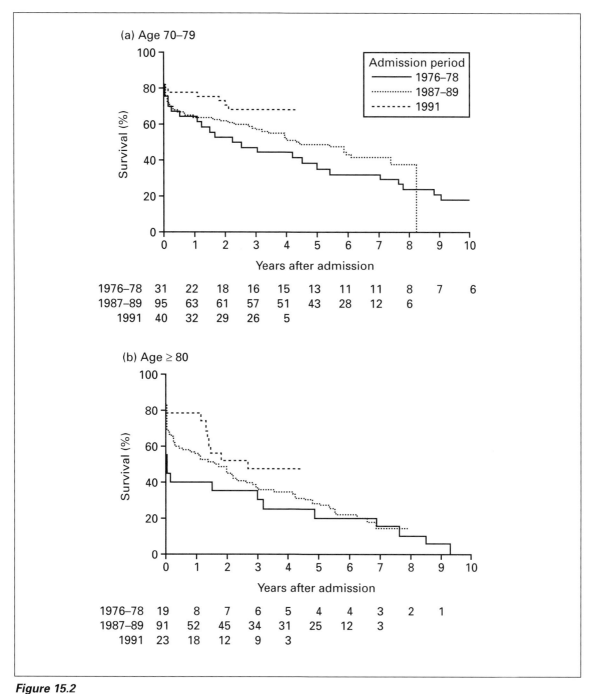

Figure 15.2
(a) Life table survival in patients 70–79 years. During the period of this study, there was little difference in short-term survival but improved long-term survival (P = 0.05). (b) In contrast to patients 70–79 years, in patients 80 years and older, there was improvement in 30-day survival but no significant improvement in longer-term survival after hospital discharge. (From Daida et al[7])

evaluated in the National Registry of Myocardial Infarction (NRMI).[11] These investigators found that over the period of their study that the absolute increase in use of thrombolytic therapy in patients 75 to 84 years was 2.7% from 18.7 to 21.4%; in patients at least 85 years, the increase was 2.1% from 7.0 to 9.1%. Even though there has been an increase, application of thrombolysis remains low.

Increased mortality rate

As previously mentioned, the mortality rate for acute myocardial infarction is markedly increased in older patients.[6,14–20] From the standpoint of the number of lives saved, however, older patients may have the greatest potential benefit. For example, a strategy that results in a 30% reduction in mortality will save more lives per 1000 patients treated if the baseline mortality is 25% than if the baseline mortality is only 6%. From a population standpoint, reperfusion strategies may be even more important in older patients. The recent joint ACC/AHA clinical practice guideline concluded that the weight of evidence favors thrombolytic therapy in patients 75 years and over provided that they meet selection criteria.

Delay in time to treatment

Older patients have a longer delay from the time of the onset of symptoms of acute myocardial infarction to medical evaluation. In the GUSTO I trial this was statistically significantly longer.[3,6] The time from presentation was 1.76 hours in patients under 65 years contrasted to 2.06 hours in patients over 85 years. Given the crucial importance of the 'golden hour of opportunity,' this can dramatically affect outcome. Boersma et al[21] evaluated this 'golden hour' in a meta-analysis of 22 trials with 50 246 patients. The absolute reduction

in mortality was greatest in those patients who presented within 1 hour of symptom onset; this reduction in mortality progressively declined the longer the interval from onset to presentation. Some of the increased mortality in older patients may be the result of the time delays in these patients.

There have been no randomized studies of reperfusion limited to the elderly. Given the small samples of the randomized trials of PTCA versus thrombolysis, the elderly subgroups may not even be able to be studied individually. There are data, however, on thrombolysis in the elderly.

The Fibrinolytic Therapy Trialists Collaborative Group[17] evaluated all nine randomized trials that included more than 1000 patients which compared the outcome of fibrinolytic therapy versus control treatment. Their review found that in patients with acute myocardial infarction and either ST segment elevation or bundle branch block, there were 15 ± 4 lives saved per 1000 patients treated under the age of 55 years ± 14 lives saved per 1000 patients treated over the age of 75 years. Therefore, thrombolytic therapy should not be withheld in this older group of patients.

In the GUSTO I trial, 12% of the enrolled patients were older than 75 years.[3,6] There were 4625 patients from 75 to 85 years and 412 patients older than 85 years of age. Older patients uniformly had more adverse baseline characteristics including more hypertension, more prior infarction, higher incidence of anterior infarction, more advanced Killip class and longer time to presentation and treatment (Table 15.1). In-hospital mortality was strikingly increased at 27.9% of patients over 85 years compared with 2.8% in patients under 65 years. Cardiogenic shock, reinfarction and heart failure were also significantly more frequent in older patients. Additional revascularization procedures either with PTCA or coronary bypass

	Age group (years)			
	<65 (N = 24 708)	65–74 (N = 11 201)	75–85 (N = 4625)	>85 (N = 412)
Age (years)	53.2 ± 8.1	69.6 ± 2.8	78.7 ± 2.6	87.4 ± 2.5
Men	20 386 (83%)	7500 (67%)	2569 (56%)	181 (44%)
Weight (kg)	82.6 ± 15.8	76.4 ± 14	71.1 ± 13.4	65.7 ± 12.5
Height (cm)	172.8 ± 8.9	169.6 ± 9.3	167.2 ± 9.5	164.6 ± 9.3
Diabetes mellitus	3143 (13%)	2017 (18%)	790 (17%)	55 (13%)
Hypertension	8318 (34%)	4929 (44%)	2099 (46%)	186 (45%)
Current smoker	13 925 (57%)	2948 (27%)	601 (13%)	25 (6%)
History				
Angina	8429 (34%)	4535 (41%)	1914 (42%)	160 (39%)
Myocardial infarction	3488 (14%)	2211 (20%)	927 (20%)	77 (19%)
Coronary angioplasty	1084 (4%)	445 (4%)	113 (2%)	4 (1%)
Coronary artery bypass				
surgery	950 (4%)	661 (6%)	167 (4%)	5 (1%)
Infarct location				
Anterior wall	9077 (37%)	4533 (41%)	2108 (46%)	224 (55%)
Inferior wall	14 705 (60%)	6258 (56%)	2344 (51%)	174 (42%)
Other	847 (3%)	381 (3%)	160 (3%)	12 (3%)
Killip class				
I	21 882 (89%)	9123 (82%)	3486 (76%)	291 (71%)
II	2399 (10%)	1707 (15%)	916 (20%)	94 (23%)
III	186 (1%)	201 (2%)	144 (3%)	16 (4%)
IV	134 (1%)	107 (1%)	64 (1%)	10 (2%)
Time to presentation (hours)	1.76 ± 1.17	1.96 ± 1.2	2.06 ± 1.22	2.06 ± 1.23
Time to treatment (hours)	3.0 ± 1.6	3.21 ± 1.62	3.35 ± 1.58	3.43 ± 1.59
Treatment				
Aspirin	24 072 (98%)	10 767 (97%)	4439 (96%)	387 (94%)
Intravenous beta-blockade	11 922 (48%)	4403 (39%)	1718 (37%)	145 (35%)

Table 15.1
Baseline characteristics of 40 946 patients with acute MI who received thrombolytic therapy.[3] The patients were divided into four age groups. All differences between groups were significant (P < 0.001) except for other locations of infarct, with age compared as a continuous variable with each baseline factor. (From Straznicky et al[3] and White et al[6])

graft surgery were less frequently used. After adjusting for all the differences in baseline characteristics, increasing age was the most powerful predictor of 30-day mortality.

Important secondary endpoints in the GUSTO trial were death or stroke, and death and nonfatal stroke. Total and hemorrhagic strokes were more frequent with increasing age. Total stroke rates for patients aged under 65, 65–74, 75–85, and over 85 years were 0.8,

2.1, 3.4 and 2.9% respectively. The endpoint of death or nonfatal disabling stroke increased from 3.3% of patients under 65 years to 31.1% of patients over 85 years.

The effect of the specific thrombolytic regimen on outcome was also assessed. For patients older than 65 years, the risk of hemorrhagic stroke increased more with tissue plasminogen activator (tPA) than with streptokinase. This has led some centers to preferentially use streptokinase in elderly patients with acute myocardial infarction.

There are limited data on primary angioplasty. Several smaller series have addressed age as a discrete variable. In these series, mortality has been very variable, ranging from 5.7 to 34%.[22-26] There has been an interesting finding that several authors have reported. Namely, this finding relates to the fact that procedural success is high but the in-hospital mortality also remains high. In a recent report by Stuckey et al,[25] even though the initial success rate was 98%, the in-hospital mortality rate remained at 21.3%. Lee et al found a success rate of 91% but an in-hospital mortality rate of 18%.

We evaluated the outcome of 127 patients 80 years of age and over undergoing primary percutaneous revascularization during acute myocardial infarction. The majority of the patients (112) were treated with conventional PTCA alone. The mean age was 83.3 years; and 53% were female. Fifty percent of the patients had three-vessel disease, which is a higher percentage than usually identified in younger patients. The presence of three-vessel disease has been found by other series to be one of the strongest predictors of in-hospital death. The mean time from the onset of symptoms to procedural performance in this patient population was 10 hours, reflecting that many of these patients were treated late. The procedural success rate in this experience was 79%

of lesions treated. The in-hospital mortality rate remained high at 21%. Congestive heart failure also occurred in 21% while cardiogenic shock occurred in 15.3%. This single-center experience was not randomized data. Whether these patients would have had a higher mortality if only thrombolytic therapy had been administered cannot be determined.

The GUSTO IIb[27] trial is the largest randomized trial of primary angioplasty versus thrombolysis. This study allows assessment of the effect of age on outcome in patients who could have had either treatment. Age was assessed as a continuous variable as well as a discrete variable by 10-year increments. In the 1138 patients in this trial, 565 were randomized to PTCA and 573 to tPA. The patient groups were similar with respect to baseline patient characteristics. Of the patients treated with PTCA, 14.5% were over 75 years compared to 13.8% of patients treated with thrombolysis. As age increased, so did the risk of death, death or myocardial infarction, or death, stroke or myocardial infarction. For each 10-year increment of age, the adjusted rate of death or myocardial infarction increased by a factor of 1.32. The most important finding was that the linear relationship between age and outcome was the same, irrespective of whether the patient was treated with primary angioplasty or thrombolytic therapy. Primary angioplasty for each age group was associated with improved outcome, but tests for interaction between patient age and specific treatment selected, that is PTCA versus thrombolysis, were nonsignificant.

Summary

Acute myocardial infarction is a major problem for older patients, with high rates of morbidity and mortality. Some of the adverse outcome is the result of comorbid disease and, as such, will be difficult to modify. However, some of the adverse outcome is related to the extent and severity of coronary artery disease as well as to the delay in presentation. The optimal revascularization strategy in this group is not yet clear. Both strategies currently have problems, but both are significantly better than alternative conservative care. Vigorous attempts have to be made to improve early detection and treatment, to improve achievement of full revascularization, and to effect minimization of myocardial necrosis to optimize the long-term outcome.

References

1. Kashyap M. Cardiovascular disease in the elderly: current considerations. *Am J Cardiol* (1989) **63**:311–14.

2. Roig E, Castaner A, Simmons B et al. In hospital mortality rates from acute myocardial infarction by race in US hospitals: findings from the National Hospital Discharge Survey. *Circulation* (1987) **76**:280–8.

3. Straznicky I, White HD, Granger CB et al. Effects of four thrombolytic regimens in elderly patients. *Cardiol Rev* (1998) **15**:22–8.

4. Gillum RF. Trends in acute myocardial infarction and coronary heart disease death in the United States. *J Am Coll Cardiol* (1993) **23**: 1273–7.

5. Lee KL, Woodlief LH, Topol EJ et al. Predictors of 30 day mortality in the era of reperfusion for acute myocardial infarction: results from an international trial of 41 021 patients. *Circulation* (1995) **91**:1659–68.

6. White HD, Barbbash GI, Califf RM et al for the GUSTO I Investigators. Age and outcome with contemporary thrombolytic therapy: results from the GUSTO I trial. *Circulation* (1996) **94**:1826–33.

7. Daida H, Kottke TE, Backes RJ, Gersh MB et al. Are coronary-care unit changes in therapy associated with improved survival of elderly patients with acute myocardial infarction? *Mayo Clin Proc* (1997) **72**:1014–21.

8. Weaver WD, Simes RJ, Betrice A et al. Comparison of primary coronary angioplasty and intravenous thrombolytic therapy for acute myocardial infarction: a quantitative review. *JAMA* (1997) **278**:2093–9.

9. Chandra H, Yarzebski J, Goldberg RJ et al. Age related trends (1986–1993) in the use of thrombolytic agents in patients with acute myocardial infarction. *Arch Intern Med* (1997) **147**:741–6.

10. Krumholz HM, Murillo JE, Chen J et al. Thrombolytic therapy for eligible elderly patients with acute myocardial infarction. *JAMA* (1997) **277**:1683–8.

11. Gurwitz JH, Gore JM, Goldberg RJ et al. Recent age-related trends in the use of thrombolytic therapy on patients who have had acute myocardial infarction. *Ann Intern Med* (1996) **124**:283–91.

12. Weaver WE, Litwin PE, Martin JS et al. Effect of age on the use of thrombolytic therapy and mortality in acute myocardial infarction. *J Am Coll Cardiol* (1991) **18**:657–62.

14. ISIS-2 (Second International Study of Infarct Survival) Collaborative Group. Randomized trial of intravenous streptokinase, oral aspirin, both or neither among 17 187 cases of suspected acute myocardial infarction. ISIS-2. *Lancet* (1988) **ii**:349–60.

13. Krumholz HM, Friesinger GC, Cook EF et al. Relationship of age with eligibility for thrombolytic therapy and mortality among patients with suspected acute myocardial infarction. *J Am Geriatr Soc* (1994) **42**:127–31.

15. Gruppo Italiano per lo Studio della Streptokinase nell' Infacto Miocardio (GISSI). Long-term effects of intravenous thrombolysis in acute myocardial infarction: final report of the GISSI study. *Lancet* (1987) **ii**:871–4.

16. The GUSTO Investigators. An interventional randomized trial comparing four thrombolytic strategies for acute myocardial infarction. *N Engl J Med* (1993) **329**:673–82.

17. Fibrinolytic Therapy Trialists (FTT) Collaborative Group. Indications for fibrinolytic therapy in suspected acute myocardial infarction: collaborative overview of early mortality and major morbidity results from all randomized trials of more than 1000 patients. *Lancet* (1994) **343**:311–22.

18. Ellerbeck EF, Jencks SF, Radford MJ et al. Treatment of Medicare patients with acute myocardial infarction: report on a four-state pilot of the Cooperative Cardiovascular Project. *JAMA* (1995) **273**:1509–14.

19. Goldberg RJ, Gore JM, Gurwitz JH et al. The impact of age on the incidence and prognosis of initial acute myocardial infarction: the Worcester Heart Attack Study. *Am Heart J* (1989) **117**:543–9.

20. Krumholz HM, Pasternak BC, Weinsein MC et al. Cost effectiveness of thrombolytic therapy with streptokinase in elderly patients with suspected acute myocardial infarction. *N Engl J Med* (1992) **327**:7–13.

21. Boersma E, Maas ACP, Deckers JW, Simoons ML. Early thrombolytic treatment in acute myocardial treatment: reappraisal of the golden hour. *Lancet* (1996) **348**:771–5.

22. Brodie BR, Weintraub RA, Stuckey TD et al. Outcomes of direct coronary angioplasty for acute myocardial infarction in candidates and non-candidates for thrombolytic therapy. *Am J Cardiol* (1991) **67**:7–12.

23. Holland KJ, O'Heioll WW, Bates ER et al. Emergency percutaneous transluminal coronary angioplasty during acute myocardial infarction for patients more than 70 years of age. *Am J Cardiol* (1989) **63**:399–403.

24. Lee TC, Laramee LA, Rutherford BD et al. Emergency percutaneous transluminal coronary angioplasty for acute myocardial infarction in patients 70 years of age and older. *Am J Cardiol* (1990) **66**:663–7.

25. Stuckey T, Brodie B, Hansen C et al. Primary angioplasty for acute myocardial infarction in elderly thrombolytic candidates: is it the best option? *J Am Coll Cardiol* (1995) 47A.

26. Stone GW, Grines CL Browne KF et al. Acute outcome after primary angioplasty in acute myocardial infarction: the Primary Angioplasty in Myocardial Infarction Trial (PAMI). *J Am Coll Cardiol* (1993) **21**:331.

27. Holmes DR, White HD, Pieper KS et al. Effect of age on outcome with primary angioplasty versus thrombolysis: the GUSTO IIb Randomized Trial. *Am Coll Cardiol* In press.

16

Coronary artery bypass surgery in octogenarians
Charles J Mullany

Introduction

By the year 2025, 5–9% of the population of developed nations will be at least 80 years of age and 68% of those over the age of 65 years will live in third world countries.[1] Within this 'older' group, octogenarians represent the most rapidly expanding segment of the population. In the United States and the United Kingdom, the population over 80 years will rise from 2.7% and 3.7% respectively in 1990, to 4.5% and 6.2% in the year 2025.[1] These changes in demographics present considerable challenges in the provision of health care for the elderly, including the management of symptomatic cardiovascular disease.

Although coronary artery disease is not an inevitable result of aging, the most important risk factor for developing symptomatic coronary artery disease continues to be increasing age. Up to 80% of individuals over the age of 60 years can be demonstrated to have significant coronary atherosclerosis at autopsy.[2] Moreover, coronary artery disease remains an important and major cause of death in elderly patients, despite a general decline in coronary artery disease mortality in all age groups.

Consequently, an increasing number of octogenarians are now undergoing myocardial revascularization by either coronary artery bypass grafting (CABG) or percutaneous transluminal coronary angioplasty (PTCA). It has been estimated that if the rate of CABG in octogenarians remains constant at 1990 levels, which is unlikely, then the number of these procedures in this age group in the US will increase from 8000/year to 30 000/year by 2050.[3] This trend has considerable financial implications for society. Other issues which must be considered when providing care for this patient group include quality of life, patient and family expectations, and long-term survival.

In reviewing the literature related to octogenarians, many publications group elderly patients as those 75 years of age and over. Where possible, most information relating to mortality, morbidity and survival has been obtained from publications relating to patients 80 years of age and over. However, in this chapter, some data related to coronary pathology, clinical symptoms and comorbidity have been obtained from publications concerning patients 75 years of age and over.

Symptoms

Elderly patients often present with significant unstable angina pectoris and more than 50% of all patients admitted to hospital for myocardial infarction are older than 65 years.[4] Many of these patients have more extensive coronary artery disease than their younger counterparts and often have severe angina pectoris that is refractory to medical therapy.[3,5–7] In patients over 80 years of age undergoing

CABG at the Mayo Clinic,[8] 86% had triple vessel disease and 41% had greater than 50% luminal narrowing of the left main coronary artery. Elderly patients are also more likely to have diffuse and distal disease as well as a greater number of complicated coronary stenoses than their younger counterparts. Coronary and aortic calcification is also particularly common in this age group.

In addition to the extensive nature of the coronary artery disease and the high incidence of unstable class III–IV angina, the elderly often have other significant cardiac and non-cardiac comorbid conditions that have to be taken into consideration when selecting the most appropriate therapy. Older patients are more likely to be female, and to have hypertension, heart failure, ST depression on the resting ECG, peripheral vascular disease, cerebrovascular disease, chronic pulmonary disease, renal impairment, and coexisting malignancy.[3,5–7,9,10] Diabetes mellitus, although present in up to 29% of this elderly group,[11] seems to be less common than in younger patients.[3,5,10] This decline in frequency, as Hannan and Burke[5] have suggested, may be due to earlier mortality from diabetes-related illness. Treatment of the octogenarian has to be carefully individualized because chronological age may be a poor predictor of both functional capacity and physiological function of the patient. Many elderly individuals remain vigorous and are in excellent physical and mental health apart from their symptomatic coronary artery disease.

Patient selection for surgery

The primary treatment aim for most octogenarians should be symptom relief, discharge from acute hospital care, improvement in quality of life, and return to independent living. In certain instances, prolongation of life

may be obtained. However, reliable data regarding this are lacking, since randomized controlled trials comparing medical treatment with revascularization (CABG/PTCA) have been confined to patients less than 80 years. A nonrandomized survival analysis of octogenarian patients with coronary artery disease managed by elective CABG versus conventional medical treatment was published by Ko et al.[12] They reported a 3-year survival of 77% in surgical patients compared with 54% in medical patients. In addition, the surgical patients had a significant improvement in their New York Heart Association functional class, whereas the medical group had no significant change at follow-up.

For octogenarians with significant left main coronary stenosis, triple vessel disease and decreased left ventricular function or severe ischemia, it may be reasonable to assume that improved survival can be obtained if they are revascularized, so long as they do not have other significant comorbidity that may increase operative mortality or may limit long-term survival. The decision to revascularize an asymptomatic or minimally symptomatic patient in this age group has to be very carefully individualized and depends a great deal upon patient expectations, physiological age, anticipated activities, comorbidity and a clear understanding by the patient and family of possible surgical complications (e.g. stroke).

The high incidence of unstable or post-infarction angina, rest angina and admission to the coronary care unit seen in many of these patients attests to the severity of their illness and the need to control disabling symptoms.[3,5,8] In part, this may have been due to a reluctance to either investigate or to revascularize the patient several years earlier because, at that time, they were thought 'too old' to undergo invasive therapy, particularly CABG. Failure to control symptoms with intensive medical therapy usually requires a decision regarding coronary angiography and subsequent revascularization. The decision to perform coronary angiography is often difficult and is done in the hope that the patient will have a 'dilatable culprit lesion'. Moreover, it is often hoped by the attending physician, as well as the patient and family, that PTCA will be the preferred treatment in such patients. However, many elderly patients will be unsuitable for PTCA because of significant left main coronary artery stenosis, chronic occlusions, calcified vessels or the extensive nature of the coronary artery disease. Additionally, in a recent review of CABG versus PTCA in 310 octogenarians, CABG had a lower mortality (5.8%) than PTCA (8.6%) and a better 5-year survival (66% versus 55%).[13] Nevertheless, PTCA may be a viable option in those patients where the risk of surgery is considered too high and where PTCA, although not optimal, may resolve the patient's acute problem.

Operative technique

CABG in the elderly follows the usual principles of myocardial revascularization undertaken in younger patients. Special attention has to be paid to the aorta because of the significant incidence of aortic calcification and atheroma that is present in the elderly patient (Figures 16.1 and 16.2). Occasionally aortic cannulation may not be possible and femoral cannulation will be needed. Aortic cross-clamping may also be unwise, and on such occasions surgery can be performed during cardiopulmonary bypass and ventricular fibrillation.

Complete revascularization should be undertaken, but need not necessarily be as extensive as in a younger patient. Although the internal mammary artery (IMA) is a particularly useful conduit for the elderly and is

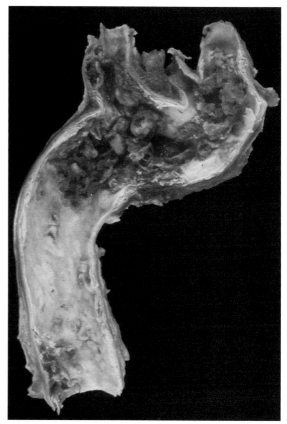

Figure 16.1
Extensive atheroma involving the ascending aorta, aortic arch, and great vessels in an elderly patient who underwent coronary artery bypass surgery.

not used as often as in younger patients, it should be used more frequently.[9,14] The quality of the saphenous vein may be poor and the use of the IMA avoids an extra aortic anastomosis; this is a valuable strategy in the presence of aortic calcification. Additionally, there is no evidence that use of the IMA in octogenarians significantly increases postoperative mortality or morbidity. To the contrary, there are data

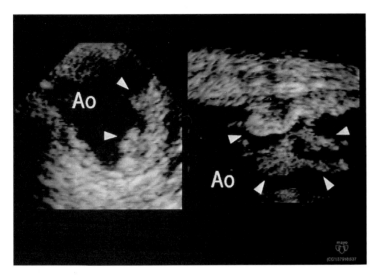

Figure 16.2
Intra-operative transesophageal echo showing extensive atheromatous debris within the lumen of the aorta (Ao). From Click et al[30] (From Click et al[30] with permission)

that suggest that long-term survival is significantly better in octogenarians when the IMA is used compared with the survival of those patients who receive saphenous veins only (Figure 16.3).[14] Since the primary aim of surgery is symptom relief, rarely do the elderly require more than three bypasses to the major vessels of the coronary circulation (left anterior descending, circumflex and right). An expeditious operation is important since prolonged cardiopulmonary bypass can be a risk factor for postoperative stroke in these patients.[15]

Elderly tissues are particularly fragile and tear easily (Figure 16.4). Careful handling of all tissues, particularly the right atrium, aortic cannulation site and the lateral wall of the left ventricle is essential. Extensive atrial tears may require repair with autologous pericardium. A fragile aortic cannulation site can be reinforced with a Teflon felt strip placed circumferentially around the aorta. For patients with

a recent myocardial infarction, poor left ventricular function and difficulty in being weaned from cardiopulmonary bypass, an intra-aortic balloon pump should be used. However, femoral insertion of a balloon may not be possible because of the presence of extensive peripheral vascular disease. On a rare occasion an intra-aortic balloon pump can be placed through the ascending aorta. Use of more sophisticated left ventricular devices is most probably not indicated in this age group.

Operative mortality

The reported operative mortality for octogenarians undergoing CABG ranges from 4.7% to 15% (Table 16.1).[3,5,8,10,11,13,14,16–25] In the largest reported series, collected from 24 461 US Medicare records for patients undergoing CABG from 1987–1990, operative mortality

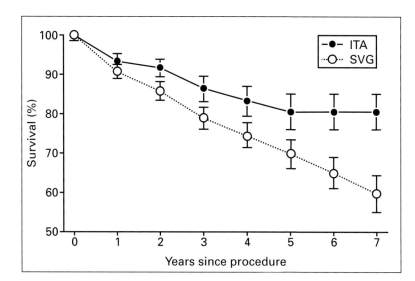

Figure 16.3
Survival of octogenarians undergoing coronary artery bypass surgery with internal thoracic artery (ITA) versus saphenous vein graft (From Morris et al[14] with permission).

was 11.5%.[3] During 1995–96, the mortality for 5184 patients 81–90 years of age, contained within the Society of Thoracic Surgeons (STS) database, was 4.7%.[26] These differences in mortality between the STS database and Medicare may be due to improvement in results over time, or to incomplete reporting to the STS database. Not all cardiac surgical units in the US report results to the STS database.

Important factors that increase operative mortality in this age group include recent myocardial infarction,[3] rest pain,[8] admission to the coronary care unit,[8] congestive heart failure,[3] poor left ventricular function,[8] cerebrovascular disease,[3] peripheral vascular disease,[3] and diabetes mellitus with complications.[10] Particular caution has to be taken in deciding whether to operate upon very elderly patients who have had a recent myocardial infarction and who have a significant reduction in ejection fraction with acute pulmonary edema. If possible, these patients may be better treated with aggressive medical therapy, diuresis and possible use of an intra-aortic balloon pump. Unfortunately, medical therapy is

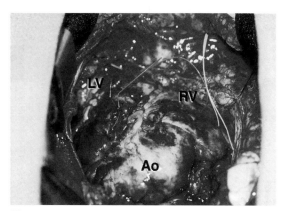

Figure 16.4
Operative photograph showing extensive bruising and hemorrhage of the anterior aspect of the heart in an octogenarian undergoing coronary artery bypass surgery (Ao, aorta; RV, right ventricle; LV, left ventricle)

Authors[ref]	N	Years	Mortality (%)	Stroke (%)	Survival
Naunheim et al[16]	71	1980–89	13.0		
Mullany et al[8]	159	1977–89	10.7	4.4	71% at 5 years
Mick et al[17]	142	1982–89	6.0	4.0	87% at 3 years Hospital survivors
Weintraub et al[10]	146	1981–89	8.3	4.1	—
Ko et al[18]	100	1985–89	12.0	—	57% at 4 years
Peterson et al[3]	24 461	1987–90	11.5	—	71% at 3 years
Curtis et al[25]	68	1978–91	14.7	—	—
Cane et al[19]	84	1982–91	5.9	—	—
Glower et al[20]	86	1983–91	13.9	9.3	64% at 3 years
Tsai et al[21]	303	1982–92	8.3	—	62% at 5 years
Hannan and Burke[5]	1372	1991–92	8.3	—	—
Talwalkar et al[22]	100	1989–92	8.0	—	73% at 4 years
Kaul et al[13]	205	1982–93	5.8	1.5	65% at 5 years
Morris et al[14]	474	1987–94	7.8	8.0	80% at 5 years IMA+ 60% at 5 years IMA–
Williams et al[11]	300	1989–94	11.0	2.3	76% at 4.5 years Hospital survivors
Akins et al[23]	292	1985–95	5.8	7.9	55% at 5 years
Ranger et al[24]	255	1991–95	8.6	—	65% at 5 years

IMA, internal mammary artery.

Table 16.1
Published results in patients ≥80 years undergoing isolated coronary artery bypass surgery (Only series with >50 patients included)

less well tolerated by the elderly than by their younger counterparts and often one is forced to opt for surgery.

Morbidity

Postoperative morbidity can be significant in these patients. The incidence of arrhythmias, particularly atrial fibrillation, may be as high as 35%.[8] Stroke is an important complication and is reported to occur in 1.9–9% of patients (Table 16.1). Although all such events may not have permanent residua, postoperative stroke is a significant cause of hospital death, prolonged hospital stay and subsequent disability. Risk factors for stroke include known cerebrovascular disease (TIA, previous stroke, carotid endarterectomy, carotid stenosis), peripheral vascular disease, calcified aorta, hypertension, diabetes mellitus, prolonged cardiopulmonary bypass and peri-operative hypotension.[10,15,27,28] Prevention of stroke is an important aspect of management. This includes minimal handling and clamping of the aorta, avoidance of cannulation at calcified plaques, maintenance of adequate perfusion pressure (>60 mmHg), use of the IMA to avoid an extra aortic anastomosis and careful evaluation of the carotid circulation in those patients who are thought to be at high risk for cerebrovascular disease.

Although it is not normal practice to advise combined carotid endarterectomy and CABG in a patient who has asymptomatic cerebrovascular disease, it may be advisable if one carotid artery is occluded and a greater than 70% stenosis exists in the other internal carotid. In this situation oculoplethysmography may be helpful in determining the adequacy of the carotid and cerebral circulations. Nevertheless, it still remains controversial as to whether a combined coronary and carotid operation reduces the incidence of postoperative cerebral accidents in such patients.

Rehabilitation and quality of life

Although the patients may have a 'technically' successful operation, social issues are important factors in returning them to normal life. Generally the elderly take longer to recover, spend a longer than average time in the intensive care unit and hospital, and often have other medical problems that require attention while hospitalized. They also require coordination of home help after discharge. Often a spouse is deceased or disabled, and other family members may not be available to provide convalescent care for the patient because of distance or other family obligations. Enlistment of social workers, home nursing, temporary nursing-home facilities, and cardiac rehabilitation services is invaluable in eventually returning patients to an independent life in the community.

For most patients, relief of angina is excellent with marked improvement in their quality of life. There is some evidence to suggest that angina relief tends to be better in older patients than in those under 65 years.[9,29] This may be due to a combination of factors including less vigorous activity in the elderly as well as different expectations by this age group. Glower et al[20] evaluated pre- and postoperative performance status (Karnofsky scores) in 86 consecutive patients between 80 and 90 years of age undergoing isolated CABG. Medium performance status Karnofsky score improved from 20 to 70% ($P = 0.0001$) with 89% of hospital survivors being discharged home. Factors associated with failure to achieve a successful functional outcome included the presence of one or more pre-operative comorbid conditions, preoperative myocardial infarction within 7 days of surgery and low cardiac output postoperatively. Others have also found a significant relief of disabling symptoms following isolated CABG.[8,19,21,22] In the Mayo experience, with a mean follow-up of 29 months, 79% of patients were angina free and 89% were in NYHA class I or II.[8] Eighty-one percent of patients thought that they were significantly improved by the surgery, 3% felt unchanged and 13% thought that they were worse. Although most patients show excellent improvement in quality of life, some patients will show no, or little, improvement. This emphasizes the need in this age group to carefully select patients prior to submitting them to extensive cardiac procedures.

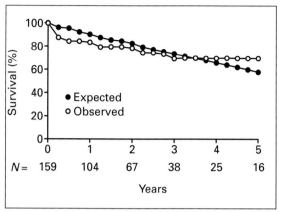

Figure 16.5
Survival curve of 159 patients aged 80 years and older undergoing coronary artery bypass surgery (Observed), compared with survival of an age- and sex-matched population (Expected). Number at risk shown by year. (From Mullany et al[8] with permission)

Survival

Long-term survival from reported series is variable and depends to some degree on whether all patients or only hospital survivors are included in the life survival analysis. At the Mayo Clinic, the 5-year survival of all patients was 71% and for hospital survivors was 80%.[8] For most series, 5-year survival is 60–70% (Table 16.1). Survival in this age group is very similar to that for the US octogenarian population as a whole (Figures 16.5 and 16.6).[3,8] Significant factors, apart from poor left ventricular function (Figure 16.7) and congestive heart failure, which negatively influence survival are co-morbid conditions, particularly chronic renal disease (Figure 16.8), peripheral vascular disease, and chronic obstructive airways disease. Patients with class

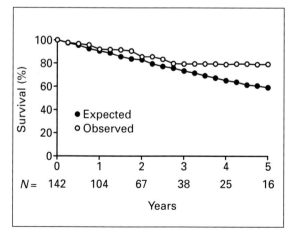

Figure 16.6
Survival curve of 142 hospital survivors aged 80 years and older undergoing coronary bypass surgery (Observed), compared with survival of age- and sex-matched population (Expected). Number at risk shown by year. (From Mullany et al[8] with permission)

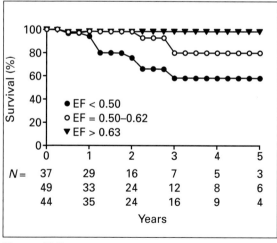

Figure 16.7
Effect of ejection fraction (EF) on survival in 130 hospital survivors aged 80 years and older undergoing coronary artery bypass surgery (P = 0.000). Number at risk shown by year. (From Mullany et al[8] with permission)

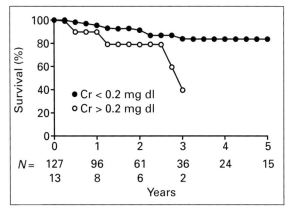

Figure 16.8
Effect of renal impairment on survival in 130 hospital survivors aged 80 years and older undergoing coronary artery bypass surgery (P = 0.04). Number at risk shown by year. Cr, creatinine.

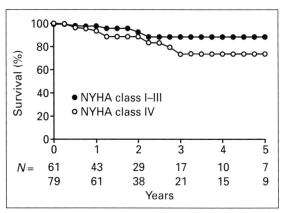

Figure 16.9
Effect of pre-operative NYHA class on survival in 130 hospital survivors aged 80 years and older undergoing coronary artery bypass surgery (P = 0.06). Number at risk shown by year.

III–IV symptoms prior to surgery also tend to have a poorer long-term survival (Figure 16.9). Given that octogenarians usually have particularly severe symptoms and disease at the time of surgery, their long-term survival is particularly gratifying. However, a bias in selecting those patients best able to tolerate surgery most probably plays an important part in their ultimate survival.

Conclusion

CABG in the octogenarian is becoming more common and is likely to increase as the population ages. However, patient selection for surgery is of utmost importance since the presence of significant comorbid conditions can result in an adverse outcome. Careful attention has to be given to associated conditions, particularly cerebrovascular, peripheral vascu-

lar and renal disease. Operative mortality for this age group is 5–10% depending on the urgency of the surgery. Significant risk factors related to operative mortality include acuteness and severity of symptoms as well as poor left ventricular function. Postoperative morbidity may be significant with reported stroke rates being 2–10%. For patients discharged from hospital, relief of angina is usually excellent and long-term survival is good. Many are able to return to active lives. The elderly often require extensive support for the first few months after surgery in order to make a satisfactory return to their community. In selecting patients for surgery, physiological age is an important consideration. The results would indicate that surgery in this age group is well worthwhile, particularly in the presence of good left ventricular function and in the absence of major comorbid conditions.

References

1. Pollock Sean R, ed., *Statistical Forecasts of the United States*, 2nd edn. (Gale Research Inc.: Detroit, MI 1995) 686.
2. White NK, Edward JE, Dry TJ. Relationship of degree of coronary atherosclerosis with age, in men. *Circulation* (1950) **1**:645–54.
3. Peterson ED, Cowper PA, Jollis JG et al. Outcomes of coronary artery bypass graft surgery in 24 461 patients aged 80 years or older. *Circulation* (1995) **92**(Suppl II):85–91.
4. Graves EJ. *Summary 1989 National Hospital Discharge Survey: Advance data from vital and health statistics No. 199*. (National Center for Health Statistics: Hyattsville, Maryland, 1991), 1–12.
5. Hannan EL, Burke J. Effect of age on mortality in coronary artery bypass surgery in New York, 1991–1992. *Am Heart J* (1994) **128**: 1184–91.
6. Salomon NW, Page US, Bigelow JC et al. Coronary artery bypass grafting in the elderly patients. Comparative results in a consecutive series of 469 patients older than 75 years. *J Thorac Cardiovasc Surg* (1990) **101**:209–18.
7. Khan SS, Kupfer JM, Matloff JM et al. Interaction of age and preoperative risk factors in predicting operative mortality for coronary bypass surgery. *Circulation* (1992) **86**(Suppl II): 186–90.
8. Mullany CJ, Darling GE, Pluth JR et al. Early and late results after isolated coronary artery bypass surgery in 159 patients aged 80 years and older. *Circulation* (1990) **82**(Suppl II): 229–36.
9. Mullany CJ, Brooks M, Kelsey S et al. Outcome of patients ≥65 years undergoing coronary revascularization: a report from bypass angioplasty revascularization investigation (BARI). *J Am Coll Cardiol* (1997) **29**(Suppl): 73A.
10. Weintraub WS, Craver JM, Jones EL, Guyton RA. Influence of age on results of coronary artery surgery. *Circulation* (1991) **84**(Suppl II): 226–35.
11. Williams DB, Carrillo RG, Traad EA et al. Determinants of operative mortality in octogenarians undergoing coronary bypass. *Ann Thorac Surg* (1995) **60**:1038–43.
12. Ko W, Gold JP, Lazzaro R et al. Survival analysis of octogenarian patients with coronary artery disease managed by elective coronary artery bypass surgery versus conventional medical treatment. *Circulation* (1992) **86** (Suppl II):191–7.
13. Kaul TK, Fields BL, Wyatt DA. Angioplasty versus coronary artery bypass in octogenarians. *Ann Thorac Surg* (1994) **58**:1419–26.
14. Morris RJ, Strong MD, Grunewald KE et al. Internal thoracic artery for coronary artery grafting in octogenarians. *Ann Thorac Surg* (1996) **62**:16–22.
15. Gardner TJ, Horneffer PJ, Manolio TA et al. Stroke following coronary artery bypass grafting: a ten-year study. *Ann Thorac Surg* (1985) **40**:574–81.
16. Naunheim KS, Dean PA, Fiore AC et al. Cardiac surgery in the octogenarian. *Eur J Cardiothorac Surg* (1990) **4**:130–5.
17. Mick MJ, Simpfendorfer C, Arnold AZ et al. Early and late results of coronary angioplasty and bypass in octogenarians. *Am J Cardiol* (1991) **68**:1316–20.
18. Ko W, Krieger KH, Lazenby WD et al. Isolated coronary artery bypass grafting in one hundred consecutive octogenarian patients. A multivariate analysis. *J Thorac Cardiovasc Surg* (1991) **102**:532–8.
19. Cane ME, Chen C, Bailey BM et al. CABG in octogenarians: early and late events and actuarial survival in comparison with a matched population. *Ann Thorac Surg* (1995) **60**: 1033–7.
20. Glower DD, Christopher TD, Milano CA et al. Performance status and outcome after coronary artery bypass grafting in persons aged 80 to 93 years. *Am J Cardiol* (1992) **70**:567–71.
21. Tsai TP, Nessim S, Kass RM et al. Morbidity and mortality after coronary bypass surgery in octogenarians. *Ann Thorac Surg* (1991) **51**:983–6.

22. Talwalkar NG, Damus PS, Durban LH et al. Outcome of isolated coronary artery bypass surgery in octogenarians. *J Card Surg* (1996) **11**:172–9.

23. Akins CW, Daggett WM, Vlahakes CG et al. Cardiac operations in patients 80 years old and older. *Ann Thorac Surg* (1997) **64**:606–14.

24. Ranger WR, Glover JL, Shannon FL et al. Coronary artery bypass and valve replacement in octogenarians. *Am Surg* (1996) **62**:941–6.

25. Curtis JJ, Walls JT, Boley TM et al. Coronary revascularization in the elderly: determinants of operative mortality. *Ann Thorac Surg* (1994) **58**:1069–72.

26. STS Database, STS on the web: http://www.sts.org

27. D'Agostino RS, Svensson LG, Neumann DJ et al. Screening carotid ultrasonography and risk factors for stroke in coronary artery surgery patients. *Ann Thorac Surg* (1996) **62**:1714–23.

28. Newman MF, Wolman R, Kanchuger M et al. Multicenter preoperative stroke risk index for patients undergoing coronary artery bypass graft surgery. Multicenter Study of Perioperative Ischemia (McSPI) Research Group. *Circulation* (1996) **94**(Suppl II):74–80.

29. Gersh BJ, Kronmal RA, Schaff HV et al. Long-term (5-year) results of coronary bypass surgery in patients 65 years old or older: a report from the Coronary Artery Surgery Study. *Circulation* (1983) **68**(Suppl II): 190–9.

30. Click RL, Espinosa RE, Khandera BK et al. Source of embolism: utility of transesophageal echocardiography. In: Freeman WK, Seward JB, Khandheria BK et al, eds, *Transesophageal Echocardiography* (Little Brown: Boston, 1994) 490.

17

Cardiac rehabilitation in the aged patient
Carl J Lavie and Richard V Milani

Introduction

Coronary heart disease (CHD) continues to be a major threat to health in older Americans, who account for over 75% of total CHD mortality and over 50% of all acute myocardial infarctions (MI) in the United States.[1–4] Older patients with MI have higher morbidity and mortality, and they often require longer hospitalizations and develop more deconditioning, which further increases their overall morbidity. Although many physicians believe that life expectancy in the elderly is short, statistics indicate otherwise. In fact, the average 65 year old patient can expect to live 15–20 more years and function independently for most of this time. Even the person older than 80 years of age can expect to live approximately 7–10 more years and will function independently for about half of this time.[5–8] Although elderly persons with CHD will probably have reduced longevity compared with elderly persons without CHD, it seems likely that even very elderly individuals with CHD are often functionally very active and should benefit from primary and, particularly, secondary prevention strategies such as cardiac rehabilitation programs.

However, despite the high prevalence of CHD among very elderly, as well as the considerable morbidity and mortality due to CHD in the very elderly, there appears to be a strong age bias in the prevention and treatment of this disease.[1,2,5] This has been

demonstrated for the treatment of acute MI, as well as for numerous preventive strategies, including cardiac rehabilitation. In fact, data from Ades et al, as well as from our institution, indicate that elderly patients are less likely to be referred for cardiac rehabilitation and exercise training programs.[9–12] In addition, studies have indicated that the strength of the physician's recommendation for cardiac rehabilitation also has a major impact on whether the referred patient will actually attend the program. Ades et al have also reported that even when the elderly are referred for cardiac rehabilitation, the strength of the recommendation is relatively weak.[10,11] Not surprisingly, therefore, elderly patients are considerably less likely to attend cardiac rehabilitation and exercise training programs.[1,2,9–13]

Background

Cardiovascular rehabilitation can be defined as the process of developing and maintaining a desirable level of physical, social and psychological function after the onset of a cardiovascular illness.[14,15] Specific goals of cardiac rehabilitation programs include stratifying risk, improving psychological and emotional well-being, modifying CHD risk factors, decreasing symptoms, and particularly in the very elderly, improving functional capacity and quality of life, as well as overall morbidity and mortality. Although cardiac rehabilitation

Phase	Type	Duration
I	Inpatient	3–7 days
II	Outpatient, immediately after hospital stay	12 weeks
III	Late recovery	6 months beyond phase II
IV	Maintenance	Lifetime

Table 17.1
Phases of cardiac rehabilitation

primarily involves nurses, exercise physiologists, dietitians and physicians, a variety of skills and expertise are often required from other health-care professionals. In addition, although the exercise component of cardiac rehabilitation is often emphasized, the benefits of cardiac rehabilitation programs are derived from the efforts directed at psychological factors, education (for both the patient and family, especially the spouse), as well as from the exercise portion of the program.

The cardiac rehabilitation process has been arbitrarily divided into four phases (Table 17.1). The in-hospital phase (phase 1) and the immediate outpatient phase (phase II) are the most important for patients following acute CHD events, particularly for the very elderly.

Phase I cardiac rehabilitation

Although the importance of inpatient cardiac rehabilitation has been decreasing, especially with the progressive increase in intensity and reduction in duration of hospital stays following an acute CHD event, this phase is probably more important for the very elderly than for younger patients with CHD events. The

physical activity portion of the inpatient program involves a range of motion exercises, self-care activities and supervised and progressive ambulation. These activities are even more important in the very elderly who are often more deconditioned at baseline and who have other medical and significant musculoskeletal limitations compared with younger CHD patients. Typically, an upper limit of heart rate of 15–20 beats per minute above the resting rate is used. Early and rapid mobilization after an uncomplicated MI does not increase infarct size, decrease ejection fraction or worsen prognosis. The short-term benefit of inpatient rehabilitation includes reduction in orthostatic symptoms, thromboembolism, joint complications and hypoventilation, all of which are extremely important in the very elderly. In addition, improvement in psychological state and sense of well-being, early return to previous activity and employment (which is, of course, less common in the very elderly), and potentially decreasing in-hospital stay are all goals of the phase I program.

Psychological problems, particularly depression, are quite prevalent in patients with CHD, including elderly patients, and are often worsened following acute events.[16–19] Careful education and encouragement are generally all that are necessary, with particular emphasis on the 'normal' psychological and emotional reactions to major cardiac events, stress education, and, at times, relaxation training. In addition, considerable data have emphasized that sexual dysfunction is quite prevalent after acute CHD events, and surprising to some, many very elderly continue to be sexually active. In this regard, education about the acute event and the energy cost of sexual activity is extremely helpful in returning elderly patients to their 'normal' sexual activity. Exercise testing and training are helpful in increasing both the patient's and, more importantly in many situations, the partner's confidence and sense of well-being. The energy used during most sexual activity is less than 5 METs (probably 3–4 METs in most elderly), which is less than climbing 1–2 flights of stairs. Therefore, most elderly patients, if they were sexually active before the CHD event, are able to return to sexual activity almost immediately following small CHD events, whereas others can generally return to their usual sexual activity within 2–3 weeks following clinical events with more significant myocardial damage.

Phase II cardiac rehabilitation

The details of the outpatient phase II cardiac rehabilitation and exercise training program, including specifics related to the elderly and very elderly, have been extensively reviewed elsewhere.[1,2,13,17,20,21] Traditionally, patients have entered outpatient programs no more than 4–6 weeks after their major CHD event, but now vigorous efforts are being made to have more patients enter the program 1–2 weeks after hospitalization, during a time when patients' 'memories' of the acute event are more fresh and when physical limitations in the elderly are more pronounced.

At our institution, patients participate in an outpatient phase II program that lasts approximately 12 weeks and consists of 36 educational and exercise sessions. Although more than 95% of elderly patients are referred for cardiac rehabilitation following major cardiac events at our institution, only 25–30% of these patients commonly attend the program. Other studies in the literature indicate that elderly patients are less likely to be referred for cardiac rehabilitation; at our center, the percentage of referrals is similar in older and younger patients. However, only 15–20% of the very elderly actually attend our program, which is considerably lower than the attendance rate for younger cardiac patients. The duration of the program is occasionally altered based on the patient's ability to progress in improving risk factors, and, more importantly in the very elderly, in developing independence in performing and monitoring the individually prescribed exercise program.

Each exercise session consists of 10 minutes of warm-up calisthenics and stretching, 30–40 minutes of continuous upright dynamic exercise consisting of various combinations of walking, bicycling, and occasionally slow jogging in the more fit elderly. Other activities combined with light isometric exercise, such as hand weights are included and these are followed by a 10-minute cool-down period of calisthenics and stretching. It has been shown that at any level of oxygen uptake, vigorous isometric exercise raises heart rate and systemic vascular resistance and lowers stroke volume and cardiac output more than dynamic exercise. For this reason, vigorous isometric exercises are contraindicated in cardiac patients. In particular the very elderly and those with significant left ventricular systolic dysfunction may have an even greater adverse response, for example exaggerated increases in systemic vascular resistance and left ventricular end-diastolic pressure with marked decreases in stroke volume, cardiac output and ejection fraction. Despite these factors, however, some isometric activity and strengthening exercises are regularly prescribed in most cardiac rehabilitation programs. This may be even more important in the more deconditioned elderly patients who may have considerably lower amounts of muscle mass. Because many daily activities involve mostly isometric exercise and because regular performance of light isometric exercise (e.g. hand weights) may decrease heart rate, systolic pressure, and oxygen consumption at submaximal isometric workloads, light isometric exercises are safe and improve the quality of life in many cardiac patients, particularly the very elderly and those with left ventricular dysfunction.

The exercise intensity for very elderly patients is prescribed on an individual basis, based on exercise stress testing results and individual patient characteristics. The patient's exercise heart rate is targeted at 65–85% of the maximal heart rate and is at least 10–15 beats per minute below the level of any exercise-induced symptomatic or silent myocardial ischemia. Initially, a conservative intensity of exercise is often prescribed for more deconditioned elderly patients, who have an average exercise capacity that is 25–50% lower than that of younger patients. In addition, longer warm-up and cool-down periods may be required due to reduced cutaneous blood flow and temperature regulation, and slow rise and fall in heart rate due to decreased catecholamine sensitivity.[2] Cardiovascular training in the very elderly should certainly take into consideration the marked differences in overall cardiovascular profile in elderly and younger patients (Table 17.2).[22] In

addition to the supervised portion of the program, patients are encouraged to exercise 1–3 times per week outside the formal program, and periodically exercise prescriptions are adjusted to encourage gradual increases in exercise performance. Dietary counseling is also employed, and patients are frequently encouraged by exercise physiologists, nurses, dietitians and physicians to comply with both the dietary and exercise portions of the program. All patients (and sometimes spouses or adult children) attend daily teaching sessions in all aspects of CHD and its prevention, including emphasis on stress management, psychological and behavioral factors, as well as sexual adaptation to cardiac disease.

Before entering the cardiac rehabilitation and exercise training program, all patients undergo symptom-limited graded exercise testing to determine the onset of myocardial ischemia, as well as to determine the individ-

1.	Increase in vascular stiffness and systolic blood pressure
2.	Left ventricular hypertrophy
3.	Diastolic dysfunction and relaxation abnormality
4.	Lower peak heart rate
5.	Slightly reduced cardiac output
6.	Increased peripheral vascular resistance
7.	Reduced peak oxygen consumption
8.	Lower plasma renin activity
9.	Reduced sensitivity to catecholamines
10.	Reduction in skin blood flow

Table 17.2
Cardiovascular adaptations in the elderly

ual's exercise prescription. From these data, exercise capacity is either estimated in metabolic equivalents (METs), or for the more recently enrolled patients, the amount of oxygen per kilogram per minute is precisely measured by cardiopulmonary exercise assessment. The majority of the patients, particularly the more recently enrolled elderly, undergo exercise testing using an intermediate ramping protocol where treadmill speed and incline are slowly increased in 15 second increments.[23,24] In some patients, an even less vigorous treadmill protocol or an upright bicycle ergometric study is performed before and after the cardiac rehabilitation program.

1.	Improves exercise capacity
2.	Improves plasma lipids
3.	Reduces indices of obesity
4.	May decrease insulin resistance
5.	Improves behavioral characteristics
6.	Improves quality of life parameters
7.	Reduces subsequent hospitalization costs
8.	Reduces subsequent morbidity and mortality

Table 17.3
Potential benefits of outpatient, phase II cardiac rehabilitation programs

Benefits of cardiac rehabilitation

Substantial evidence has now demonstrated the benefits of Phase II cardiac rehabilitation and exercise training programs in patients after major CHD events; these include significant improvements in exercise capacity, lipids, obesity indices, behavioral characteristics and quality of life (Table 17.3), and involve several studies of elderly cohorts.[1,2,10,13,14,17,20,21,25,26] Although not specifically studied in subgroups of elderly patients, Ades and colleagues demonstrated in a study of 500 patients that subsequent hospitalization costs, excluding physicians fees, were reduced by over 35% in patients attending cardiac rehabilitation programs.[27] Likewise, in a meta-analysis of mostly nonelderly groups of over 2000 patients enrolled in 22 separate randomized studies, those randomized to formal cardiac rehabilitation and exercise training programs had significant 20–25% reductions in major CHD events, including fatal MI and total mortality during a 3-year follow-up period. Sudden death was reduced significantly by 37% after 1 year with strong trends of benefit (which

were not quite significant statistically) for cardiac rehabilitation after 2 and 3 years.[28]

Although cardiac rehabilitation programs are known to improve most CHD risk factors, the most substantial benefit is noted in exercise capacity and overall levels of physical fitness. Numerous epidemiological studies have demonstrated the importance of exercise and fitness levels for reducing CHD risk factors and overall CHD events and mortality; and improvements in exercise capacity and fitness have resulted in reduction in overall cardiovascular risk, as well as all-cause mortality.[29–33] In fact, some studies have suggested that the greatest reduction in mortality with exercise training occurs in the elderly.[29–31] Several earlier studies have shown improvements in exercise capacity following exercise training programs in the elderly.[10,34] In addition, a recent study from Belgium confirmed the prognostic value of training-induced changes in peak aerobic capacity following outpatient cardiac rehabilitation programs after MI or coronary artery bypass grafting.[35]

Ochsner studies in the elderly

We recently compared the benefits of cardiac rehabilitation and exercise training in 199 elderly CHD patients and 259 younger patients.[13] At baseline, as we previously demonstrated in a similar cohort of patients,[1] elderly patients had significantly lower exercise capacity (−28%), triglycerides, body mass indices (BMI), hostility scores and overall function scores, as well as a higher percentage body fat and higher levels of high-density lipoprotein (HDL) cholesterol than did the younger patients. The two groups were statistically similar regarding all other major baseline factors.

Following formal cardiac rehabilitation and exercise training programs, this large elderly cohort demonstrated modest improvements in total and low-density lipoprotein (LDL) cholesterol (−2 and −3%, respectively), HDL-cholesterol (+3%; $P = 0.03$) and LDL/HDL ratio (−5%; $P = 0.05$). The elderly, however, showed dramatic improvements in estimated exercise capacity (+43%; $P < 0.001$) and modest improvements in obesity indices. Almost all behavioral components and the quality of life improved significantly in the elderly patients after cardiac rehabilitation. The improvements in most of the parameters that were studied were statistically similar in older and younger patients; however, the elderly actually had greater improvements in exercise capacity (+43% versus +32%; $P < 0.01$) and in mental health scores (+5 versus +2%; $P = 0.05$) than did younger patients.

In a study of a small cohort of very elderly patients aged at least 75 years ($N = 54$), we also demonstrated very significant improvements in CHD risk factors, behavioral characteristics and quality of life components.[20] Compared with patients younger than 60 years, the very elderly had greater relative improvements in exercise capacity, overall quality of life, well-being and hostility scores and had statistically similar improvements in all other parameters. These two studies further support the fact that the elderly, including groups of patients well over the age of 75 years, should not only be referred to but should be vigorously encouraged to attend formal cardiac rehabilitation and exercise training programs following major CHD events. In fact, since the very elderly had 42% lower exercise capacity at baseline compared to younger patients, the improvements may be even more 'clinically significant' in this group compared with younger patients, who had fairly good baseline exercise capacity.

In addition, elderly women are probably the largest growing segment in society and in cardiology practices, and members of this group are the least likely to be referred to and to attend cardiac rehabilitation programs.[21] We recently analyzed the results of cardiac rehabilitation in 70 elderly women (mean age 71 years) and compared the effects of this therapy with that of 574 other patients (91% men; mean age 61 years).

At baseline, elderly women had 26% lower exercise capacity and 7% higher BMI, higher percentage of body fat (+29%), and higher levels of total cholesterol, LDL-cholesterol and HDL-cholesterol than did the other patients. Both groups were statistically similar regarding other parameters studied. Following the cardiac rehabilitation and exercise training program, elderly women had significant improvements in exercise capacity (+30%), obesity indices (BMI −2% and percentage body fat −10%), and in LDL/HDL ratio (−12%) and borderline improvements in triglycerides (−13%; $P = 0.08$). For most parameters, the improvements following cardiac rehabilitation were statistically similar in the elderly women and other patients. However, elderly women had significantly greater improvements in obesity indices, including BMI (-2% versus 0%; $P < 0.03$) and percentage body fat (-10 versus -5%; $P = < 0.01$), compared with the other patients. The improvements may be particularly noteworthy since obesity seems to be a stronger CHD risk factor in women than in men. In other studies, we demonstrated the marked benefits of cardiac rehabilitation and exercise training in obese CHD patients, particularly in those who were more successful with even modest weight reduction.[25,36] Elderly women also had significant improvements in anxiety, somatization, total quality of life and six other components studied, as well as borderline improvements (-31%; $P = 0.07$) in depression scores following cardiac rehabilitation.

Numerous studies have demonstrated that depression is prevalent following CHD events and that it may be involved in the pathogenesis of CHD and affect recovery following CHD events.[16–19] We recently reported a study of 268 consecutive elderly patients following CHD events; 18% met criteria for depression by validated questionnaire.[17] Depressed elderly patients had reduced exercise capacity and lower levels of HDL-cholesterol than did other elderly. In addition, the depressed elderly patients also had significantly more symptoms of anxiety, hostility and somatization, and reduced scores for quality of life and all other components studied. Following the cardiac rehabilitation program, the depressed elderly had modest improvements in traditional CHD risk factors, but had marked improvements in depression score (-57%), anxiety (-53%), hostility (-36%) and somatization (-39%). They also had a 32% improvement in quality of life score with marked improvements noted in all of the subgroups studied. The marked improvements noted in the depressed elderly

in behavioral factors and quality of life components were statistically greater than the improvements in the other elderly patients. These data indicate that depression remains prevalent in elderly CHD patients after major cardiac events, a factor that is often unrecognized. Furthermore, elderly CHD patients enrolled in cardiac rehabilitation programs benefit from significant reductions in the prevalence and severity of depression.

Severe left ventricular dysfunction

Traditionally, congestive heart failure (CHF) was considered a contraindication to exercise training and such patients have often been encouraged to maintain a sedentary lifestyle.[14] Since CHF is the most frequent DRG diagnosis in the United States, this seems to be most applicable to the elderly population, who have high prevalence of both systolic and/or diastolic CHF. In fact, CHF patients are often not referred to cardiac rehabilitation and exercise training programs.

In the late 1980s, we reported the outcomes of 20 consecutive post-MI patients, with an average resting ejection fraction of 21%, who participated in cardiac rehabilitation and exercise training programs.[37] These patients had a nearly 40% improvement in exercise capacity, nearly 60% returned to work, and most continued to exercise long after the program had ended. More importantly, there were no complications of the exercise program in this cohort and we were encouraged by the seemingly low annualized mortality rate of only 8% over 3 years. Several other investigators have now confirmed our data regarding the ability of patients with severely reduced left ventricular contractility to improve their functional capacity, and have excellent prognosis with minimal complications due to exercise training programs.[14]

Safety of cardiac rehabilitation

A major concern regards the safety of vigorous exercise for many groups, particularly elderly patients who have survived cardiovascular events. Although almost all epidemiological studies have demonstrated the benefits of regular physical activity and physical fitness to protect against major CHD events, several studies have indicated that sudden cardiac death occurs more frequently following vigorous physical activity, particularly in subjects who are normally very sedentary.[14] These factors are often emphasized both to the lay public and by many general physicians.

Although there are no large studies in the very elderly (or even those over 65 years), the best data regarding the safety of exercise in CHD patients comes from Van Camp and Peterson, who pooled data from 167 randomly selected cardiac rehabilitation and exercise training programs.[38] Their data from over 57 000 patients and over 2 000 000 exercise hours, identified only 21 cardiac events (three fatal and eight nonfatal MIs) during exercise training. This accounts for approximately one cardiac event per over 100 000 exercise hours,

one acute MI per 300 000 exercise hours and one fatality per nearly 1 000 000 exercise hours. These data, collected before the era of increased revascularization following acute CHD events and better medical treatments as well, demonstrate the overall safety of regular physical exercise training even after major CHD events.

Summary and conclusions

Cardiac rehabilitation and exercise training programs have been shown to have numerous benefits following major CHD events, noted in several studies of elderly (and very elderly) patients. These improvements include marked improvements in exercise capacity, modest improvements in lipids and obesity indices, and marked improvements in behavioral characteristics (including subgroups of depressed elderly patients) and in quality of life and all of its components. In addition, this therapy seems to reduce subsequent medical costs and major CHD morbidity and mortality. In the future, greater effort has to be made to reduce the costs but, at the same time, maintain the effectiveness of this critical therapy.[39] In addition, improved access to this therapy, especially increasing home cardiac rehabilitation, would seem to be most appropriate for the elderly population.

References

1. Lavie CJ, Milani RV, Littman AB. Benefits of cardiac rehabilitation and exercise training in secondary coronary prevention in the elderly. *J Am Coll Cardiol* (1993) **22**:678–83.
2. Lavie CJ, Milani RV, Cassidy MM, Gilliland YE. Benefits of cardiac rehabilitation and exercise training in older persons. *Am J Geriatr Cardiol* (1995) **4**:42–8.
3. National Center for Health Statistics. *Advanced Report of Final Mortality Statistic, 1988 Monthly Vital Statistics Report.* Hyattsville, Maryland: Public Health Service (1990) **39**(Supplement 7):1–48.
4. National Center for Health Statistics *National Hospital Discharge Survey* (United States Department of Health and Human Services: Washington, DC, 1987).
5. Yusuf S, Furberg CD. Are we biased in our approach to treating elderly patients with heart disease? *Am J Cardiol* (1991) **68**:54–6.
6. Spencer G. *Projections of the Populations of the United States by Age, Sex, and Race: 1988–2080.* US Bureau of the Census. Current population reports, series P-25, No. 1018. US Governmental Printing Office: Washington, DC, 1989) 1–17.
7. Black JS, Sefeik T, Kapoor W. Health promotion and disease prevention in the elderly: comparison of house staff and attending physician attitudes and practices. *Arch Intern Med* (1990) **150**:389–92.
8. Stults BM. Preventive health care for the elderly. *West J Med* (1984) **141**:832–45.
9. Ades PA, Meacham CP, Handy MA et al. The cardiac rehabilitation program of the University of Vermont Medical Center. *J Cardiopulmon Rehab* (1986) **5**:265–77.
10. Ades PA, Waldmann ML, Pok DM et al. Referral patterns and exercise response in the rehabilitation of female coronary patients ages > 62 years. *Am J Cardiol* (1992) **69**:1422–5.
11. Ades PA, Waldmann ML, McCann WJ et al. Predictors of cardiac rehabilitation participation in older coronary patients. *Arch Intern Med* (1992) **152**:1033–5.
12. Banks BC, Lavie CJ, Milani RV. Analysis of risk status in elderly and young in-patients with acute coronary syndromes. *Chest* (1992) **102**(Supplement):57S.
13. Lavie CJ, Milani RV. Effects of cardiac rehabilitation programs on exercise capacity, coronary risk factors, behavioral characteristics, and quality of life in a large elderly cohort. *Am J Cardiol* (1995) **76**:177–9.
14. Lavie CJ, Milani RV. Cardiac rehabilitation. In: Brown DC, ed., *Textbook of Cardiac Intensive Care.* (WB Saunders: Philadelphia, 1998) 329–35.
15. Squires RW, Gau GT, Miller TD et al. Cardiovascular rehabilitation: status, 1990. *Mayo Clin Proc* (1990) **65**:731–55.
16. Milani RV, Lavie CJ, Cassidy MM. Effects of cardiac rehabilitation and exercise training programs on depression in patients after major coronary events. *Am Heart J* (1996) **132**: 726–32.
17. Milani RV, Lavie CJ. Prevalence and effects of cardiac rehabilitation on depression in the elderly with coronary artery disease. *Am J Cardiol* (1998) **81**:1233–6.
18. Milani RV, Lavie CJ. Behavioral differences and effects of cardiac rehabilitation in diabetic patients following cardiac events. *Am J Med* (1996) **100**:517–23.
19. Milani RV, Littman AB, Lavie CJ. Psychological adaptation to cardiovascular disease. In: Messerli FH, ed., *Cardiovascular Diseases in the Elderly*, 3rd edn. (Kluwer: Massachussetts, Norwell, 1993) 401–12.
20. Lavie CJ, Milani RV. Effects of cardiac rehabilitation programs in very elderly patients ≥75 years of age. *Am J Cardiol* (1996) **78**:675–7.
21. Lavie CJ, Milani RV. Benefits of cardiac rehabilitation and exercise training in elderly women. *Am J Cardiol* (1997) **79**:664–6.
22. Lavie CJ, Milani RV, Boykin C. Cardiac rehabilitation, exercise training, and preventive cardiology in the elderly. *Cardio.* September (1993) 47–52.
23. Rubin SM, Sidney S, Black DM et al. High blood cholesterol in elderly men and the excess risk for coronary heart disease. *Ann Intern Med* (1990) **113**:916–20.

24. Lavie CJ, Milani RV, Boykin C. High-density lipoprotein cholesterol is the strongest lipid risk factor in elderly coronary patients. *J Cardiopulmon Rehab* (1993) **13**:334 (abst).

25. Lavie CJ, Milani RV. Effects of cardiac rehabilitation, exercise training, and weight reduction on exercise capacity, coronary risk factors, behavioral characteristics and quality of life in obese patients with coronary artery disease. *Am J Cardiol* (1997) **79**:394–401.

26. Ades PA, Meacham CP, Handy MA et al. The cardiac rehabilitation program of the University of Vermont Medical Center. *J Cardiopulmon Rehab* (1986) **5**:265–77.

27. Ades PA, Huang D, Weaver SO. Cardiac rehabilitation participation predicts lower rehospitalization cost. *Am Heart J* (1992) **123**: 916–21.

28. O'Connor GT, Buring JE, Yusuf S et al. An overview of randomized trials of rehabilitation with exercise after myocardial infarction. *Circulation* (1989) **80**:234–44.

29. Paffenbarger RS Jr, Hyde RT, Wing AL et al. Physical activity. All-cause mortality and longevity of college alumni. *N Engl J Med* (1986) **314**:605–13.

30. Kannel WB, Balanger A, D'Agostino R et al. Physical activity and physical demand on the job and risk of cardiovascular disease and death: The Framingham study. *Am Heart J* (1986) **112**: 820–4.

31. Lavie CJ, Milani RV, Squires RW et al. Exercise and the heart: good, benign, or evil? *Postgrad Med* (1992) **91**:130–50.

32. Blair WN, Kohl HW III, Paffenbarger RS et al. Physical fitness and all-cause mortality: a prospective study of healthy men and women. *JAMA* (1989) **262**:2395–401.

33. Blair WN, Kohl HW III, Barlow CE et al. Changes in physical fitness and all-cause mortality: a prospective study of healthy and unhealthy men. *JAMA* (1995) **273**:1093–8.

34. Milani RV, Littman AB, Lavie CJ. Simplified depression index predicts functional improvement following cardiac rehabilitation and exercise program, abstract. *Clin Res* (1991) **39**:414A.

35. Vanhees L, Fagard R, Thijs L et al. Prognostic value of training-induced change in peak exercise capacity in patients with myocardial infarcts and patients with coronary bypass surgery. *Am J Cardiol* (1995) **76**:1014–19.

36. Lavie CJ, Milani RV. Effects of cardiac rehabilitation and exercise training in obese patients with coronary artery disease. *Chest* (1996) **109**:52–6.

37. Squires RW, Lavie CJ, Brandt TR et al. Cardiac rehabilitation in patients with severe ischemic left ventricular dysfunction. *Mayo Clin Proc* (1987) **62**:997–1002.

38. Van Camp SP, Peterson RA. Cardiovascular complications of outpatient cardiac rehabilitation programs. *JAMA* (1986) **256**:1160–3.

39. Lavie CJ, Milani RV. Cardiac rehabilitation and health-care reform. *Chest* (1995) **107**: 1189–90.

18

Hypertension
W Dallas Hall

Introduction
Definitions

In this chapter, 'hypertension' (HBP) is defined as a repeated (i.e. on two or more consecutive occasions after an initial reading) systolic blood pressure (BP) of 140 mmHg or over *or* a diastolic BP of 90 mmHg or more. 'Isolated systolic HBP' (ISH) is defined as a systolic BP (SBP) of 140 mmHg or over and a diastolic BP (DBP) less than 90 mmHg.[1] 'Elderly' is categorized according to the decade of age: sexagenarian (60–69 years), septuagenarian (70–79 years), octogenarian (80–89 years), nonagenarian (90–99 years) or centenarian (≥100 years) (Table 18.1).

Age range (years)	Terminology
60–69	Sexagenarian
70–79	Septuagenarian
80–89	Octogenarian
90–99	Nonagenarian
≥100	Centenarian

Table 18.1
Nomenclature of the elderly

Measurement of blood pressure
Pseudohypertension and pseudohypotension

Pseudohypertension is a condition in which the cuff BP overestimates the true (i.e. intra-arterial) BP because of a stiff, often calcified brachial artery. In previous years, it was suspected clinically by a positive Osler's sign in which the radial artery remained easily palpable despite increasing the cuff pressure above the auscultated SBP. Recent studies, however, cast serious doubt on the validity and clinical use of the Osler's maneuver.[2,3] Pseudohypertension can only be confirmed by direct and near simultaneous comparison of the cuff and intra-arterial BP. Intra-arterial measurement of BP is rarely indicated in elderly hypertensives, but the levels can be obtained easily if the patient has other indications for cardiac catheterization or renal or femoral angiography.

Pseudohypotension is a condition in which the cuff BP underestimates the true (i.e. intra-arterial) BP because of extensive unilateral atherosclerosis or chronic occlusion of the subclavian artery. It is suspected clinically by a 30 mmHg or more BP difference between the two arms, a slight unilateral decrease in the brachial artery pulsation, and an infraclavicular bruit near the arm with the lower BP. Use the value in the arm with the highest pressure for clinical management, and tell the patient to always have the BP measured in that arm.

Falsely low SBP measurements also occur in elderly patients with an auscultatory gap, especially common with valvular aortic stenosis.[4] Korotkoff sounds may be heard at 180 mmHg, and then disappear until they recur at 140 mmHg. The SBP would be thought erroneously to be 140 mmHg when it is actually 180 mmHg. The clinical and prognostic significance of an auscultatory gap was summarized recently by Cavallini et al[5] who noted the gap in 21% of older hypertensives (average age 64 years). Auscultatory gap was associated with age, female gender, increased arterial stiffness and increased prevalence of atherosclerotic carotid plaques. It may well have prognostic importance.

Variability, circadian patterns, and the 'white-coat' effect

BP is more variable in the elderly.[6] This is partly because of a higher level of SBP, which is especially variable.[7] For example, Fotherby and Potter[8] reported office (i.e. three resting measurements 2 minutes apart) and home ambulatory BP levels in 69 elderly patients (aged 66–86, average 76 years) with office SBP greater than 150 mmHg. Clinic SBP fell an average of 11 mmHg from the first to the third reading. Daytime home SBP averaged 17 mmHg below the lowest of the clinic readings! Tell the patient that it is not uncommon for the SBP to vary transiently 40–50 mmHg during normal daily activities.

A white-coat effect occurs in 15–20% of all hypertensives,[9,10] but it is even more common in older persons, especially women.[11] In some patients, BP can increase as much as 20–40 mmHg during an office visit. The white-coat phenomenon is suspected if the patient reports much lower BP at home. It can

be confirmed by home BP measurements immediately before and after the office visit, or by ambulatory BP monitoring.[12]

Most sexagenarians and septuagenarians have the usual nocturnal decrease in BP (i.e. about 7–14 mmHg systolic and 7–13 mmHg diastolic).[13,14] This pattern, however, may differ in octogenarians and nonagenarians. Few data are available, but one study of 52 very old subjects (aged 80–95, average 86 years) reported *no* difference in clinic versus daytime home ambulatory SBP, and a marked blunting of the usual nocturnal decrease in BP, especially in women.[15] The persistence of elevated nocturnal BP levels in the very old is not readily explained by altered sleeping patterns.[16] There is some evidence, however, that the diurnal variation in BP is related to autonomic nervous system function whereby dippers have lower sympathetic nervous system activity and nondippers have lower parasympathetic nervous system activity and higher plasma catecholamines.[17,18] Interesting are reports of more silent cerebrovascular disease (i.e. lacunae and periventricular hyperintensity on magnetic resonance imaging) in nondippers,[19] and loss of the nocturnal decrease in BP after stroke.[20]

Orthostatic hypotension

Orthostatic hypotension is defined as a decrease in SBP of 20 mmHg or more on rising from the supine (or seated) to the standing position. When measured after 1 and 3 minutes of standing, it is present before therapy in one of every six elderly (aged 60–96 years) patients with hypertension.[21] Orthostatic hypotension is a common and often unrecognized cause of dizziness or syncope in the elderly. Be cautious with the use of alpha-blockers or higher diuretic doses in these patients. Reduction of BP by therapy with most other antihypertensive agents can be associated with a decrease in the prevalence of orthostatic hypotension in elderly hypertensives.[22]

Postprandial hypotension

Postprandial hypotension also occurs in elderly hypertensives.[23] Decreases in SBP of 20 mmHg or more can occur 30–120 minutes after a meal and can be associated with dizziness, syncope or falls. It may be caused by vasodilation related to an exaggerated insulin response to a glucose load.[24] In elderly hypertensives, make decisions about BP control or titration of drug doses in context of whether the patient has eaten breakfast or lunch in the 1 or 2 hours just preceding the office visit.

Clinical evaluation
Physical examination

Physical examination of hypertensive individuals aged 80 or more is essentially the same as for sexagenarians and septuagenarians with a few exceptions. The high likelihood of advanced atherosclerosis makes it even more important to:

- Initially measure BP in both arms and use only the arm with the highest BP for all subsequent determinations;
- measure the 1 to 3 minute standing BP (at least initially);
- detect sinus bradycardia of 55 beats per minute or less because this may influence the use of beta-blockers or nondihydropyridine calcium channel antagonists (CCAs), and will certainly curtail the combined use of these two drug classes; and
- give special attention to the detection of carotid, renal or femoral bruits. The presence of carotid bruits may slow the desired rapidity with which BP control is achieved. High-pitched upper abdominal bruits that

radiate laterally are of special interest because of the high prevalence of renal artery stenosis in patients 80 or more years of age,[25,26] and the risk of precipitating acute renal failure with the use of angiotensin-converting enzyme (ACE) inhibitors in patients with bilateral renal artery stenosis.[27]

Laboratory evaluation
Routine

Laboratory evaluation of hypertensive individuals age 80 or more is the same as that for those aged 60–79 years. The clinician, however, should focus specifically on five values:

- BUN-to-creatinine ratio. An abnormally high (e.g. >20) ratio is an indicator of pre-renal azotemia related to either dehydration or a low ejection fraction.[28] Use caution in beginning diuretic therapy or increasing diuretic doses in these patients;
- Serum potassium. The high prevalence of ventricular arrhythmias and the frequent use of digoxin in the elderly demands a vigilant watch for hypokalemia (i.e. serum potassium below 3.5 mmol/l). Remember also that there is normally a large diurnal variation in the serum potassium level such that values between 8 pm and midnight average 0.6 mmol/l below those obtained between 8 am and noon;[29]
- Serum sodium. A decrease in the ability of the kidney to concentrate or dilute urine is well documented with aging.[30] Baseline serum sodium levels of 135 mmol/l or less should flag concern about the risk of the relatively rare but often disastrous thiazide-induced acute hyponatremia in elderly women.[31] In patients with congestive heart failure (CHF), hyponatremia can be a clue to high renin levels with an increased risk of hypotension shortly after starting therapy

with the usual cautious dose of an ACE inhibitor;[32]

- Serum creatinine. In the Systolic Hypertension in the Elderly Program (SHEP), the average creatinine level for a 73 year old with ISH was 1.0 mg/dl (88 μmol/l). Levels of 1.2–1.4 mg/dl are deceptively abnormal in the elderly because of low muscle mass, but these levels typically reflect impaired renal function with a creatinine clearance below 40–60 ml/minute.[33] Use the Cockcroft and Gault[34] formula to make a quick and useful estimation of glomerular filtration rate (GFR) without having to obtain a 24-hour urine collection.

$$\frac{[140 - \text{age (years)}] \times \text{body weight (kg)}}{72 \times \text{serum creatinine (mg/dl)}}$$

The above formula applies to men; multiply the result by 0.85 in women. Knowing the approximate GFR is important for clinicians treating geriatric patients, particularly with regard to potential toxicity from commonly prescribed drugs that are excreted by the kidney. Examples include allopurinol, aminoglycosides, digoxin, nadolol, potassium supplements, quinidine, tetracycline, theophylline, trimethoprim-sulfamethoxazole and verapamil;

- Proteinuria. Dipstick values of 2-plus or more should provoke a re-evaluation for diabetic nephropathy although this degree of proteinuria can also occur with CHF. If the patient is anemic, also reconsider the possibility of multiple myeloma because the prevalence is so high in patients age 80 or more.

Screening tests for secondary causes

Patients aged 80 or more rarely present with primary aldosteronism; most present in the third or fourth decade and about 70% are diagnosed before age 50.[35] Only one case of pheochromocytoma is known to have presented at 80 years of age.[36] Of much greater concern is the possibility of atherosclerotic renal artery stenosis, the risk of which increases progressively with advancing age.[37] Renovascular HBP is associated with an increase in both SBP and DBP. As such, it rarely or never causes ISH with normal levels of DBP. Hence, renal arteriography is not indicated in an 84 year old women who has a treated BP that remains 230/78 mmHg. Aortic and renal artery atherosclerosis may well be present, but are unlikely to contribute to elevation of only the SBP. In contrast, new-onset DBP elevation (especially in the range 110–130 mmHg) in a previously well-controlled patient is a reason to pursue the diagnosis *if* angioplasty or surgery would be recommended should a greater than 75% narrowing of the renal artery be found. Noninvasive screening tests include a nuclear medicine ACE-enhanced renal scan, duplex Doppler flow studies and magnetic resonance angiography.[1] Select the test that has the most local experience because all three are technique- and operator-dependent. The definitive diagnosis requires renal angiography, which carries an increased risk of contrast-induced acute renal failure or atheroembolism in older patients.[38]

Epidemiology
Clinical trials in the very old

The majority of the major HBP clinical trials in the elderly include few or no individuals age 80 or more. Table 18.2 emphasizes this point. Note, for example, that essentially no octogenarians or nonagenarians were included in the MRC-elderly,[39,40] VA elderly,[41] HOT,[42,43] HDFP[44] or TONE[45,46] trials (see Table 18.3). Five clinical trials (SHEP,[47,48] SYST-EUR,[49,50]

Trial*	BP category	Age range (years)	Total number	Number aged ≥ 80
SHEP[47,48]	ISH	60–96	4736	650
SYST-EUR[49,50]	ISH	60–100	4695	441[†]
STOP-H[51,52]	HBP	70–84	1627	269
EWPHE[53–55]	HBP	60–97	840	155
HYVET[56–58]	HBP	≥ 80	2100 (goal)	2100 (goal)
MRC ELDERLY[39,40]	HBP	65–74	4396	0
VA ELDERLY[41]	HBP	60–88	690	<20
HOT[42,43]	HBP	50–80	19 736	0
HDFP[44]	HBP	30–69	5485	0
TONE[45,46]	HBP	60–80	975	0

NA, not applicable.
*See Table 18.3.
† JA Staessen, personal communication.

Table 18.2
Inclusion of the very old (≥80 years) in clinical trials on hypertension

Abbreviation	Trial name
ALLHAT	Antihypertensive and Lipid Lowering Treatment to Prevent Heart Attack Trial
EWPHE	European Working Party on Hypertension in the Elderly
HDFP	Hypertension Detection and Follow-up Program
HOT	Hypertension Optimal Treatment study
HYVET	HYpertension in the Very Elderly Trial
MRC	Medical Research Council trial of treatment of hypertension in older adults
NHANES	National Health And Nutrition Examination Survey
NHBPEP	National High Blood Pressure Education Program
SHEP	Systolic Hypertension in the Elderly Program
STOP-H	Swedish Trial in Old Patients with Hypertension
SYST-EUR	SYSTolic hypertension in elderly in EURope trial
TONE	Trials Of Non-pharmacologic Intervention in the Elderly

Table 18.3
Trial name abbreviations

STOP-H[51,52] EWPHE[53–55] and HYVET[56–58]), however, provide some data on hypertensives over age 80, although the number of such patients in each completed trial varies from 155 to 650, most of whom (i.e. 64–90%) are women. These studies cannot provide evidence-based definitive recommendations (with adequate statistical power) for the management of combined systolic–diastolic HBP in patients age 80 or more.

However, the SHEP data supporting treatment of ISH in hypertensives age 80 or more are convincing (Table 18.4).[48] The study used 12.5–25 mg daily of chlorthalidone with addition of 25–50 mg daily of atenolol as necessary to reduce SBP to less than 160 mmHg and by at least 20 mmHg. The relative risk of stroke in sexagenarians, septuagenarians and octogenarians/nonagenarians was decreased in the treatment group by 29%, 30% and 49%,

respectively. Note the *increased* benefit in the highest age group.

These data run counter to results on 155 patients aged 80 or more (90% women) in the EWPHE trial where no benefit was documented.[54,55] The EWPHE study, however, included patients with baseline DBP 90–119 mmHg, and used HCTZ (25–50 mg daily) plus triamterene (50–100 mg daily) with addition of methyldopa (250–2000 mg daily) as necessary to reduce BP to 160/90 mmHg or less. These differences between the two studies might partly explain the apparent discrepancy in the results. In addition, the SHEP results had much greater statistical power because of inclusion of 650 rather than 155 patients.

The overall SHEP results have also been analyzed for the 583 non-insulin-dependent diabetics in the trial, 58 of whom were age 80 or more.[59] The major cardiovascular disease

Age (years)	Active therapy			Placebo			Relative risk‡	Confidence interval
	N	Stroke events[†]	5-Year rate/100	N	Stroke events[†]	5-Year rate/100		
60–69	972	34	3.9	992	47	5.2	0.71	0.45–1.11
70–79	1062	48	5.4	1060	74	8.6	0.70	0.48–1.02
80+	331	21	7.5	319	38	14.0	0.51	0.29–0.89

* Modified from the SHEP Cooperative Research Group.[48]
† Fatal or nonfatal.
‡ Adjusted for age, sex, race, smoking, baseline SBP and DBP, baseline cholesterol, history of myocardial infarction.

Table 18.4
Benefit of antihypertensive therapy according to decade of age*

(CVD) event rate was reduced by 34% by active treatment in either diabetics or non-diabetics, and the absolute risk reduction was twice as great (i.e. 101 versus 51/1000) in diabetics.

The ongoing 6-year ALLHAT trial plans to enroll 40 000 high-risk hypertensives (22 000 men and 18 000 women, 55% African American) age 55 or more.[60] As of December 1997 38 500 have been randomized and 2502 (6.5%) were aged 80 or more, representing the largest such cohort of hypertensive octogenarians and nonagenarians.

Blood pressure and mortality in the very old

In 1988, Mattila et al[61] reported observational data on 561 residents of Tampere, Finland (82% women) aged 85 or more (average, 88.4 years). The 5-year mortality (72% in normotensives and 41% in hypertensives) was paradoxically highest in those with the lowest baseline stratum of either SBP (i.e. <120 mmHg) or DBP (i.e. <70 mmHg). Mortality was lowest in those with baseline SBP 160 mmHg or more or DBP 90 mmHg or more! The authors concluded that HBP in persons aged 85 or more was an indicator of an adequately functioning cardiovascular system.

Three subsequent studies from the Rancho Bernardo, California retirement community focused on this observation.[62–64] In a 10-year follow-up of 1159 men (39% mortality) and 1109 women (23% mortality) aged 65 or more, men aged 75 or more with the lowest stratum of diastolic BP (i.e. <75 mmHg) had the highest CVD and all-cause mortality, whereas higher DBP predicted greater survival, similar to the Finland study.[62] The Rancho Bernardo study, however, did not find the paradoxical association for SBP, or for women (recall that the Finland study had 82%

women). One interpretation was that the mean age (78.3 years) of the California women was lower than the Finnish cohort (88.4 years) and that the typically later onset of CVD in women[65,66] might have accounted for the absence of the paradoxical relationship in 'younger' Rancho Bernardo women.

Subsequent 3-year follow-up on the survival of 795 men and women aged 75–96 (average, 80.6 years) confirmed that men (but not women) aged 80 or more had increased survival with higher baseline levels of DBP.[63] This increased survival was not explained by lower CVD risk factors. Indeed, the inverse relation between DBP and mortality occurred primarily in the oldest men *without* a history of coronary heart disease. The question arose again whether the results for the women may have differed from the Finnish study because of an average age of 80 rather than 88. A somewhat longer (i.e. 5-year) follow-up on these 795 patients addressed the association between mortality and the 5-year change in BP.[64] Men, but not women, whose DBP fell by 5 mmHg or more over the 5 years had significantly more CVD as well as all-cause mortality (68% of the total mortality was from CVD).

Taken together, both the Finland and Rancho Bernardo studies suggest that higher DBP may be an indicator of a good prognosis for survival in the majority of patients age 80 or more.

The J-curve

There is concern that excessive reduction of the DBP in hypertensive patients with evidence of ischemic heart disease might reduce coronary blood flow and cause cardiac events, the so-called J-curve.[67,68] Although the SHEP study found no evidence of a J-curve for CVD events in treated patients with ISH,[48] a recent population-based cohort study[69] reported a four-fold increase in the risk of myocardial infarction (MI) in elderly men with treated DBP of 90 mmHg or less, even after adjustment for smoking habits, BP, duration of HBP, other cardiovascular diseases, lipids, diabetes mellitus, obesity and hypercreatininemia. Therefore, how far to reduce elevated DBP for optimal benefit remains unclear. This issue is under evaluation in the HOT study, which has randomized 19 196 patients with HBP (aged 50–80 years) to three DBP goals: 90, 85 or 80 mmHg with or without the addition of aspirin.[42,43]

Treatment

There is incontrovertible evidence that treatment of HBP decreases the risk of stroke by 33–36% and CVD by 19–22% in patients aged 60 or more.[70–72] As mentioned previously, however, few of these clinical trials included many patients aged 80 or more. Cutpoints in the national guidelines for the levels of DBP and SBP that should be treated, however, have decreased progressively over the last two decades from 115 to 105, then 90 mmHg for

DBP and from 'individualized therapy' to 160, then 140 mmHg for SBP (Figure 18.1). A recent report from a large HMO included 75 hypertensives (i.e. SBP ≥160 and/or DBP ≥95 mmHg) aged 75 or more. Of the 75, 43 (57%) were being treated, but only 28 (37%) were controlled to a level of SBP less than 160 mmHg and DBP less than 90 mmHg.[73]

Lifestyle modifications

Lenfant[74] as well as the National HBP Education Program (NHBPEP) guidelines for treatment of HBP in the elderly[75] have emphasized that lifestyle modifications and low-dose diuretics should be first choices for the management of HBP in the elderly. Lifestyle modifications include salt restriction, weight reduction, moderation of alcohol intake and increased physical activity.

Salt restriction

Advancing age is generally associated with increased salt sensitivity whereby salt loading increases and salt restriction decreases BP.[76,77]

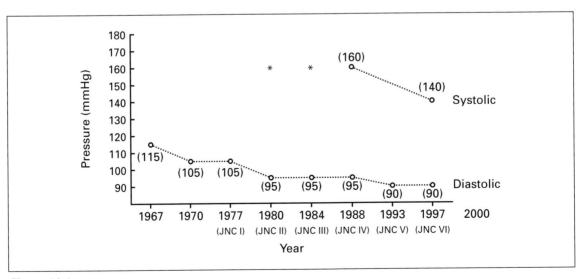

Figure 18.1
Secular trends (1967–97) in US hypertension treatment guidelines. *Individualized therapy.

Few data are available for hypertensives age 80 or more.[78] Palmer and associates[79] conducted a 16-week double-blind, placebo-controlled, randomized crossover trial on seven hypertensive patients aged 78–96 (average, 85 years). Reduction of sodium intake from 175 to 43 mmol per day was associated with an 11.0/9.1 mmHg decrease in BP, somewhat more than the 6.3/2.2 and 5.8/2.5 mmHg average reductions reported in two meta-analyses of primarily nonelderly hypertensives.[80,81] Hyponatremia or orthostatic hypotension did not occur. These data suggest that dietary sodium restriction may be as, or perhaps even more effective for reducing BP in very old hypertensives. Moderate sodium restriction is safe; any theoretical concerns are not supported by the combined evidence from multiple randomized trials of reduced sodium intake.[82] Advise most of your elderly HBP patients to maintain a sodium intake of 2400 mg daily or less.

Weight reduction, moderation of alcohol intake and increased physical activity

The Trial of Nonpharmacologic Intervention in the Elderly (TONE) included more than 900 elderly (aged 60–80 years) stage 1–2 hypertensives and documented the efficacy of weight reduction (as well as salt restriction, or both) in reducing the need to begin antihypertensive drugs.[46] There were, however, no hypertensives aged 80 or more. Similarly, there are no clinical trials of the efficacy of reduced alcohol intake or increased physical activity on the level of BP in hypertensives aged 80 or more. Data from the NHANES show a strong interaction between the level of SBP and alcohol consumption of 2 ounces or more daily.[83] Tell your very old patients with uncontrolled ISH to decrease the amount of alcohol they imbibe in the evenings.

Antihypertensive drug therapy

General

As mentioned previously, there is strong rationale for drug therapy in patients aged 80 or more with ISH (see Table 18.4).[48,84] Similar data are not yet available for patients aged 80 or more with combined systolic–diastolic HBP,[85–87] although the ALLHAT and HYVET trials are well underway. The absolute benefit of treatment, however, may be relatively small because of many competing risks for death.[88]

Adverse effects

Whatever the choice of drug therapy may be, it is safe to follow the time-tested adage, 'start low, go slow.' This is because any benefits of therapy must be balanced against drug-induced side-effects, more so for those hypertensives who have already survived to age 80 or more. These patients typically have altered drug distribution, metabolism and excretion,[89–91] but available data do not confirm the notion that adverse drug reactions increase with advancing age.[92] For example, in the diuretic- and beta-blocker-based SHEP trial, the treatment and placebo groups did not differ in overall quality of life, cognition or depression after an average follow-up period of 4.5 years.[93] Caution remains appropriate, however, especially for old patients who weigh 50 kg or less.[94] In one study of 39 free-living centenarians, the average body weight was 46.9 kg.[95] A randomized, controlled trial by Hanlon and associates[96] reported improved appropriateness of prescriptions with use of a clinical pharmacist educational program for 208 elderly (average age, 70 years) patients who were receiving five or more medications.

Diuretics

The 1994 NHBPEP Working Group on Hypertension in the Elderly recommended diuretics as the preferred initial class of drug in elderly patients.[75] JNC VI recommended that, if a diuretic was not chosen as the first drug, it was usually indicated as a second-step agent. Diuretic therapy for HBP has been defended by experts in the field.[97,98] It is supported strongly by the excellent results in patients age 80 or more in the SHEP trial.

Even very low diuretic doses (such as 12.5 mg/day HCTZ, 15 mg/day chlorthalidone, or 1.25 mg/day indapamide) are now documented to have BP-reducing efficacy.[99–103] Adverse metabolic effects such as hypokalemia, hypomagnesemia, hyperuricemia and hyperglycemia are uncommon because these are dose related. Chronic use of thiazide diuretics does not increase the risk of falling in the elderly.[104] In fact, users for 10 years or more have a significantly higher bone mass and a trend for fewer hip and wrist fractures than nonusers of similar age. This positive effect is probably related to the direct effect of thiazides to increase the renal reabsorption of calcium.

Thiazide or thiazide-like diuretics are not appropriate choices for initial therapy in certain clinical settings. These include patients who are hypokalemic or have uncontrolled hyperglycemia, gout, clinical volume depletion, severe orthostatic hypotension, hypercalcemia, symptomatic bladder outlet obstruction or a history of thiazide-induced hyponatremia, photosensitivity or allergy.

Beta-blockers

Atenolol was used as the second-line drug in the SHEP trial that included 650 octogenarians and nonagenarians with ISH. Beta-blockers are clearly the drugs of choice for elderly patients with HBP and previous MI.[105–107] They are much too underused (i.e. in only about 20%) in elderly survivors of acute MI.[108]

The initial dose should be low in elderly patients, equivalent to the 25 mg starting dose of atenolol used in SHEP. Beta-blockers are, of course, relatively contraindicated in patients with bronchospasm, significant sinus bradycardia, sick sinus syndrome or heart block greater than first degree. They are relatively contraindicated in patients with diabetes and receiving insulin and patients with significant depression. As much as 80% of topical ophthalmic medications (including beta-blockers) can be absorbed into the circulation through the nasolacrimal duct and nasal mucosa.[109] Consider this possibility in elderly patients who have unusual degrees of sinus bradycardia.

Calcium channel antagonists

Calcium channel antagonists (CCAs) are very effective for decreasing BP in elderly patients with HBP.[110,111] They may have additional beneficial effects on migraine headaches, bronchospasm, esophageal spasm and Raynaud's phenomenon.[112,113] Left ventricular (LV) diastolic dysfunction may improve after treatment with nondihydropyridine CCAs such as verapamil or diltiazem.[114] Amlodipine and felodipine (used in addition to ACE inhibitors, diuretics or digoxin) have been used safely for HBP or angina in patients with advanced LV systolic dysfunction.[115,116]

Adverse effects include dizziness, constipation, and, especially with the dihydropyridine derivatives, edema. In addition, verapamil and diltiazem can decrease cardiac contractility and conduction, especially when used in conjunction with beta-blockers in elderly patients with coronary disease. There are no adverse effects on lipids or glucose metabolism, but severe rashes and gingival hyperplasia may be more frequent than was anticipated initially.

A recent controversy has highlighted concerns that therapy with the older, short-acting formulations of CCAs might be associated with an increased risk of MI or an increased risk of death if given in high doses in patients with MI.[117,118] The short-acting form of nifedipine can cause precipitous decreases in BP. It is not approved by the FDA for hypertensive urgencies or emergencies, but the long-acting forms of nifedipine and several other CCAs are approved for the treatment of HBP. Indeed, the recently published results of the SYST-EUR trial showed 42% and 27% reductions in the 2-year risk of stroke and CVD mortality, respectively, using nitrendipine in elderly patients with HBP.[119] JNC VI thus specifically recommended long-acting dihydropyridine CCAs (as well as diuretics) for the treatment of ISH in the elderly.

Angiotensin-converting enzyme inhibitors
ACE inhibitors reduce BP effectively in elderly patients with HBP, including ISH.[111,120] Both normotensive and hypertensive sexagenarians and septuagenarians have levels of plasma renin activity (PRA) that are about 50% less than that of younger individuals.[111,120] The BP-lowering effect of ACE inhibitors is not reduced, however, suggesting that either plasma PRA levels do not accurately reflect tissue levels of ACE or angiotensin II, or that the hypotensive action of ACE inhibitors includes stimulation of vasodilatory prostaglandins and kinins. Moreover, Trenkwalder et al[121] reported that PRA (1.5–1.7 ng/ml per hour) was *not* suppressed in 91 very old (average age 79, range 69–94) normotensives or hypertensives. Thus, HBP in the 'elderly' is not necessarily a low renin state.

ACE inhibitors are the drugs of choice if HBP is complicated by CHF caused by systolic dysfunction with a low ejection fraction,[122] or if given shortly after an MI if the ejection fraction is less than 35–40%.[123] Other positive effects of ACE inhibitors for the treatment of HBP in the elderly include regression of LVH[124] and slowing the rate of progression of renal disease in insulin-dependent, proteinuric diabetics with a serum creatinine level of 2.5 mg/dl (221 µmol/l) or less.[125]

The ACE inhibitors have fewer adverse effects than do the alpha-blockers, diuretics, beta-blockers or central agents. A persistent dry cough, however, occurs especially in older women.[126,127] Uncommon adverse effects of ACE inhibitors include first-dose hypotension, rash, taste disturbance, hyperkalemia, acute renal failure in the presence of bilateral renal artery stenosis, and rarely (0.2%), angioneurotic edema. The risk of hyperkalemia deserves special attention in the elderly because of the lower GFR. Be cautious with the use of potassium supplements, and monitor the serum creatinine and potassium levels frequently after initial therapy with ACE inhibitors in elderly patients with HBP.

Elderly patients often use nonsteroidal anti-inflammatory drugs (NSAIDs). Because prostaglandin stimulation can contribute to the BP-reducing efficacy of many ACE inhibitors, NSAIDs, which reduce prostaglandin synthesis, can interfere with control of BP.

Angiotensin receptor blockers
Angiotensin receptor blockers (ATBs) such as irbesartan, losartan and valsartan are the most recently introduced class of antihypertensive drugs and little to no data are available on hypertensive patients age 80 or more.[128] Adverse effects are similar to those of ACE inhibitors except for absence of the cough that plagues many patients (especially elderly women) receiving ACE inhibitors. Caution with use of these compounds (e.g. hyperkalemia) is similar to that with the use of ACE inhibitors. They should not be used in patients with a history of angioedema.[129–131]

Miscellaneous

A sometimes useful option in some old patients with recalcitrant levels of SBP is to add progressive doses of nitrates. Duchier et al[132] compared placebo with oral sustained-release isosorbide dinitrate (20 mg twice daily) in 40 elderly (average age, 80 years) patients with HBP. After 4 months of therapy, SBP was reduced by 14 mmHg with placebo and by 30 mmHg with nitrates.

References

1. Joint National Committee on Prevention, Detection, Evaluation and Treatment of High Blood Pressure. The sixth report of the JNC on prevention, detection, evaluation, and treatment of high blood pressure. *Arch Intern Med* (1997) **157**:2413–46.

2. Lewis RR, Evans PJ, McNabb WR, Padayachee TS. Comparison of indirect and direct blood pressure measurements with Osler's manoeuvre in elderly hypertensive patients. *J Hum Hypertens* (1994) **8**:879–85.

3. Belmin J, Visintin J-M, Salvatore R et al. Osler's maneuver: absence of usefulness for the detection of pseudohypertension in an elderly population. *Am J Med* (1995) **98**:42–9.

4. Robard S. The clinical utility of the arterial pulses and sounds. *Heart Lung* (1972) **1**: 776–84.

5. Cavallini MC, Roman MJ, Blank SG et al. Association of the auscultatory gap with vascular disease in hypertensive patients. *Ann Intern Med* (1996) **124**:877–83.

6. Floras JS, Hassan MO, Jones JV et al. Factors influencing blood pressure and heart rate variability in hypertensive humans. *Hypertension* (1988) **11**:273–81.

7. Parati G, Frattola A, Rienzo MD et al. Broadband spectral analysis of blood pressure and heart rate variability in very elderly subjects. *Hypertension* (1997) **30**:803–8.

8. Fotherby MD, Potter JF. Variations of within visit blood pressure readings at a single visit in the elderly and their relationship to ambulatory measurements. *J Hum Hypertens* (1994) **8**:107–11.

9. Pickering TG. Ambulatory monitoring and the definition of hypertension. *Hypertension* (1992) **20**:401–9.

10. Cox JP, Amery A, Clement D et al. Relationship between blood pressure measured in the clinic and by ambulatory monitoring and left ventricular size as measured by electrocardiogram in elderly patients with isolated systolic hypertension. *J Hypertens* (1993) **11**:269–76.

11. Wiinberg N, Høegholm A, Christensen HR et al. 24-hour ambulatory blood pressure in 352 normal Danish subjects, related to age and gender. *Am J Hypertens* (1995) **8**:978–86.

12. Appel LJ, Stason WB. Ambulatory blood pressure monitoring and blood pressure self-measurement in the diagnosis and management of hypertension. *Ann Intern Med* (1993) **118**:867–82.

13. Rutan GH, McDonald RH, Kuller LH. Comparison of ambulatory and clinic blood pressure and heart rate in older persons with isolated systolic hypertension. *Am J Hypertens* (1992) **5**:880–6.

14. Sega R, Cesana G, Milesi C et al. Ambulatory and home blood pressure normality in the elderly. Data from the PAMELA population. *Hypertension* (1997) **30**(1 Pt 1):1–6.

15. Fotherby MD, Potter JF. Twenty-four-hour ambulatory blood pressure in old and very old subjects. *J Hypertens* (1995) **13**(12 Pt 2): 1742–6.

16. Piexoto Filho AJ, Mansoor GA, White WB. Effects of actual versus arbitrary awake and sleep times on analysis of 24-h blood pressure. *Am J Hypertens* (1995) **8**:676–80.

17. Kario K, Motai K, Mitsubashi T et al. Autonomic nervous system dysfunction in elderly hypertensive patients with abnormal diurnal blood pressure variation: relation to silent cerebrovascular disease. *Hypertension* (1997) **30**:1504–10.

18. Kohara K, Nishida W, Maguchi M, Hiwada K. Autonomic nervous system function in non-dipper essential hypertensive subjects: evaluation by power spectral analysis of heart rate variability. *Hypertension* (1995) **26**:808–14.

19. Kario K, Matsuo T, Kobayashi H et al. Relation between nocturnal fall of blood pressure and silent cerebrovascular damage in elderly hypertensives: advanced silent cerebrovascular damage in extreme-dippers. *Hypertension* (1996) **27**:130–5.

20. Kario K, Shimada K. Change in diurnal blood

pressure rhythm due to small lacunar infarct. *Lancet* (1994) **344**:200.

21. Applegate WB, Davis BR, Black HR et al. Prevalence of postural hypotension at baseline in the systolic hypertension in the elderly (SHEP) cohort. *J Am Geriatr Soc* (1991) **39**:1057–64.

22. Masuo K, Mikami H, Ogihara T, Tuck ML. Changes in frequency of orthostatic hypotension in elderly hypertensive patients under medications. *Am J Hypertens* (1996) **9**:263–8.

23. Jansen RWMM, Lipsitz LA. Postprandial hypotension: epidemiology, pathophysiology, and clinical management. *Ann Intern Med* (1995) **122**:286–95.

24. Masuo K, Mikami H, Ogihara T, Tuck ML. Mechanisms mediating postprandial blood pressure reductions in young and elderly subjects. *Am J Hypertens* (1996) **9**:536–44.

25. Olin JW, Vidt JG, Gifford RW, Novick AC. Renovascular disease in the elderly: an analysis of 50 patients. *J Am Coll Cardiol* (1985) **5**:1232–8.

26. Vetrovec GW, Landwehr DM, Edwards VL. Incidence of renal artery stenosis in hypertensive patients undergoing coronary arteriography. *J Intervent Cardiol* (1987) **2**:69–76.

27. Hrick DE, Browning PJ, Kopelman R et al. Captopril induced functional renal insufficiency in patients with bilateral renal artery stenosis or renal artery stenosis in a solitary kidney. *N Engl J Med* (1983) **118**:712–9.

28. Badr KF, Ichikawa I. Prerenal failure: a deleterious shift from renal compensation to decompensation. *N Engl J Med* (1988) **319**:623–9.

29. Solomon R, Weinberg MS, Dubey A. The diurnal rhythm of plasma potassium: relationship to diuretic therapy. *J Cardiovasc Pharmacol* (1991) **17**:854–9.

30. Lindeman RD. Changes in renal function with aging. Implications for treatment. *Drugs Aging* (1992) **2**:423–31.

31. Ashouri OS. Severe diuretic-induced hyponatremia in the elderly. A series of eight patients. *Arch Intern Med* (1986) **146**:1355–7.

32. Packer M, Medina N, Yushak M. Relation between serum sodium concentration and the hemodynamic and clinical responses to converting enzyme inhibition with captopril in severe heart failure. *J Am Coll Cardiol* (1984) **3**:1035–43.

33. Friedman JR, Norman DC, Yoshikawa TT. Correlation of estimated renal function parameters versus 24-hour creatinine clearance in ambulatory elderly. *J Am Geriatr Soc* (1989) **37**:145–9.

34. Cockcroft DW, Gault MH. Prediction of creatinine clearance from serum creatinine. *Nephron* (1976) **16**:31–41.

35. Conn JW, Knopf RF, Nesbit RM. Clinical characteristics of primary aldosteronism from an analysis of 145 cases. *Am J Surg* (1964) **107**:159–72.

36. Eisenberg AA, Wallerstein H. Pheochromocytoma of the suprarenal medulla (paraganglioma). *Arch Pathol* (1932) **14**:818–36.

37. Schwartz CJ, White TA. Stenosis of renal artery: an unselected necropsy study. *BMJ* (1964) **ii**:1415–21.

38. Vidt DG. Cholesterol emboli: a common cause of renal failure. *Annu Rev Med* (1997) **48**:375–85.

39. MRC Working Party. Medical Research Council trial of treatment of hypertension in older adults: principal results. *BMJ* (1992) **304**:405–12.

40. Hansson L. Future goals for the treatment of hypertension in the elderly with reference to STOP-Hypertension, SHEP, and the MRC trial in older adults. *Am J Hypertens* (1993) **6**(3 Pt 2): 40–3S.

41. Materson BJ, Cushman WC, Goldstein G et al. Treatment of hypertension in the elderly: I. Blood pressure and clinical changes. Results of a Department of Veterans Affairs Cooperative Study. *Hypertension* (1990) **15**:348–60.

42. Hansson L, Zanchetti A, for the HOT Study Group. The Hypertension Optimal Treatment (HOT) study–patient characteristics: randomization, risk profiles, and early blood pressure results. *Blood Press* (1994) **3**:322–7.

43. Hansson L, Zanchetti A, for the HOT Study Group. The Hypertension Optimal Treatment (HOT) Study: 24-month data on blood pressure and tolerability. *Blood Press* (1997) **6**: 313–17.

44. Hypertension Detection and Follow-up Program Cooperative Group. Five-year findings

of the Hypertension Detection and Follow-up Program. II. Mortality by race, sex, and age. *JAMA* (1979) **242**:2572–7.

45. Appel LJ, Espeland M, Whelton PK et al. Trial of non-pharmacologic intervention in the elderly: design and rationale of a blood pressure control trial. *Ann Epidemiol* (1995) **5**:119–29.

46. Whelton PK, Appel LJ, Espeland MA et al. Sodium reduction and weight loss in the treatment of hypertension in other persons: a randomized controlled trial of non pharmacologic interventions in the elderly (TONE). TONE Collaborative Research Group. *JAMA* (1998) **279**:839-46.

47. SHEP Cooperative Research Group. Prevention of stroke by antihypertensive drug treatment in older persons with isolated systolic hypertension. Final results of the Systolic Hypertension in the Elderly Program (SHEP). *JAMA* (1991) **265**:3255–64.

48. Systolic Hypertension in the Elderly Program Cooperative Research Group. Implications of the Systolic Hypertension in the Elderly Program. *Hypertension* (1993) **21**:335–43.

49. Staessen JA, Fagard R, Thijs L et al for the SYST-EUR trial investigators. Randomized double-blind comparison of placebo and active treatment for older patients with isolated systolic hypertension. *Lancet* (1997) **350**:757–64.

50. Antikainen R, Tuomilehto J, Thijs L et al. Therapy in old patients with isolated systolic hypertension: fourth progress report on the SYST-EUR trial. *J Hum Hypertens* (1997) **11**:263–9.

51. Dahlof B, Lindholm LH, Hansson L et al. Morbidity and mortality in the Swedish Trial in Old Patients with Hypertension (STOP-Hypertension). *Lancet* (1991) **338**:1281–5.

52. Ekbom T, Dahlof B, Hansson L et al. Antihypertensive efficacy and side effects of three beta-blockers and a diuretic in elderly hypertensives: a report from the STOP-Hypertension study. *J Hypertens* (1992) **10**:1525–30.

53. Amery A, Birkenhäger W, Brixko P et al. Mortality and morbidity results from the European Working Party on High Blood Pressure in the Elderly trial. *Lancet* (1985) i:1349–54.

54. Amery A, Birkenhäger W, Brixko P et al.

Influence of antihypertensive drug treatment on morbidity and mortality in patients over the age of 60 years. EWPHE results: subgroup analysis based on entry stratification. *J Hypertens* (1986) **4**(Supplement 6):S642–7.

55. Amery A, Birkenhäger W, Brixko P et al. Efficacy of antihypertensive drug treatment according to age, sex, blood pressure, and previous cardiovascular disease in patients over the age of 60. *Lancet* (1986) ii:589–92.

56. Bulpitt CJ, Fletcher AE, Amery A et al. The hypertension in the very elderly trial (HYVET). *J Hum Hypertens* (1994) **8**:631–2.

57. Bulpitt CJ. Hypertension in the very elderly. *J Hum Hypertens* (1994) **8**:603–5.

58. Bulpitt CJ, Fletcher AE, Amery A et al. The Hypertension in the Very Elderly Trial (HYVET). Rationale, methodology and comparison with previous trials. *Drugs Aging* (1994) **5**:171–83.

59. Curb JD, Pressel SL, Cutler JA et al. Effect of diuretic-based antihypertensive treatment on cardiovascular disease risk in older diabetic patients with isolated systolic hypertension. *JAMA* (1996) **276**:1886–92.

60. Davis BR, Cutler JA, Gordon DJ et al for the ALLHAT Research Group. Rationale and design for the antihypertensive and lipid lowering treatment to prevent heart attack trial (ALLHAT). *Am J Hypertens* (1996) **9**:342–60.

61. Mattila K, Haavisto M, Rajala S, Heikinhiemo R. Blood pressure and five year survival in the very old. *BMJ* (1989) **296**:887–9.

62. Langer RD, Ganiats TG, Barrett-Connor E. Paradoxical survival of elderly men with high blood pressure. *BMJ* (1988) **298**:1356–7.

63. Langer RD, Ganiats TG, Barrett-Conner E. Factors associated with paradoxical survival at higher blood pressures in the very old. *Am J Epidemiol* (1991) **134**:29–38.

64. Langer RD, Criqui MH, Barrett-Conner EL et al. Blood pressure change and survival after age 75. *Hypertension* (1993) **22**:551–9.

65. Wenger NK, Speroff L, Packard B. Cardiovascular health and disease in women. *N Engl J Med* (1993) **329**:247–56.

66. Wenger NK. Hypertension and other cardiovascular risk factors in women. *Am J Hypertens* (1995) **8**(12 Pt 2):94–9S.

67. Cruickshank JM, Thorb JM, Zacharias FJ.

Benefits and potential harm of lowering high blood pressure. *Lancet* (1987) i:531–84.

68. Kaplan NM. The appropriate goals of antihypertensive therapy: neither too much nor too little. *Ann Intern Med* (1992) **116**:686–90.

69. Merlo J, Ranstam J, Liedholm H et al. Incidence of myocardial infarction in elderly men being treated with antihypertensive drugs: population-based cohort study. *BMJ* (1996) **313**:457–61.

70. MacMahon S, Rodgers A. The effects of blood pressure reduction in older patients: an overview of five randomized controlled trials in elderly hypertensives. *Clin Exp Hypertens* (1993) **15**:967–78.

71. Psaty BM, Smith NL, Siscovick DS et al. Health outcomes associated with antihypertensive therapies used as first-line agents: a systematic review and meta-analysis. *JAMA* (1997) **277**:739–45.

72. Mulrow CD, Cornell JA, Herrera CR et al. Hypertension in the elderly. Implications and generalizability of randomized trials. *JAMA* (1994) **272**:1932–8.

73. Barker WH, Mulloony JP, Linton KLP. Trends in hypertension prevalence, treatment, and control in a well-defined older population. *Hypertension* (1998) **31**(1 Pt 2): 552–9.

74. Lenfant C. Lifestyle changes, low-dose diuretics should be first choice for treating hypertension in the elderly. *JAMA* (1994) **272**:842.

75. National High Blood Pressure Education Program Working Group. National high blood pressure education working group report on hypertension in the elderly. *Hypertension* (1994) **23**:275–85.

76. Luft FC, Weinberger MH, Fineberg NS et al. Effects of age on renal sodium homeostasis and its relevance to sodium sensitivity. *Am J Med* (1987) **82**(Supplement 1B):9–15.

77. Shimamoto H, Shimamoto Y. Time course of hemodynamic responses to sodium in elderly hypertensive patients. *Hypertension* (1990) **16**:387–97.

78. Applegate WB, Miller ST, Elam JT et al. Nonpharmacologic intervention to reduce blood pressure in older persons with mild hypertension. *Arch Intern Med* (1992) **152**:1162–6.

79. Palmer RM, Osterweil D, Loon-Lustig G, Stern N. The effect of dietary salt ingestion on blood pressure of old-old subjects. A double-blind, placebo-controlled crossover trial. *J Am Geriatr Soc* (1989) **37**:931–6.

80. Midgley JP, Matthew AO, Greenwood CMT, Logan AG. Effect of reduced dietary sodium on blood pressure: a meta-analysis of randomized controlled trials. *JAMA* (1996) **275**:1590–7.

81. Cutler JA, Follmann D, Allender PS. Randomized trials of sodium reduction: an overview. *Am J Clin Nutr* (1997) **65**(Supplement): 643–51S.

82. Kumanyika SK, Cutler JA. Dietary sodium reduction: is there a cause for concern? *J Am Coll Nutr* (1997) **16**:192–203.

83. Welte JW, Greizerstein HB. Alcohol consumption and systolic blood pressure in the general population. *Subst Alcohol Actions Misuse* (1985) **5**:299–306.

84. Hall WD. Management of systolic hypertension in the elderly. *Semin Nephrol* (1996) **16**:299–308.

85. Applegate WB, Rutan GH. Advances in management of hypertension in older persons. *J Am Geriatr Soc* (1992) **40**:1164–72.

86. Zanchetti A. Hypertension in the elderly. *Am J Geriatr Cardiol* (1993) **2**:13–21.

87. Bulpitt CJ, Fletcher AE. Prognostic significance of blood pressure in the very old. Implications for the treatment decision. *Drugs Aging* (1994) **5**:184–91.

88. Welch HG, Albertsen PC, Nease RF et al. Estimating treatment benefits for the elderly: the effect of competing risks. *Ann Intern Med* (1996) **124**:577–84.

89. Curb JD, Borhani NO, Blaszkowski TP et al. Long-term surveillance for adverse effects of antihypertensive drugs. *JAMA* (1985) **253**: 3263–8.

90. Cohen JL. Pharmacokinetic changes in aging. *Am J Med* (1986) **80**(Supplement 5A):31–8.

91. Grodzicki T, Messerli FH. Cardiovascular drug therapy in the elderly. In: Messerli FH, ed., *Cardiovascular Drug Therapy*, 2nd edn. (WB Saunders: Philadelphia, 1996) 225–33.

92. Gurwitz JH, Avorn J. The ambiguous relation between aging and adverse drug reactions. *Ann Intern Med* (1991) **114**:956–66.

93. Applegate WB, Pressel S, Wittes J et al.

Impact of the treatment of isolated systolic hypertension on behavioral variables: results from the Systolic Hypertension in the Elderly Program. *Arch Intern Med* (1994) **154**:2154–60.

94. Campion EW, Avorn J, Reder VA, Olins NJ. Overmedication of the low-weight elderly. *Arch Intern Med* (1987) **147**:945–7.

95. Chan Y-C, Suzuki M, Yamamoto S. Dietary, anthropometric, hematological and biochemical assessment of the nutritional status of centenarians and elderly people in Okinawa, Japan. *J Am Coll Nutr* (1997) **16**:229–35.

96. Hanlon JT, Weinberger M, Samsa GP et al. A randomized, controlled trial of a clinical pharmacist intervention to improve inappropriate prescribing in elderly outpatients with polypharmacy. *Am J Med* (1996) **100**: 428–37.

97. Freis ED. The efficacy and safety of diuretics in treating hypertension. *Ann Intern Med* (1995) **122**:223–6.

98. Gifford RW Jr, Kaplan NM. Thiazides and hypertension in the elderly. *Hypertension* (1995) **25**:1052 (edit).

99. Berglund G, Anderson O. Low doses of hydrochlorothiazide in hypertension: antihypertensive and metabolic effects. *Eur J Clin Pharmacol* (1976) **10**:177–82.

100. Vardan S, Mehrota KG, Mookherjee S et al. Efficacy and reduced metabolic side effects of a 15-mg chlorthalidone formulation in the treatment of mild hypertension: a multicenter study. *JAMA* (1987) **258**:484–8.

101. Hall WD, Weber MA, Ferdinand K et al. Lower dose diuretic therapy in the treatment of patients with mild to moderate hypertension. *J Human Hypertens* (1994) **8**:571–5.

102. Weir MR, Flack JM, Applegate WB. Tolerability, safety, and quality of life and antihypertensive therapy: the case for low-dose diuretics. *Am J Med* (1996) **101**(Supplement): 83–92S.

103. Kaplan NM. Diuretics: cornerstone of antihypertensive therapy. *Am J Cardiol* (1996) **77**: 3–5B.

104. Cauley JA, Cummings SR, Seeley DG et al. Effects of thiazide diuretic therapy on bone mass, fractures, and falls. *Ann Intern Med* (1993) **118**:666–73.

105. Yusef S, Peto R, Lewis J et al. Beta blockade during and after myocardial infarction: an overview of the randomized trials. *Prog Cardiovasc Dis* (1985) **27**:335–71.

106. Yusef S, Wittes J, Probstfield J. Evaluating effects of treatment in subgroups of patients within a clinical trial: the case on non-Q-wave myocardial infarction and beta-blockers. *Am J Cardiol* (1990) **66**:220–2.

107. Kendall MJ, Lynch KP, Hjalmarson A, Kjekshus J. β-Blockers and sudden cardiac death. *Ann Intern Med* (1995) **123**:358–67.

108. Soumeral SB, McLaughlin TJ, Spiegelman D et al. Adverse outcomes of underuse of β-blockers in elderly survivors of acute myocardial infarction. *JAMA* (1997) **277**: 115–21.

109. Shiuey Y, Eisenberg MJ. Cardiovascular effects of commonly used ophthalmic medications. *Clin Cardiol* (1996) **19**:5–8.

110. Materson BJ, Reda OJ, Cushman WC et al. Single-drug therapy for hypertension in men: a comparison of six antihypertensive agents with placebo. *N Engl J Med* (1993) **328**:914–21.

111. Hall WD. Hypertension in the elderly with a special focus on treatment with angiotensin-converting enzyme inhibitors and calcium antagonists. *Am J Cardiol* (1992) **69**:33–42E.

112. Weiner DA. Calcium channel blockers. *Med Clin North Am* (1988) **72**:83–115.

113. Black HR. Therapeutic considerations in the elderly hypertensive: the role of calcium channel blockers. *Am J Hypertens* (1990) **3**(Supplement): 347–54S.

114. Giles TD, Sander GE. Aspects of the use of angiotensin-converting-enzyme inhibitors and calcium antagonists in treatment of heart failure in the older patient. *Am J Geriatr Cardiol* (1993) **2**:51–4.

115. Packer M, O'Connor CM, Ghali JK et al for the Prospective Randomized Amlodipine Survival Evaluation Study Group. Effect of amlodipine on morbidity and mortality in severe chronic heart failure. *N Engl J Med* (1996) **335**:1107–14.

116. Cohn JN, Ziesche S, Smith R et al for the Vasodilator-Heart Failure Trial. Effect of the calcium antagonist felodipine as supplementary vasodilator therapy in patients with chronic heart failure treated with enalapril: V-HeFT III. *Circulation* (1997) **96**:856–63.

117. Psaty BM, Heckbert SR, Koepsell TD et al. The risk of myocardial infarction associated with antihypertensive drug therapies. *JAMA* (1995) **274**:620–5.

118. Furberg CD, Psaty BM, Meyer JV. Nifedipine. Dose-related increase in mortality in patients with coronary heart disease. *Circulation* (1995) **92**:1326–31.

119. Staessen JA, Fagard R, Thijs L et al. Randomised double-blind comparison of placebo and active treatment for older patients with isolated systolic hypertension. *Lancet* (1997) **350**:757–64.

120. Israili ZH, Hall WD. ACE inhibitors: differential use in elderly patients with hypertension. *Drugs Aging* (1995) **7**:355–71.

121. Trenkwalder P, James GD, Laragh JH, Sealey JE. Plasma renin activity and plasma prorenin are not suppressed in hypertensives surviving to old age. *Am J Hypertens* (1996) **9**:621–7.

122. SOLVD Investigators. Effect of enalapril on mortality and the development of heart failure in asymptomatic patients with reduced left ventricular ejection fractions. *N Engl J Med* (1992) **327**:685–91.

123. Pfeiffer MA, Braunwald E, Moye LA et al. Effect of captopril on mortality and morbidity in patients with left ventricular dysfunction after myocardial infarction. *N Engl J Med* (1992) **327**:669–77.

124. Liebson PR. Clinical studies of drug reversal of hypertensive left ventricular hypertrophy. *Am J Hypertens* (1990) **3**:512–17.

125. Lewis EJ, Hunsicker LG, Bain RP, Rhode RD for the Collaborative Study Group. The effect of angiotensin-converting-enzyme inhibition on diabetic nephropathy. *N Engl J Med* (1993) **329**:1456–62.

126. Israili ZH, Hall WD. Cough and angioneurotic edema associated with angiotensin converting enzyme inhibitor therapy: a review of the literature and pathophysiology. *Ann Intern Med* (1992) **117**:234–42.

127. Os I, Bratland B, Dahlof B et al. Female preponderance for lisinopril-induced cough in hypertension. *Am J Hypertens* (1994) **7**: 1012–15.

128. Burrell LM, Johnston CI. Angiotensin II receptor antagonists. Potential in elderly patients with cardiovascular disease. *Drugs Aging* (1997) **10**:421–34.

129. Acker CG, Greenberg A. Angioedema induced by the angiotensin II blocker losartan. *N Engl J Med* (1995) **333**:1572 (letter).

130. Boxer M. Accupril- and Cozaar-induced angioedema in the same patient. *J Allergy Clin Immunol* (1996) **98**:471 (letter).

131. Sharma PK, Yium JJ. Angioedema associated with angiotensin II receptor antagonist losartan. *South Med J* (1997) **90**:552–3.

132. Duchier J, Iannascoli F, Safar M. Antihypertensive effect of sustained-release isosorbide dinitrate for isolated systolic systemic hypertension in the elderly. *Am J Cardiol* (1987) **60**:99–102.

19

Valve disease in the octogenarian

Melvin D Cheitlin

Introduction

The patient who reaches the late years of life has obviously weathered the dangers of premature demise from coronary artery disease, and also most probably has not had severe, untreated valve disease from childhood or young adulthood. Many of these patients may have had mild valve disease for many years, the severity of which has increased recently because of progressive fibrosis and calcification of the already-diseased valve.[1] Although any type of valve disease can be seen in the octogenarian, the most frequent problems are calcific aortic stenosis and mitral regurgitation, the latter due either to a myxomatous mitral valve or to coronary artery disease.[2,3] Mitral regurgitation as a result of calcified mitral annulus, or any disease resulting in left ventricular dilation and failure, usually does not, in this age group, cause mitral regurgitation sufficient to consider surgery. Other valve problems, such as severe aortic insufficiency or mitral stenosis, are less commonly seen in this age group. Infective endocarditis is always a problem, even in this age group, but is infrequent, and is dealt with in Chapter 26.

Problems in the diagnosis of valve disease in the octogenarian

The diagnosis and estimation of the severity of valve disease can be a problem in the octoge-narian. First, the incidence of systolic murmurs in this age group is high, in the order of 50% of patients.[4] Lindroos and colleagues[5] reported the prevalence of aortic valve calcification and disease in the elderly in a randomly selected group of 577 men and women, aged 75–86, who were participants in the Helsinki Aging Study. These patients were studied with echo-Doppler. Mild calcification of the aortic valve was present in 40% of the patients and severe calcification in 13%. Critical valve stenosis was present in 12 patients, or 2.2%. The prevalence of critical aortic stenosis was 2.9% (95% confidence limits: 0.4–5.1%) in this 75–86 year age group. Aortic regurgitation, mostly mild, was present in 29% of the entire study population. In a second paper, Lindroos and colleagues[6] described the association of age, hypertension and low body mass with the presence of aortic valvular calcification. Older age and increased serum ionized calcium were associated with significant aortic stenosis.

The diagnosis of severe aortic stenosis can be a problem, since a murmur is generated by the entire stroke volume ejected through a large gradient by the left ventricle; with a normal chest wall, this results in a very loud systolic ejection murmur. The absence of a grade III or IV systolic murmur in such a patient is good evidence against aortic stenosis requiring surgery. However, two things occur as the patient ages: (1) there is progressive kyphosis and deepening of the antero-posterior (AP) diameter of the chest, resulting in more air between the place where the murmur originates and the body surface; (2) many elderly patients with severe aortic stenosis present with pulmonary edema, or at least with a decreased stroke volume. This decreased stroke volume and deep AP diameter of the chest results in a grade I or II systolic ejection murmur, or even absence of a murmur, if the patient is in pulmonary edema. Another problem in the diagnosis of aortic stenosis is that there is a decrease in compliance of the aorta, resulting in a brisker upstroke of the carotid arterial pulse for any given stroke volume.[7] This can mask the delayed and small impulse (the pulsus parvus and tardus), which is classic for severe aortic stenosis. The diagnosis should be suspected in the patient who presents in left heart failure when a systolic ejection murmur is heard, or even in the absence of a systolic ejection murmur when the carotid pulses are small and delayed in upstroke, or when there is unexplained left ventricular hypertrophy (LVH) on the electrocardiogram (ECG). Another worthwhile study to perform when the diagnosis of severe aortic stenosis is in doubt is fluoroscopy, looking for calcification of the valve. It is extremely unusual in this age group that severe aortic stenosis is present without some calcification seen on fluoroscopy.

A similar problem exists in the diagnosis and estimation of the severity of mitral stenosis. Most patients with mitral stenosis who have lived to the ninth decade are in atrial fibrillation. With a rapid ventricular response rate, there is a decrease in stroke volume; together with a deep AP diameter of the chest, a murmur may be inaudible. Another reason for inaudibility of the murmur is the fact that this low-frequency, rumbling diastolic murmur is best heard at the point of maximum impulse, where the left ventricle contacts the chest wall. The murmur becomes inaudible as one moves away from the apical impulse. With increase in AP diameter of the chest, or with dilation of the right ventricle, as occurs with pulmonary hypertension and right ventricular failure, the left ventricle no longer contacts the chest wall and the murmur cannot be heard, even with the patient in the rolled-over left lateral position. In most of these very old patients, the valve is fibrotic and calcified, so that there are no longer the hallmark heart sounds of mitral stenosis, the loud first heart sound and opening snap. Pulmonary hypertension and its consequences (the loud second heart sound, right heart failure, right-sided S3 or S4, pulmonic and tricuspid regurgitation) may be the only clues to mitral stenosis. In patients with pulmonary hypertension, it is obviously important to rule out mitral stenosis, since this is a potentially correctable cause of pulmonary hypertension.

The etiology of aortic regurgitation in this age group can be rheumatic, but can also be due to a congenital abnormality of the aortic valve such as bicuspid aortic valve, due to infective endocarditis, atherosclerosis and dilation of the aorta, or to ascending aortic aneurysm or dissection of the aorta.[8] With aortic regurgitation, a murmur may be difficult to hear because of the increased AP diameter of the chest. In these patients, if the point of maximal impulse is formed by the left ventricle, sometimes the murmur is best detected at the apex, with the patient rolled into the left lateral position. The severity of the aortic regurgitation is usually best appreciated by the hemodynamic effects of the aortic regurgitation on the peripheral vasculature. The wide pulse pressure, which causes many of the peripheral signs of aortic regurgitation, can be seen in elderly patients with very stiff aortas, so that the wide pulse pressure and many of the peripheral signs may be the result of an atherosclerotic aorta rather than severe aortic regurgitation. In my experience, in severe aortic regurgitation, the Duroziez's sign and the collapse of the carotid pulse due to ventricularization of the aortic pressure remain and are different from the patient with simply a stiff aorta. However, many of the signs and the consequences of left ventricular afterload, such as LVH, useful in determining the severity of aortic stenosis and aortic insufficiency in younger patients, can be caused by the patient's having many years of systolic hypertension. Stiffness of the left ventricle caused by hypertrophy is seen in the aging heart. Therefore, the presence of an S4 is of no help in elderly patients with a murmur of aortic stenosis in determining severity, whereas in a younger patient with the murmur of aortic stenosis, an S4 is usually associated with LVH due to severe aortic stenosis.

Tricuspid regurgitation in this age group is commonly related to right ventricular failure, mainly due to pulmonary hypertension secondary to left ventricular disease. Of course, pulmonary hypertension can be a consequence of lung disease, right heart failure or cor pulmonale. Primary tricuspid valve problems are much less often seen in the octogenarian, since they are the result of infective endocarditis, and usually seen primarily in the intravenous drug user. The elderly, at this age, are rarely intravenous drug users. Trauma, both penetrating and nonpenetrating, is another etiology for primary tricuspid valve disease, to which the elderly can be susceptible. Other, rarer causes of tricuspid regurgitation: right atrial myxoma, eosinophilic myocarditis and serotonin-producing drugs, such as Phen-Fen, all relatively rare in this age group.

Pulmonary stenosis is seen occasionally in the very elderly patient, at which time the valve will always be calcified and easily seen on fluoroscopy. These cases are rare.

Pulmonic valve insufficiency is frequent with pulmonary hypertension, but primary pulmonary valve regurgitation is rare indeed in the octogenarian. Occasionally, it can be seen as a result of former surgery across the right ventricular outflow tract, such as performed in tetralogy of Fallot repair. Since definitive surgery for tetralogy of Fallot has been available only since the mid-1950s, we are only now approaching 50-year follow-up for the earliest operated patients. We have not yet seen these patients in the octogenarian age group, but I have no doubt we will start seeing such patients in the future.

Congenital etiologies for aortic valve disease in this age group include bicuspid aortic valve. If the bicuspid valve becomes calcified, it usually does so at age 40–50; but if allowed to proceed, it may not be discovered until the patient reaches age 80.

Although rare, patients with Ebstein's disease can be seen in the octogenarian age group.

The differential diagnosis of various valve diseases in octogenarians is similar to that in younger patients. For instance, hypertrophic cardiomyopathy can present as a murmur and be mistaken for valvular aortic stenosis, mitral regurgitation or ventricular septal defect. Left atrial myxoma may masquerade as mitral stenosis or mitral regurgitation. Patients with atrial septal defect can be seen in the very elderly age group, and have many of the same findings on ECG, X-ray and physical examination as patients with mitral stenosis. Fortunately, at the present time, Doppler echocardiography has become extremely important in making the definitive diagnosis, that is, hypertrophic cardiomyopathy rather than aortic stenosis, left atrial myxoma rather than mitral regurgitation, atrial septal defect rather than mitral stenosis, etc.

Treatment

The medical treatment of octogenarians with severe valvular disease is similar to that of younger patients. Patients with aortic stenosis, aortic regurgitation and mitral regurgitation who enter in congestive heart failure are treated with digoxin, diuretics and, in patients with valvular insufficiency, angiotensin-converting enzyme (ACE) inhibitors. There are, however, problems with medication in the octogenarian that are different compared to the younger patient. For instance, with mitral stenosis and atrial fibrillation, patients have an extremely high incidence of systemic emboli, and most importantly, stroke. Proper anticoagulation can markedly reduce the incidence of stroke. Even though there is increased incidence of hemorrhagic stroke with anticoagulants in the octogenarian, the balance of therapeutic value seems to fall on the side of anticoagulation, keeping the patient with an INR of between 2 and 3.[9,10]

Valve repair/replacement

Making a decision to operate in the very elderly patient with valve disease is extremely difficult, and must be considered on a patient-by-patient basis. Certain generalities, however, do apply. Thoracotomy and cardiopulmonary bypass surgery in octogenarians is associated with a higher morbidity and mortality than in patients less than 75 years of age.[11] This is especially true of central nervous system injury with cardiopulmonary bypass surgery. Also, the elderly have more problems after valve replacement, especially with mechanical valves, because of the complications of anticoagulant therapy. The increased comorbidity in elderly patients, especially coronary artery disease but also carotid and pulmonary disease and renal insufficiency, is another reason for the higher morbidity and mortality seen with cardiopulmonary bypass surgery.[12–14]

The goal of valve surgery in the octogenarian must be to relieve symptoms not controlled by medical management, rather than the hope of increasing lifespan. The best reason for taking the risk of surgery in the octogenarian is that the patient will have an improved quality of life after surgery rather than without it. In general, this means that surgery should not be undertaken for a theoretical benefit, that is prolongation of life, but for a definite benefit, that is reduction of symptoms. Therefore, it is rare for a patient who reports no symptoms and has a satisfactory physical activity level to be offered surgery. Finally, there are no studies of severe valvular disease where elderly patients are randomized to continued medical management versus surgery. There are a large number of reports of many elderly patients who were operated upon, and of peri-operative as well as late morbidity and mortality in patients surviving surgery. There are a few studies comparing those who were operated upon and those who refused surgery, especially for patients with aortic valve disease.[15] It is difficult to find series of patients that looked only at the octogenarian. Frequently the 'elderly' are defined as those above age 65; sometimes above age 75. Results with patients younger than 75 years are extrapolated to those over 80 only with some trepidation.

Aortic stenosis

In patients with calcific aortic stenosis, two retrospective studies using echo-Doppler suggest that sudden death as the first symptom in adult patients with severe aortic stenosis is rare, and is certainly less than the operative mortality.[16,17] For this reason, after a careful history is elicited and in cases with no symptomatology suggesting heart failure, angina or exertional syncope, and no deterioration of ventricular function, the elderly patient should be followed closely, but not sent to surgery.

Once symptoms appear, the patient falls into a high-risk category, with one-fifth to one-quarter of patients who die, dying suddenly.[18] Therefore, if there are no contraindications to surgery, aortic stenosis is the major problem, and there is minimal comorbidity, surgery can be offered with success.

Aortic valve replacement

In general, this is recommended for octogenarians who have severe aortic stenosis or aortic regurgitation, with either symptoms or signs of deteriorating left ventricular function, usually manifested by an increasing left ventricular end-diastolic volume, end-systolic volume and decreasing ejection fraction. As stated, there are no controlled studies in the elderly; however, there are studies that followed all patients who were offered surgery, most of whom accepted and some of whom refused.[15] Within 1 year, those with aortic stenosis who continued medical management had a significantly worse survival than those who were operated upon. Other studies indicating that surgery benefits patients with aortic stenosis that compare them to an age-matched general population, show that those with aortic valve replacement have a similar survival to the age-matched general population.[19,20]

A number of studies have examined patients with aortic valve replacement at over age 80. Logeais et al[21] reported 675 patients at 75 years of age and over who had surgery at a mean age of 78.5 ± 3 years. Associated lesions were present in 226 patients, and concomitant surgical procedures were done in 133 patients. Surgical mortality overall was 12.4%. Compared with 2196 patients operated on for aor-

tic stenosis who were less than 75 years of age in the same period, the operative mortality was 6.6% ($P < 0.0001$). In the overall series of 2871 cases, the surgical mortality varied from 2.2 to 12.4%, depending on the age group. In the 675 elderly patients, mortality did not increase after the age of 90.

In most series, peri-operative mortality in the age group 70 years and over varied from 2.4% to 12.4%, depending on the era in which an operation occurred (before or after 1980) and the presence of other lesions and concomitant procedures (coronary artery bypass surgery, mitral valve replacement, etc.). Glock et al[14] reported 96 patients 80 years of age or over, operated on from 1985 to 1992. Forty-five had aortic valve replacement and coronary artery bypass surgery, and 70% were in New York Heart Association (NYHA) class III or IV. The operative mortality was 9.8%. Elayda et al[22] reported 171 patients aged 80 and above with aortic valve replacement operated on between 1975 and 1991. Peri-operative mortality in isolated aortic valve replacement was only 5.2%; with additional procedures, the mortality was 27.7%. The overall mortality was 17.5%. Akins et al[23] reported 105 patients with isolated aortic valve replacement, with a peri-operative mortality of 7.6% and 111 patients with aortic valve replacement and coronary artery bypass surgery with a similar peri-operative mortality of 6.3%. Aranki et al[24] reported 188 octogenarians and 529 septuagenarians. The average age of the entire group was 77 years. Of these, 386 (56%) had aortic valve replacement and coronary artery bypass surgery. The overall mortality was 6.6%. For aortic valve replacement alone, it was 4.2%; with additional coronary artery bypass surgery, it was 8.8%.

The predictors of peri-operative mortality and late mortality have also been examined. In general, in-hospital mortality increases after age 70.[19] The factors predictive of peri-operative mortality by multivariate logistic regression analysis are poor left ventricular function and chronic heart failure, the presence of comorbid disease (lung disease, renal disease and diabetes) and concomitant procedures (coronary artery bypass surgery, mitral valve replacement), nonsinus rhythm and urgency of surgery. The predictors of late mortality are the presence of comorbid diseases (chronic obstructive pulmonary disease, chronic renal disease and diabetes) and poor left ventricular function.[19]

The choice of mechanical versus biological valves is easy in octogenarians, since there is an increased problem with anticoagulation in elderly patients with a higher occurrence of intracranial hemorrhage and subdural hematoma than in younger patients.[9,10] Biological valves are preferred over mechanical valves since the former do not need long-term anticoagulation in the absence of atrial fibrillation. Since significant failure of biological valves does not occur before 5–10 years, the longevity of biological valves is sufficient to ensure that they will last for the natural life of the patient.[25,26] Anticoagulation is usually recommended for the first 3 postoperative months until the sewing ring is endothelialized. After this, aspirin 0.3 g/day is used. The incidence of thromboemboli is one or two episodes per 100 patient years off anticoagulants.[26,27] If the patient is in atrial fibrillation, careful anticoagulation should be continued, with the INR between 2 and 3.[10]

The long-term results of aortic valve replacement in the octogenarian with aortic stenosis also appear to be good. Late death may be valve-related, but also has to be compared to the total mortality of the age-matched general population. Five-year actuarial survival in several large series has been reported. Elayda et al,[22] with 171 patients with aortic stenosis aged 80–91 operated on between 1975 and 1991, had a 5-year actuarial survival of 76%. Akins et al's[23] 105 patients aged 80 and above with isolated aortic valve replacement had a 5-year survival of 67%. With additional coronary artery bypass surgery, it was 59%. Glock et al[14] reported 96 patients 80 years of age and older operated on between 1985 and 1992. Forty-five had aortic valve replacement and coronary artery bypass surgery; 70% were in NYHA class III and IV. The 1-year actuarial survival was 76%, but dropped to 46% in 4 years. Verheul et al,[19] in patients older than 70, had a 5-year survival of 76% with isolated aortic valve replacement and 55% in those with additional CABG. Tseng et al[28] reported 247 patients aged 70–89, with a mean age of 76.2 years. The 5-year survival was 68%, the 10-year survival 41%.

The sicker the patients, the higher the operative mortality and the higher the late mortality. This appears to be especially true when the patient is operated on for aortic regurgitation, especially if the patient is symptomatic, with decreased left ventricular function.[19] Verheul et al[19] evaluated the observed late mortality and, using the mortality of the age-matched general population, assessed excess mortality. Excess mortality was the mortality that was related to the aortic valve disease, or was valve-related. Risk factors for observed mortality were related to previous myocardial infarction, coronary disease, congestive heart failure and atrial fibrillation. Age 70 years and over was a risk factor for observed mortality (hazard-rate ratio = 2.4; 95% confidence interval 1.6–3.7%), but was not a risk factor for excess mortality. With isolated aortic regurgitation, congestive heart failure was a risk factor for excess late mortality (hazard-rate ratio = 3.8; 95% confidence interval 1.3–11.2%). Late mortality was valve-related in 22% of the patients, and congestive heart failure the main cause of death in 38%. Chocron et al[20] reported 95 patients older than 75 years of age with calcific aortic stenosis, mean age 80 years. Fourteen needed coronary artery bypass surgery, 67% were NYHA class III or IV and 9% needed urgent surgery. Actuarial survival was similar to the survival for the age-matched general population.

It appears that age itself is not an important risk factor for excess mortality, but the observed mortality is higher because of comorbid diseases and pre-operative left ventricular dysfunction.

If survival is good, is quality of life improved? This is a more difficult question to answer. However, in Chocron's[20] patients, who were operated on for calcific aortic stenosis at a mean age of 80 years, 67% were in NYHA class III or IV; on follow-up 78.6% were in functional class I and were living autonomously and free of operative sequelae. Glock et al[14] reported 96 consecutive patients aged 80 and above, 70% of whom were in NYHA class II or IV. At 4 years postoperatively, 87% were class I or II. Straumann et al[29] reported 93 patients 60 years of age and older, and 47 patients older than 70, with aortic stenosis. At 51 months, 96% were in NYHA class I or II. Tseng et al[28] reported 247 patients 70–89 years of age, with a mean age of 76 years. By using an instrument to assess quality of life, the patients scored comparably to the age-matched population norms in seven of eight dimensions of overall health. The exception was in mental health.

In summary, pre-operative mortality is higher than in younger patients, but probably is mainly due to higher pre-operative incidence of comorbidity and poor left ventricular function. The late survival is good, and the patients survive with good quality of life.

Mitral valve replacement/repair

There is less information about mitral valve replacement. Lee et al[30] reported 190 patients at least 70 years of age and 424 patients younger than 70 who were consecutively operated upon. The elderly patients had more degenerative mitral regurgitation, coronary artery disease, left ventricular dysfunction and class III or IV symptomatology. Operative mortality was 3.7% in the elderly versus 3.5% in the younger group. Seven-year survival was poorer in the elderly, $49 \pm 6\%$ versus $72 \pm 3\%$ in the younger. Freedom from complication-related death was poorer in the elderly, $57 \pm 7\%$ versus $79 \pm 3\%$, and freedom from death due to myocardial failure lower, $66 \pm 6\%$ versus $86 \pm 3\%$. By multivariate analysis, there was better survival with the younger age in mitral valve repair versus replacement, better NYHA pre-operative class and better left ventricular function. However, the 7-year freedom from complication-related death was excellent, and similar, for elderly patients $(90 \pm 7\%)$ and younger patients $(93 \pm 3\%)$ if the surgery was done only while the patient was in class I or II, with a left ventricular ejection fraction greater than 40%.[30] Akins et al[23] operated on patients 80 years of age and older and reported an in-hospital mortality of 6.3% with aortic valve replacement and coronary artery bypass surgery. With mitral valve replacement with or without coronary artery bypass surgery, the in-hospital mortality was 9.5%.

Arom et al[10] reported 610 patients with aortic valve replacement and 186 patients with mitral valve replacement, operated on from 1977 to 1992, either with or without coronary artery bypass grafts. Operative mortality was 6.4% with aortic valve replacement and 16% with mitral valve replacement. The mean follow-up time was 4.9 years for aortic valve replacement and 4.2 years for mitral valve replacement. Late death was 30% for aortic valve replacement and, similarly, 33% for mitral valve replacement. Freedom from thromboembolism was 91.6% ± 1.8%; from valve thrombosis, 98.8% ± 0.7%; from anticoagulant-related hemorrhage, 95.9% ± 1.1%; and from operative death, valve-related death and all complications, 78.8% ± 2.4%.

It appears that peri-operative mortality, and possibly late survival, is related to the presence of ischemic heart disease. Bolling et al[31] reported 100 consecutive patients aged 65–86 years, with a mean age of 73 years, operated from 1990 to 1995. Pre-operative functional class was III or IV, with an ejection fraction of 32 ± 2%. The average number of bypass grafts was 2.7 ± 0.2 grafts. All the patients had 4+ mitral regurgitation. A flexible annuloplasty ring was placed, and 54 patients had additional complex mitral valve repair. After surgery, no patient had greater than 1+ mitral regurgitation; peri-operative mortality was 4%, and late mortality 6%. There was a mean follow-up of 25 months, with congestive heart failure (CHF) occurring in nine patients, a transient ischemic episode (TIA) in one patient, infective endocarditis in one patient and respiratory failure in five patients. There were one early and two late mitral valve replacements. All the remaining patients were NYHA class I or II.

Mitral valve replacement in the presence of severe valvular and annular calcification can present major technical problems to the surgeon. In these situations, valve repair is usually not possible, and valve replacement is necessary. The calcification can result in a high incidence of paraprosthetic leaks, and special techniques have been designed to solve this problem.[32]

Balloon valvuloplasty

In 1986, balloon valvuloplasty was introduced as a possible nonsurgical way of dealing with aortic stenosis. It has been quite successful in congenital valvular aortic stenosis in children, increasing valve area and reducing systolic gradient; and presently it is the procedure of choice. In older patients with valvular aortic stenosis, however, balloon valvuloplasty has not been successful in relieving aortic stenosis on a long-term basis.[33] Otto et al[33] reported predictors of long-term outcome after balloon aortic valvuloplasty in 674 adults, mean age 78 ± 9 years. The mean aortic valve area was 0.3 cm²; overall survival was 55% at 1 year, 35% at 2 years and 23% at 3 years. Rehospitalization was common (64%), although 61% of survivors at 2 years reported improved symptoms. At 6 months, repeat echocardiography showed restenosis from a post-procedural valve area of 0.78 ± 0.31 cm² to 0.65 ± 0.25 cm² ($P < 0.0001$). With stepwise multivariate analysis, the model identified independent predictors of decreased survival as decreased baseline functional status, decreased cardiac output, decreased renal function, cachexia, female gender, decreased left ventricular systolic function and mitral regurgitation. Patients with the lowest risk were defined by normal left ventricular systolic function and mild clinical functional limitations. However, even their survival at 3 years was only 36%, compared with 17% in the remainder of the patients. Others have reported similar grim statistics.[34]

It is obvious that balloon aortic valvuloplasty is not an alternative to aortic valve replacement. However, it is possible to enlarge the valve opening in those patients who are poor candidates for aortic valve surgery because of their clinical condition. In such patients, balloon aortic valvuloplasty has been useful as a temporizing procedure to improve ventricular function and cardiac output, perfuse peripheral organs better and improve the overall functional status of the patient.[35,36] Once the patient has improved, aortic valve surgery should be done before valve restenosis occurs and the patient again becomes a high risk for surgery.

Another time when balloon aortic valvuloplasty is useful in the elderly patient with severe aortic stenosis is when the patient is not a candidate for surgery because of coexisting medical problems and is repeatedly hospitalized for problems related to the aortic stenosis, such as repeated congestive heart failure. Here the palliative effect of doubling the aortic valve area by valvuloplasty can be very helpful in improving the patient's quality of life and keeping the patient more functional and out of the hospital.[35,37]

Balloon valvuloplasty for mitral stenosis in the adult was introduced in 1984, and has been much more successful long-term. There have been large numbers of patients reported, with relatively short average follow-up times, from 1 to 3 years. The majority of patients have marked clinical improvement, and hemodynamic and clinical improvement persists at long-term follow-up.[38,39]

A randomized trial of balloon valvuloplasty versus surgical closed and open mitral commissurotomy has been reported, with a 7-year follow-up. There were 30 patients in each group.[40] The mitral area increased more with balloon valvuloplasty or open commissurotomy than with closed commissurotomy. There was no early or late mortality in any of the groups. The valve area at 7 years was still larger with balloon valvuloplasty or open commissurotomy than with closed commissurotomy. Restenosis was present in 6.6% after balloon valvotomy or open commissurotomy, versus 37% after closed commissuro-

tomy. Of the patients, 87% after balloon valvotomy, and 90% after open commissurotomy, were NYHA class I, versus 33% after closed commissurotomy ($P < 0.0001$). Freedom from reintervention was 90% after balloon valvotomy, 93% after open commissurotomy and 50% after closed commissurotomy. It appears that the results of balloon valvotomy are equivalent to open commissurotomy and better than closed commissurotomy.

However, in the older patient there is more calcification of the valve, which makes it less likely that balloon valvotomy would be successful. Le Feuvre et al[41] reported 280 patients treated with balloon mitral valvuloplasty; 28 (10%) were at least 70 years of age. The older patients were clinically sicker than the younger patients (NYHA class III or IV, 84 versus 67%; $P < 0.007$), had a higher echocardiographic score (9.3 ± 2 versus 8 ± 1.6; $P < 0.0004$), and greater incidence of atrial fibrillation (61 versus 36%; $P < 0.0001$). Complications of the procedure, that is, perforation of the left ventricle, embolism, severe mitral regurgitation or left-to-right shunt through the atrial septum, were greater in the older than in the younger patient (27 versus 9%), and 30-day mortality was higher (12 versus 0.8%; $P < 0.005$).

Complete success (mitral valve area increased $> 25\%$, and postmitral valve area > 1.5 cm^2) was present in 72% of the older, compared with 81% of the younger patients ($P = 0.1$). At 6 months, 20 of 21 surviving patients who had not crossed over to surgery had an improvement of at least one functional class, and 13% remained improved after a mean follow-up of 28 ± 17 months. It appears that balloon valvuloplasty can be effective in patients 70 years of age and over, but there is an increased morbidity and mortality compared to younger patients. Still, the hemodynamic success rate and midterm follow-up in those with good initial results, are similar to those seen in younger patients.

Summary

The most common valve problems in the octogenarian requiring surgery are aortic stenosis and mitral regurgitation. Valve surgery is possible in the patient whose major limitations are due to valve disease, albeit at a somewhat higher risk of morbidity and mortality than in the younger patient. Functional improvement is good, and appears to be sustained similarly to that seen in younger patients. However, because it is less a question of prolongation of life, surgery should be done only where there is a reasonable expectation that the result will improve the quality of the patient's life. Age alone is not a contraindication to valve surgery.

References

1. Beppu S, Suzuki S, Matsuda H et al. Rapidity of progression of aortic stenosis in patients with congenital bicuspid aortic valves. *Am J Cardiol* (1993) **71**:322–7.

2. Angelini A, Basso C, Grassi G et al. Surgical pathology of valve disease in the elderly. *Aging* (1994) **6**:225–37.

3. Sugiura M, Ohkawa S, Hiraoka K et al. A clinicopathological study on valvular diseases in 1000 consecutive autopsies of the aged. *Jpn Heart J* (1981) **22**:1–13.

4. Constant J. Clinical findings with elderly heart patients. In: Messerli FH, ed., *Cardiovascular Disease in the Elderly*, 3rd edn. (Kluwer Academic: Boston, 1993) 67.

5. Lindroos M, Kupari M, Heikkilä J, Tilvis R. Prevalence of aortic valve abnormalities in the elderly: an echocardiographic study of a random population sample. *J Am Coll Cardiol* (1993) **21**:1220–5.

6. Lindroos M, Kupari M, Valvanne J et al. Factors associated with calcific aortic valve degeneration in the elderly. *Eur Heart J* (1994) **15**:865–70.

7. Lakatta EG, Mitchell JH, Pomerance A, Rowe GG. Human aging: changes in structure and function. *J Am Coll Cardiol* (1987) **10**(Supplement A):42–7A.

8. Olson LJ, Subramanian R, Edwards WD. Surgical pathology of pure aortic insufficiency: a study of 225 cases. *Mayo Clin Proc* (1984) **59**:835–41.

9. Hylek EM, Singer DE. Risk factors for intracranial hemorrhage in outpatients taking warfarin. *Ann Intern Med* (1994) **120**: 897–902.

10. Arom KV, Emery RW, Nicoloff DM, Petersen RJ. Anticoagulant related complications in elderly patients with St Jude mechanical valve prostheses. *J Heart Valve Dis* (1996) **5**:505–10.

11. Merrill WH, Stewart JR, Frist WH et al. Cardiac surgery in patients age 80 years or older. *Ann Surg* (1990) **211**:772–5.

12. Naunheim KS, Dean PA, Fiore AC et al. Cardiac surgery in the octogenarian. *Eur J Cardiothorac Surg* (1990) **4**:13–15.

13. Rich MW, Sandza JG, Kleiger RE, Connors JP. Cardiac function in patients over 80 years of age. *J Thorac Cardiovasc Surg* (1985) **90**:56–60.

14. Glock Y, Faik M, Laghzaoui A et al. Cardiac surgery in the ninth decade of life. *Cardiovasc Surg* (1996) **4**:241–5.

15. Schwarz F, Baumann P, Manthey J et al. The effect of aortic valve replacement on survival. *Circulation* (1982) **66**:1105–10.

16. Pellikka PA, Nishimura RA, Bailey KR, Tajik AJ. The natural history of adults with asymptomatic, hemodynamically significant aortic stenosis. *J Am Coll Cardiol* (1990) **15**: 1012–17.

17. Kelly TA, Rothbart RM, Cooper CM et al. Comparison of outcome of asymptomatic to symptomatic patients older than 20 years of age with valvular aortic stenosis. *Am J Cardiol* (1988) **61**:123–30.

18. Rapaport E. Natural history of aortic and mitral valve disease. *Am J Cardiol* (1975) **35**:221–7.

19. Verheul HA, van den Brink RB, Bouma BJ et al. Analysis of risk factors for excess mortality after aortic valve replacement. *J Am Coll Cardiol* (1995) **26**: 1280–6.

20. Chocron S, Etievent JP, Clement F et al. Is surgery for aortic stenosis justified in patients over 75 years of age? *J Cardiovasc Surg* (1996) **37**:255–9.

21. Logeais Y, Langanay T, Roussin R et al. Surgery for aortic stenosis in elderly patients. A study of surgical risk and predictive factors. *Circulation* (1994) **90**:2891–8.

22. Elayda MA, Hall RJ, Reul RM et al. Aortic valve replacement in patients 80 years old and older. Operative risks and long-term results. *Circulation* (1993) **88** (Suppl II):11–16.

23. Akins CW, Daggett WM, Vlahakes GJ et al. Cardiac operations in patients 80 years old and older. *Ann Thorac Surg* (1997) **64**:606–14.

24. Aranki SF, Rizzo RJ, Couper GS et al. Aortic valve replacement in the elderly. Effect of gender and coronary artery disease on operative mortality. *Circulation* (1993) **88** (Suppl II):17–23.

25. Jamieson WRE, Tyers GFO, Janusz MT et al. Age as a determinant for selection of porcine bioprostheses for cardiac valve replacement: experience with Carpentier-Edwards standard biprosthesis. *Can J Cardiol* (1991) **7**:181–8.

26. Orszulak TA, Schaff HV, Mullany CJ et al. Risk of thromboembolism with the aortic Carpentier-Edwards bioprosthesis. *Ann Thorac Surg* (1995) **59**:462–8.

27. Cohn LH, Collins JJ Jr, DiSesa VJ et al. Fifteen-year experience with 1678 Hancock porcine bioprosthetic heart valve replacements. *Ann Surg* (1989) **210**:435–42.

28. Tseng EE, Lee CA, Cameron DE et al. Aortic valve replacement in the elderly. Risk factors and long-term results. *Ann Surg* (1997) **225**:793–802.

29. Straumann E, Kiowski W, Langer I et al. Aortic valve replacement in elderly patients with aortic stenosis. *Br Heart J* (1994) **71**:449–53.

30. Lee EM, Porter JN, Shapiro LM, Wells FC. Mitral valve surgery in the elderly. *J Heart Valve Dis* (1997) **6**:22–31.

31. Bolling SF, Deeb GM, Bach GS. Mitral valve reconstruction in elderly, ischemic patients. *Chest* (1996) **109**:35–40.

32. McEnany MT. Mitral valve replacement in the presence of severe valvular and annular calcification. *J Card Surg* (1993) **8**:117–24.

33. Otto CM, Mickel MC, Kennedy JW et al. Three-year outcome after balloon aortic valvuloplasty. Insights into prognosis of valvular aortic stenosis. *Circulation* (1994) **89**:642–50.

34. Kvidal PD, Stahle E, Nygren A et al. Long-term follow-up study on 64 elderly patients after balloon aortic valvuloplasty. *J Heart Valve Dis* (1997) **6**:480–6.

35. Cribier A, Jolly N, Letac B. The role of balloon aortic valvuloplasty in current practice. *Coron Artery Dis* (1993) **4**:943–6.

36. Smedira NG, Ports TA, Merrick SH, Rankin JS. Balloon aortic valvuloplasty as a bridge to aortic valve replacement in critically ill patients. *Ann Thorac Surg* (1993) **55**:914–16.

37. Cheitlin MD. Severe aortic stenosis in the sick octogenarian. A clear indicator for balloon valvuloplasty as the initial procedure. *Circulation* (1989) **80**:1906–8.

38. Iung B, Cormier B, Ducimétrière P et al. [5 year results of percutaneous mitral commissurotomy. Apropos of a series of 606 patients; late results after mitral dilatation.] *Arch Mal Coeur Vaisseux* (1996) **89**:1591–8.

39. Dean LS, Mickel M, Bonan R et al. Four-year follow-up of patients undergoing percutaneous balloon mitral commissurotomy. A report from the National Heart, Lung, and Blood Institute Balloon Valvuloplasty Registry. *J Am Coll Cardiol* (1996) **28**:1452–7.

40. Ben Farhat M, Ayari M, Maatouk F et al. Percutaneous balloon versus surgical closed and open mitral commissurotomy: seven-year follow-up results of a randomized trial. *Circulation* (1998) **97**:245–50.

41. Le Feuvre C, Bonan R, Lachurie ML et al. Balloon mitral commissurotomy in patients aged ≥70 years. *Am J Cardiol* (1993) **71**:233–6.

20

Surgery for valvular heart disease in octogenarians

Sary F Aranki, Meena Nathan and Lawrence H Cohn

Introduction

With the marked increases in life expectancy, survival beyond the ninth decade of life has become increasingly achievable. The life expectancy has increased by an astonishing 30 years since the beginning of this century. The average life expectancy by the year 2000 is expected to be almost 77 years.[1] By the year 2010 it is expected that well over 12 million people will be over the age of 80 in the United States alone.[2] This is roughly equivalent to the population of New York City, or the entire population of New England.

The socio-economic impact of such a large number of older people is significant. What is more significant is the impact posed by a sick octogenarian population.[3] Since cardiovascular disease is by far the most prevalent disease in the elderly population,[4] it becomes a major determinant in formulating the interaction between old age and survival.

General characteristics of octogenarians

Because women tend to outlive men by an average of 6–9 years, a large proportion of octogenarians are women and as a result are likely to be widowed and living alone. Life tables of the US population show that the life expectancy is 8.1 years and 6 years for an 80 and 85 year old respectively.[1] Independent living for this age group is the ultimate goal to achieve. However, in reality, some form of dependence is the norm rather than the exception.

Due to a multitude of factors, sick elderly patients occupy a large percentage of available hospital beds and the majority of available rehabilitation facilities. Consequently healthcare costs are disproportionately higher for older patients when compared to their younger cohorts.[5]

The pathophysiology of aging

Although natural selection may have allowed a person to reach the age of 80 and beyond, certain pathophysiological characteristics are prevalent in this age group. Increasing age is associated with a marked decrease in cell mass and with an accompanying increase in connective tissue formation. As a result there is a progressive linear loss of function with increasing age.[6] Therefore, diminished multisystem organ reserve and the presence of chronic comorbid conditions such as diabetes and chronic lung disease are more likely at this age. Such limitations may be adequate at baseline but can lead to rapid decompensations under stressful conditions such as major surgery. This can be further amplified when subjected to non-physiological conditions that can occur during cardiopulmonary bypass.[7]

Cardiovascular physiology in the elderly

Cardiac physiology tends to change with age. The myocardium tends to be stiffer due to a marked reduction in cell mass and its replacement with fibrous tissues. As a result, there is prolongation of myocardial relaxation time that leads to retardation of ventricular filling and cardiac output. There is also elevation of left ventricular end-diastolic pressure at rest and during exercise. Therefore pulmonary and systemic venous congestion occur easily and congestive heart failure (CHF) can occur even in the absence of systolic dysfunction. The elderly tend to have a higher afterload because of decreased arterial compliance. Left ventricular hypertrophy (LVH) can therefore occur even in the absence of hypertension due to diastolic dysfunction. This further increases the incidence of congestive heart failure.[8] Signs and symptoms of CHF are atypical in the elderly. They often present with somnolence, fatigue, confusion, disorientation, weakness and anorexia. There is also cognitive impairment that makes them poor historians which adds to the diagnostic dilemma.[9]

Cardiovascular disease in the elderly

Over the age of 80 there is an over 50% prevalence of heart disease that accounts for over 40% of all deaths at this age group. Coronary artery disease accounts for 85% of all deaths due to heart disease.[4] It is therefore inevitable that with the increase in the population of the elderly, there is a parallel increase in the number requiring major cardiac surgery for acquired disease such as valvular disease, coronary disease or a combination of the two.

Because coronary artery disease is by far the leading cardiac pathology at any age, this is even more pronounced in the elderly. It is inevitable that elderly patients are more likely to undergo combined valvular and coronary bypass operations than their younger cohorts. Therefore the results of valvular surgery in the elderly should be analyzed with this in mind.

Valvular heart disease in the elderly

Aortic stenosis

Aortic stenosis is the commonest valvular lesion in the elderly. The usual pathology is calcification of a tricuspid aortic valve. Less commonly a congenital bicuspid valve or rheumatic pathology may be the cause of stenosis.[10] The delay in carotid upstroke may be absent in the older patients because of the noncompliant vasculature. In very severe cases where the cardiac output is very diminished, the ejection systolic murmur may disappear altogether. Surgery is indicated when symptoms develop because of the extremely poor prognosis under this circumstance.[11,12]

Aortic regurgitation

Aortic regurgitation can present either acutely or chronically. The chronic form is by far the most common etiology. It is usually associated with hypertension, atherosclerosis, valvular deformity (sclerosis, congenital or infective) and aortic root dilation. Chronic aortic regurgitation is often asymptomatic for long periods and is well tolerated. Surgery is indicated when symptoms develop or if there is increased left ventricular dilation and worsening left ventricular function on serial echocardiographic follow up.[13]

Acute aortic regurgitation is usually secondary to infective endocarditis or acute ascending aortic dissection. It usually presents with acute congestive heart failure secondary to sudden volume overload. Surgical intervention is usually done on a nonelective basis, in contrast to the chronic lesions.[14]

Mitral regurgitation

Mitral regurgitation is secondary to leaflet, annular or subannular abnormalities or a combination of these lesions. The predominant pathology in the elderly is mitral valve prolapse or annular dilation secondary to left ventricular dysfunction. Coronary insufficiency is usually responsible for left ventricular dysfunction and papillary muscle dysfunction.[10] These pathophysiological mechanisms lead to the development of mitral insufficiency of ischemic origin (ischemic mitral regurgitation); less commonly, mitral regurgitation may be acute following papillary muscle rupture due to acute ischemic infarction of this muscle. Under these circumstances the presentation is more dramatic and surgical intervention is usually performed in a timely fashion after optimal medical management of cardiogenic shock.[15]

Mitral stenosis

Mitral stenosis, usually rheumatic in origin, is acquired at a young age. Silent mitral stenosis should be considered when dyspnea and/or atrial fibrillation are present. Surgery can be postponed for many years by maintenance of sinus rhythm alone. Indications for surgery include increasing symptoms, and signs of progressive pulmonary hypertension. Unlike younger patients, the mitral valve annulus and leaflets are usually heavily calcified in older patients. Consequently open mitral commissurotomy and mitral valve repair are rarely performed. Mitral valve replacement is the treatment of choice.[15]

Tricuspid regurgitation

Tricuspid regurgitation is due to left-sided valvular lesions in the majority of cases. Surgical correction should be considered in the presence of severe regurgitation and preserved right ventricular function. Caution should be exercised in the presence of moderate to severe right ventricular dysfunction and fixed pulmonary hypertension.[16] In the majority of cases, valve repair can be accomplished successfully. For the remainder, tricuspid valve replacement, usually with a bioprosthesis, is performed. For both techniques, the results (short and long term) are similar.[17]

Infective endocarditis

Infective endocarditis is not uncommon in the elderly and in fact the elderly are the second most common group affected after intravenous drug abusers. Elderly patients tend to have more silent valvular pathology and as a result proper endocarditis prophylaxis may be significantly underpracticed. In addition, there is an increasing number of older patients with prosthetic heart valves, with an inevitable increase in the number of cases of prosthetic valve endocarditis. Therefore, any unexplained fever warrants prompt fever workup and immediate treatment with intravenous broad spectrum antibiotics and surgery if indicated.[18]

The results of valvular surgery in octogenarians

Advances in cardiac surgery have contributed markedly to the results of cardiac surgery in general and to those of elderly patients in particular. A multitude of factors has contributed to these improvements. Refinements in surgical techniques, better myocardial protection and advances in the care of the critically ill patients are perhaps the leading responsible factors. Other equally important factors include advances in cardiac anesthesia, the technology of cardiopulmonary bypass, and the development of strategies to reduce blood loss.

Before discussing the results of cardiac surgery in octogenarians it is prudent to discuss the role of balloon valvuloplasty in this age group. This technique is not readily performed for rheumatic mitral valve stenosis due to the reasons mentioned earlier. Aortic balloon valvuloplasty for aortic stenosis, on the other hand, was widely practiced for a brief period that peaked in the late 1980s. The failure rate of this procedure[19] has relegated its use to the bare minimum as a supporting role (if any) to surgical intervention. The attraction of balloon valvuloplasty as a minimally invasive approach to valvular heart disease was the driving force behind its use. However, the recent development of minimally invasive cardiac surgical techniques[20] has revived this concept in order to minimize the trauma of surgery and shorten the rehabilitation period.

The results of valvular surgery in octogenarians should be compared to the aggregate survival in unselected 80 year olds. Data from the 1980 United States census estimate the 1-, 5- and 10-year survival for this age group to be 91%, 55%, and 21% respectively.[21] More importantly, the impact of surgery on the natural history of the valvular pathology should be carefully examined. For instance, the survival of patients (at any age) after the onset of symptoms with severe aortic stenosis is 57%, 37%, and 25% at 1, 2, and 3 years, respectively.[22] The results of surgery can therefore be compared to these statistics to determine the inherent risk/benefit probabilities of these procedures.

Old age and cardiac surgery have undergone a major evolution in recent years. The definition of old age was the centerpiece of such an evolution. Reports on patients over 65 years of age appeared in the literature in the early 1970s. Barnhorst et al[23] from the Mayo Clinic reported on the results of cardiac surgery in patients older than 65 years. None of the 305 patients in that report were older than age 80, and 70% of the patients were younger than 70 years. Double digit mortality was reported for valvular procedures, with isolated aortic valve replacement having the lowest mortality. Jamieson et al[24] reported on 320 consecutive patients older than 65 years with a mean age of 68 years. The operative mortality for isolated aortic valve replacement was 4.7% compared to double digit mortality for other procedures. The authors contributed a table to compare the early mortality for various valvular procedures that gives clear information about the risk of surgery in older patients for that particular time.

Continued improvements in cardiac surgical techniques were mirrored by improved results in older and sicker patients. This is evidenced by the next generation of reports that focused primarily on patients older than 70 years of age. The results of these various reports were summarized by Aranki et al[25] and give an indication about the mortality rates for isolated valve surgery and for patients requiring concomitant CABG. The focus then shifted to the older elderly patients, and multiple reports appeared in the literature on octogenarians and cardiac valvular surgery.[25–33] Table 20.1 summarizes the results of these reports. It appears that the majority of these patients underwent aortic valve surgery. In addition, there is an equal gender distribution and a higher rate of requirement for a concomitant CABG procedure. Isolated valve procedures have lower operative mortality than valve and concomitant procedures. The 5-year actuarial survival is in line with or even better than the natural life tables for a matched age group,

Study	Year	Number of patients	Mean age (years)	Male (%)	CABG (%)	AVR (%)	MVR (%)	OM (%)	LOS (days)	Survival (%)
Rich et al[26]	1984	15	83	64	80	60	40	7	19.5	NS
Tsai et al[27]	1985	25	82	49	60	58	42	21	23	NS
Fiore et al[28]	1989	25	82	44	56	68	32	20	18	NS
Levinson et al[29]	1989	64	82	58	45	100	—	9	NS	67
Deleuze et al[30]	1990	60	82	45	10	100	—	28	15	61
Guilford et al[31]	1991	71	83	49	60	100	—	12.7	NS	NS
Freeman et al[32]	1991	113	82	51	50	87	27	15	16.4	60
MacArthur et al[33]	1993	171	82	50	44	100	—	17.5	NS	76
Aranki et al[25]	1993	188	83	40	56	100	—	6.4	NS	NS

CABG, coronary artery bypass grafts; AVR, aortic valve replacement; MVR, mitral valve replacement; OM, operative mortality; LOS, mean length of hospital stay in days; NS, not stated.

Table 20.1
Summary of published results on valvular surgery in octogenarians

and certainly better than that of the natural history of the underlying pathology.

Current results of valvular surgery in octogenarians

Most published results to date have focused on aortic valve replacement in the octogenarian. Data on the results of mitral valve surgery are scarce in comparison. The reason for this discrepancy perhaps relates to the fact that aortic valve surgery is more common in this age group and the results are more gratifying.

Data from the Cleveland Clinic presented recently reviewed the results of aortic valve replacement in 248 octogenarians (mean age 82.6 ± 2.3 years) who were operated on between 1980 and 1995. Myocardial revascularization was required in 60% of the patients. Bioprostheses were used in 92% of the patients and 26% of the patients required a size 19 mm valve. In-hospital mortality was 8.9% overall. The mortality for isolated valve surgery was 5% and for that combined with CABG was 11.9%. Hospital survivors were followed for a mean of 9.7 years. Survival was 85%, 60% and 30% and freedom for cardiovascular events was 80%, 49% and 30% at 1, 5, and 10 years, respectively. Multivariate analysis and Cox regression analysis identified triple vessel coronary artery disease and congestive heart failure to be independent predictors of early and late mortality.[34]

We reviewed our recent results in valvular heart surgery in octogenarians at the Brigham and Women's Hospital. Two recent distinct periods, separated by an interval of 5 years, were chosen to determine the trend in our practice and the results achieved. All valvular surgery procedures in octogenarians for the years 1992 and 1997 were analyzed. Octogenarians accounted for 12% and 15% of the total valvular procedures performed in 1992 and 1997 respectively. Table 20.2 summarizes the profile of these patients, their operative mortality and their length of hospital stay. There is a trend for a significant reduction in operative mortality that appears to be due to improvement in the results of mitral valve surgery. Patients who underwent more complicated procedures were grouped under 'other' in Table 20.2. These included double or triple valve replacements with or without CABG, with half of these patients requiring a reoperative procedure. Of the five deaths in 1992, two were re-operations (40%), three had a concomitant CABG (60%) and three (60%) were from the 'other' category. Of the seven deaths in 1997, three (43%) were re-operations, four had a concomitant CABG (57%) and four (57%) were from the 'other' category.

The other striking difference between these two periods was the marked reduction in the length of hospital stay (LOS). There has been about a 40% reduction in the LOS overall, and about 50% reduction for aortic and mitral valve surgery. For the higher risk and complicated procedures there was no meaningful reduction of LOS (Table 20.2). The type of prostheses used are listed in Tables 20.3 and 20.4 for those used in the aortic and mitral positions respectively. Another major difference between the two periods appears to be an increase in the use of bovine pericardial valves in the aortic position, and a modest use of the recently introduced stentless porcine valve. For the mitral position there was a marked increase in mitral valve repair compared to replacement. The rate of use of mechanical valves in the mitral position was double that of the aortic position, probably because these patients were already anticoagulated for atrial fibrillation.

For the 1992 group, 36 patients were dis-

	AVR		MVR		Other		All	
	1992	*1997*	*1992*	*1997*	*1992*	*1997*	*1992*	*1997*
Number (%)	27 (66%)	56 (62%)	8 (19%)	26 (29%)	6 (15%)	8 (9%)	41	90
Mean age	83.5	83.5	82.5	83	82	82	82.8	83.4
Males (%)	49	48	12.5	35	50	80	39	44
Reop (%)	7	11	36	19	33	38	17	17
CABG (%)	67	54	38	65	50	63	59	59
OM (%)	3.7	3.5	12.5	0	50	50	12.2	7.7
LOS (days)	14.7	8.9	28.6	12.6	17	16	17.3	10.6

AVR, aortic valve replacement; MVR, mitral valve replacement; other, patients who had two or more valvular procedures; CABG, coronary artery bypass grafts; OM, operative mortality; LOS, mean length of hospital stay in days; reop, reoperations or redo surgery.

Table 20.2
The profile and results of patients requiring valvular surgery in 1992 and 1997

	Number (percentage) of prostheses	
Type of prosthesis	*1992*	*1997*
Porcine	22 (70%)	22 (37%)
Pericardial	7 (22%)	30 (50%)
Mechanical	3 (9%)	4 (8%)
Stentless	0	3 (5%)
Total	32	59

Table 20.3
The type of prostheses used in the aortic position for octogenarians in 1992 and 1997

charged from the hospital and at the end of 5 years of follow-up 21 patients were alive. Mean New York Heart Association Functional Class at 5 years was 1.4, decreased from a pre-operative value of 3.1. Survival at yearly intervals is shown in Figure 20.1. Overall 5-year survival was 51% and the survival for discharged patients was 58%. Overall 5-year survival for patients who underwent aortic valve surgery was 67%, and survival for discharged patients was 70%.

Type of prosthesis	Number (percentage) of prostheses	
	1992	1997
Porcine	12	7
Mechanical	2	5
Rings (for repair)	0	20
Total	14	32

Table 20.4
The type of prostheses used in the mitral position for octogenarians in 1992 and 1997

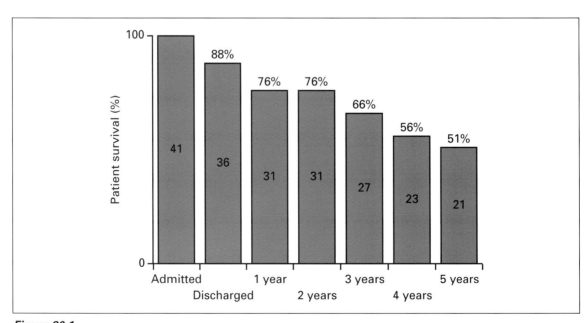

Figure 20.1
Survival at yearly intervals for octogenarian patients requiring valvular heart surgery at the Brigham and Women's Hospital operated on in 1992.

Summary

With the continuing expansion of the octogenarian population and the prevalence of acquired heart disease, the need for valvular heart surgery for this group is on the increase. Advances in cardiac surgery have allowed for continuously improved short- and long-term results. Such results are comparable to the life tables and certainly superior to the natural history of the underlying pathology. Of the various valvular lesions, the results of surgery for aortic valve pathology appear to be the most gratifying in the long term. The results of surgery for complicated multivalvular lesions, especially in the presence of coronary artery disease, are the least gratifying.

Acknowledgements

The authors thank Kathleen LaMae and Sam Sears for their valuable assistance with preparation of the manuscript.

References

1. US Bureau of the Census. Statistical Abstract of the United States 1991 (111 edition). Washington, DC, 1991.

2. National Center for Health Statistics. Vital Statistics of the United States, 1998 vol 11, Section 6, Washington, DC, 1990.

3. Butler RN. The challenge of geriatric medicine. In: Wilson JD, Braunwald E, Issellbacher KJ, Petersdof RG, Martin JB, Fauci AS, Root RK, eds, *Harrison's Principles of Internal Medicine*, 12th edn. (McGraw Hill: New York, 1991) 16–19.

4. Wei JY. Heart disease in the elderly. *Cardiovasc Med* (1989) 9:971–82.

5. Siegal JS. Recent and prospective demographic trends for the elderly population and some complications for health one. In: *Second Conference on the Epidemiology of Aging.* (National Institutes of Health: Bethesda, MD, 1980).

6. Harman D. The aging process. *Proc Natl Acad Sci USA* (1981) 78:7124–8.

7. Aranki SF. Cardiovascular surgery in the elderly. In: Homberger F, ed., *The Rationale Use of Advanced Medical Technology in the Elderly.* (Springer Publishing Company: New York, 1994) 132–45.

8. Avolio AP, Fa-Quan D, Wei-Qiang L et al. Effects of aging on arterial distensibility in populations with high and low prevalence of hypertension: comparison between urban and rural communities in China. *Circulation* (1985) 71:202–10.

9. Folstein MF, Folstein ME, McHugh PR. Minimental state: a practical method for grading the cognitive state of patients for the clinician. *J Psychiatr Res* (1975) 12:189–98.

10. Pomerance A. Cardiac pathology in the elderly. In: Noble RJ, Rothbaum DA, eds, *Geriatric Cardiology, Cardiovascular Clinics.* (F.A. Davis: Philadelphia, PA, 1981) 9–21.

11. Roberts WC, Perloff JK, Costantino T. Severe valvular aortic stenosis in patients over 65 years of age. *Am J Cardiol* (1971) 27:497–506.

12. Hwang MH, Hammermeister KE, Oprian C et al. Pre-operative identification of patients likely to have left ventricular dysfunction after aortic valve replacement: participants in the Veterans Administration Cooperative Study on Valvular Heart Disease. *Circulation* (1989) 80(Suppl 3): I65–70.

13. Bonow RO, Rosing DR, Maron BJ et al. Reversal of left ventricular dysfunction after aortic valve replacement for chronic aortic regurgitation. Influence of duration of preoperative left ventricular dysfunction. *Circulation* (1984) 70:570–9.

14. Wei JH, Gersh BJ. Heart disease in the elderly. *Curr Probl Cardiol* (1987) 12:1–65.

15. Hochberg MS, Derkae WM, Conkle DM et al. Mitral valve replacement in elderly patients. Encouraging post operative clinical and hemodynamic results. *J Cardiovasc Thorac Surg* (1979) 77:422–6.

16. Cohn LH. Valvular surgery. *Curr Opin Cardiol* (1991) 6:235–45.

17. McGrath LB, Gonzalez-Lavin L, Bailey BM et al. Tricuspid valve operations in 530 patients. Twenty five year assessment of early and late phase events. *J Thorac Cardiovasc Surg* (1990) 99:124–33.

18. Weiner G, Schultz R, Fuchs J et al. Infective endocarditis in the elderly in the era of transesophageal echocardiography. Clinical features and prognosis compared with younger patients. *Am J Med* (1996) 100:90–7.

19. Bernardo Y, Etievent J, Mourad JL et al. Long-term results of percutaneous aortic valvuloplasty compared with aortic valve replacement in patients more than 70 years old. *J Am Coll Cardiol* (1992) 20:796–801.

20. Cohn LH, Adams DH, Couper GS et al. Minimally invasive cardiac valve surgery improves patient satisfaction while reducing costs of cardiac valve replacement and repair. *Ann Surg* (1997) 226:421–8.

21. National Center for Health Statistics: United States Life Tables; US Decennial Life Tables

for 1979–1981. Vol 1, No 1. (DHHS Publication no (PHS) 85-1158-1) (US Government Printing Office: Washington DC, 1985).

22. O'Keefe JH, Vlietstra RE, Bailey KR, Holmes DR. Natural history of candidates for balloon aortic valvuloplasty. *Mayo Clin Proc* (1987) **62**:986–91.

23. Barnhorst DA, Guiliani ER, Pluth JR et al. Open-heart surgery in patients more than 65 years old. *Ann Thorac Surg* (1974) **18**:81–90.

24. Jamieson WR, Dooner J, Munro AI et al. Cardiac valve replacement in the elderly: a review of 320 consecutive cases. *Circulation* (1981) **64**(Supplement II):II177–83.

25. Aranki SF, Rizzo RJ, Couper GS et al. Aortic valve replacement in the elderly: effect of gender and coronary artery disease on operative mortality. *Circulation* (1993) **88**(Pt 2):17–23.

26. Rich MW, Sandza JG, Kleiger RE, Connors JP. Cardiac operations in patients over 80 years of age. *J Thorac Cardiovasc Surg* (1985) **90**:56–60.

27. Tsai TP, Matloff MJ, Gray RJ et al. Cardiac surgery in the octogenarian. *J Thorac Cardiovasc Surg* (1986) **91**:924–8.

28. Fiore AC, Naunheim KS, Barner HB et al. Valve replacement in the octogenarian. *Ann Thorac Surg* (1989) **48**:104–8.

29. Levinson JR, Akins CW, Buckley MJ et al. Octogenarians with aortic stenosis. *Circulation* (1989) **80**(Suppl I):I49–56.

30. Deleuze PH, Loisance DY, Besnainou F et al. Severe aortic stenosis in octogenarians: is operation an acceptable alternative? *Ann Thorac Surg* (1990) **50**:226–9.

31. Culliford AT, Galloway AC, Colvin SB et al. Aortic valve replacement for aortic stenosis in persons aged 80 years and over. *Am J Cardiol* (1991) **67**:1256–60.

32. Freeman WK, Schaff HV, O'Brien PC et al. Cardiac surgery in the octogenarian: perioperative outcome and clinical follow-up. *J Am Coll Cardiol* (1991) **18**:29–35.

33. Elayda MA, Hall RJ, Reul RM et al. Aortic valve replacement in patients 80 years and older: operative risks and long-term results. *Circulation* (1993) **88**:11–16.

34. Medalion B, Lytle BW, McCarthy P et al. Abstract book of the *34th Annual Meeting of the Thoracic Society of Thoracic Surgery*. 1998 New Orleans, 120.

21

Arrhythmias and conduction disturbances in the octogenarian: epidemiology and progression

Jerome L Fleg

Introduction

The aging of the American population that has occurred over the past half century has been most pronounced among the oldest old. Thus, the number of individuals aged 85 and older increased from 0.6 million in 1950 to 2.7 million in 1985, while the number older than 65 years only doubled over this period. Although it is widely recognized that the prevalence of cardiac arrhythmias and conduction disturbances generally increases with age, information specific to persons in their 80s and beyond is relatively sparse. This chapter briefly reviews the epidemiology and prognostic significance of arrhythmias and conduction disorders in older adults, with a focus on octogenarians when specific data are available.

Supraventricular arrhythmias

The prevalence of supraventricular arrhythmias, whether assessed at rest, during routine activity, or during strenuous aerobic exercise, rises dramatically with advancing age. Isolated atrial ectopic beats (AEB) are observed on the resting ECG in 5–10% of subjects over 60 years old and are not generally associated with organic heart disease. In healthy volunteers older than 60 years from the Baltimore Longitudinal Study of Aging (BLSA), such AEB occurred on resting ECG in 6%, during 24-hour ambulatory monitoring in 88%[1] and during or after maximal treadmill exercise in 39%.[2] Isolated AEB were found at rest in 17% of 350 Finns at least 85 years old who were free of cardiac symptoms and in 13% of 238 heart failure patients in this age group.[3] Similarly, Golden and Golden found AEB in 16 of 100 nursing-home patients older than 90 years.[4] Ambulatory monitoring detected isolated AEB during 24-hour monitoring in 89% of institutionalized elderly with a mean age of 82 years[5] and in all 50 apparently healthy subjects 80–100 years old studied by Kantelip et al.[6] Over a mean follow-up of 10 years, such isolated AEB, even if frequent, did not presage increased cardiac risk in 98 clinically normal older BLSA subjects.[7]

Short runs of paroxysmal supraventricular tachycardia (PSVT), although rarely observed on a standard 12-lead ECG, are commonly detected during 24-hour ambulatory monitoring of older subjects. In predominantly healthy subjects aged at least 65 years from the Cardiovascular Health Study (CHS), such PSVT runs were observed in 50% of 643 men and 48% of 729 women and nearly doubled in prevalence from the late 60s to the 80s.[8] Short runs of PSVT occurred in 28% of healthy 80–100 year old subjects[6] and 36% of 453 nursing home patients aged 82 ± 8 years.[5] Runs of PSVT 3–32 beats in length were found in 13% of healthy BLSA subjects at least 60 years old[1] and had no prognostic significance for coronary events over a 10-year mean follow-up period.[7] Even more common than classical PSVT in these older BLSA volunteers were short runs of benign slow atrial tachycardia, defined by an abrupt decrease in RR interval of more than 30% that persisted for at least three beats at a rate of 80–140/minute;[9] this arrhythmia occurred in 28% of the subjects and appeared to have no prognostic significance. Although the mean age of PSVT patients presenting to referral centers was 44 years in 17 published series, a recent population-based study has demonstrated that the relative risk of seeking medical attention for this arrhythmia was 5.3 in persons at least 65 years old compared with younger persons.[10]

Maximal treadmill exercise induced short runs of PSVT in 3.5% of more than 3000 tests on clinically normal BLSA subjects 20–94 years old; similar to PSVT detected during routine activity, most of these episodes were asymptomatic 3–5 beat salvos.[11] The prevalence of PSVT increased from less than 1% below age 50 to approximately 10% in the over 80s. In older subjects, exercise-induced PSVT occurred twice as frequently in men as in women. Although no differences in coronary risk profile or coronary event incidence over the subsequent 5.7 ± 3.9 years was observed in these subjects with exercise-induced PSVT compared with control subjects matched for age and sex, 10% of the former group subsequently developed a spontaneous atrial tachyarrhythmia versus only 2% of the controls.[11]

Treatment of PSVT in the elderly resembles that in younger patients. Drugs that slow atrioventricular conduction such as beta-blockers, heart-rate-limiting calcium antagonists or digoxin represent the first line of therapy. Although type 1 anti-arrhythmic

drugs may be used in patients refractory to the above agents, radiofrequency ablation is being increasingly used in such patients. This procedure was successful in 67 of 68 patients 70 years old or over with refractory PSVT or atrial fibrillation, with excellent safety and long-term results.[12]

Atrial fibrillation (AF) is undoubtedly the most clinically important supraventricular arrhythmia in the octogenarian, due to its high prevalence and major prognostic significance. In the Framingham Study and in the CHS, AF was found in 3–4% of subjects older than 60–65 years, a prevalence 10-fold higher than in the general adult population.[8,13] Past the age of 85, AF was present at rest in 14% of asymptomatic Finns and 24% of those with heart failure.[3] In the CHS, approximately two-thirds of the AF detected on ambulatory ECG was sustained and one-third was intermittent.[8] Chronic AF is most often secondary to coronary and hypertensive heart disease, mitral valve disorders, thyrotoxicosis and sick sinus syndrome. Thus, the high prevalence of AF in the elderly can be explained in large part by the high prevalence of these associated conditions. The association between thyrotoxicosis and AF occurs almost exclusively in the elderly, and AF may be the sole manifestation of so-called 'apathetic' hyperthyroidism in this age group.[14]

A minority of older patients with AF have no identifiable cause for the arrhythmia. Such individuals with 'lone AF' comprised 17% of men and 6% of women with AF in the Framingham Study with mean ages of 71 and 68 years, respectively.[15] The proportion of all AF cases represented by lone AF was more than twice as high in subjects older than 80 years than in those younger than 60. Over a mean follow-up of 11 years, individuals with lone AF suffered over four times as many strokes as controls, matched for age and sex. However, their incidence of congestive heart failure and coronary events was not increased.[15] This higher risk of strokes in older patients with lone AF differs from the benign prognosis associated with this arrhythmia in younger populations.[16]

The importance of AF as a cause of stroke appears to escalate with age; the incidence of stroke in patients with AF increases from 6.7% in the sixth decade to 26.2% in the ninth decade.[17] This high stroke risk in older AF patients has led to several large randomized trials of anticoagulants and antiplatelet drugs for nonrheumatic AF.[18–21] The consensus from these trials is that coumadin markedly reduces the risk for stroke in these older AF cohorts; in patients at high risk of bleeding on coumadin, aspirin is a reasonable alternative.

In younger patients with newly diagnosed AF, an attempt at medical or direct current cardioversion is usually recommended. Whether cardioversion versus rate control of AF is predictive of a better long-term outcome in AF patients older than 65 years must await the results of the multicenter Atrial Fibrillation Follow-up Investigation of Rhythm Management (AFFIRM) trial. In the meantime, the relatively high morbidity associated with this arrhythmia in the elderly, as well as the frequent complications from long-term anticoagulation and anti-arrhythmic drugs, make it reasonable to attempt cardioversion in most elderly patients with recent onset AF, including those older than 80 years.

Ventricular arrhythmias

Both the prevalence and density of ventricular ectopic beats (VEB) increase dramatically with advancing age, both in unselected populations in acute hospital or in chronic care facilities and in those without clinical heart disease. In asymptomatic BLSA men with a normal exercise ECG, the prevalence of VEB on a resting ECG increased from 0.5% below age 40 to 11.5% in those 80 years old or over. Of interest, no age-associated increase was observed in healthy BLSA women.[2] In Finns over 85 years old, VEB were found on resting in ECG in 5% of those without heart disease, 13% of those with coronary artery disease and 28% of those with heart failure.[3]

Ambulatory 24-hour ECG studies in older patients have consistently shown a high prevalence of both simple and complex VEB. In asymptomatic elderly, VEB have been reported in 69–96% of subjects.[2,6,8,22] Furthermore, the density and complexity of VEB on ambulatory ECG increases with age. Among 101 subjects ages 10–69 years who were free of heart disease by rigorous screening, both the prevalence and absolute number of VEB in 24-hours varied directly with age.[23] In asymptomatic subjects 65 years old or over, ventricular couplets have been reported in 4–11% and short runs of ventricular tachycardia in 2–7%;[2,6,8,22] such complex VEB forms are rare in young populations. The prevalence of both simple and complex VEB was higher in men than women in the 1372 older subjects from the CHS who underwent 24-hour ECG recording.[8] In 453 institutionalized elderly of mean age 82 years, nonsustained VT was observed in 9% and VEB couplets in another 19%, probably reflecting the high prevalence of cardiac disease in these patients.[5] Exercise testing also elicits a striking age-associated increase in the prevalence and complexity of VEB. In BLSA volunteers without apparent heart disease, isolated VEB during or after maximal treadmill exercise increased in prevalence from 11% in the third decade to 57% in the ninth decade.[2] The prevalence of frequent exercise-induced VEB or nonsustained ventricular tachycardia also increased markedly with age (Figure 21.1), although this increase was

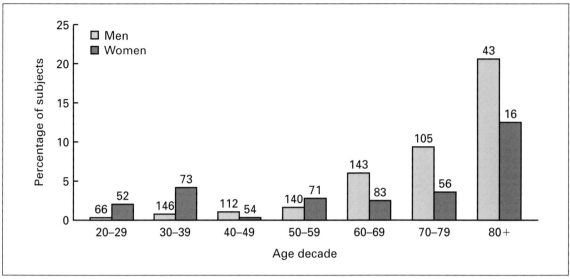

Figure 21.1
Prevalence of frequent VEB (≥10% of beats in any minute) or nonsustained VT during maximal treadmill exercise testing in 1160 clinically healthy BLSA volunteers. The numbers above each bar indicate the number of subjects tested in each decade. In both sexes, a striking increase in prevalence is observed beyond 80 years of age. (From Busby et al[24] with permission)

statistically significant only in men.[24] Possible mechanisms for the marked age-associated increase in VEB, even in apparently healthy subjects, include undetected organic heart disease, increased LV mass, higher plasma catecholamine levels, more frequent electrolyte abnormalities, longer QT intervals, or intrinsic age changes in cardiac muscle.[25]

The prognostic significance of VEB in older individuals is controversial and depends in large part on the presence or absence of underlying cardiovascular disease. On the resting ECG, VEB were associated with a 3.3-fold risk of cardiac death in Busselton[26] but no increase in Framingham[27] or in MRFIT study subjects older than 50 years;[28] in contrast, younger

MRFIT subjects with VEB on a 2-minute rhythm strip suffered a 14-fold relative risk of sudden cardiac death compared with arrhythmia-free age peers. In 1153 nursing-home residents, VEB on resting ECG were associated with a 1.6-fold risk of cardiac events over a mean follow-up of 45 months; however, multivariate analysis was not performed, leaving the independent role of VEB uncertain.[29]

In carefully screened healthy BLSA subjects 60 years old and over, VEB detected on 24-hour ambulatory ECG, even if frequent or complex, did not predict coronary events over the next 10 years.[7] A smaller study of community-dwelling healthy elders aged

79 ± 7 years reached a similar conclusion.[30] In contrast, a 5-year follow-up study by Martin et al reported an almost doubled crude mortality among individuals aged 75 years and over with at least 10 VEB/hour on 24-hour ECG.[31] About 40% of the original cohort were taking cardioactive drugs, raising the possibility that underlying cardiac disease rather than VEB per se explained these findings. Aronow et al reported a doubled risk of subsequent coronary events in elderly nursing home residents with heart disease and complex VEB on ambulatory ECG compared with similar patients without such VEB. However, the event risk was not increased in the group with complex VEB but no heart disease.[32] Long-term follow-up of 80 predominantly older (age 64 ± 13 years) asymptomatic BLSA subjects with frequent or repetitive VEB induced by treadmill exercise testing demonstrated no increase in cardiac morbidity or mortality.[24] Thus, the conclusion to be drawn from these follow-up studies is that VEB in clinically healthy elderly subjects, whether detected by resting ECG, ambulatory 24-hour monitoring or treadmill exercise, do not predict increased cardiac risk. Whether the apparent increased cardiac mortality in octogenarians with frequent or complex VEB and heart disease is due to the arrhythmia or the underlying substrate remains unclear.

Treatment of individuals with complex VEB, regardless of their age, has steered away from conventional anti-arrhythmic drugs after the Cardiac Arrhythmia Suppression Trial demonstrated excess mortality in postmyocardial infarction patients less than 80 years old treated with encainide, flecainide or moricizine.[33,34] In an elderly nursing-home population (age 82 ± 7 years), Aronow et al found no significant effect of quinidine on either cardiac or total mortality in patients with heart disease and complex VEB, defined by frequent

paired, or multiform VEB or nonsustained VT.[35] A subsequent study in this population, however, demonstrated a 47% reduction in sudden cardiac death, a 37% decrease in total cardiac death and a trend toward reduced total mortality in patients with complex VEB and ejection fraction at least 40% who were treated with propranolol.[36] Although propranolol reduced the occurrence of VEB and VT by 71%, multivariate analyses revealed that the reduction in mortality by propranolol was more closely related to its anti-ischemic effect than its anti-arrhythmic effect.[37] Whether class III anti-arrhythmic drugs such as amiodarone or sotalol can reduce arrhythmia endpoints or total mortality in octogenarians remains unclear; the potent side-effects associated with the latter drugs dictate that they be reserved for those with life threatening ventricular arrhythmias who are unresponsive to, or intolerant of, beta-blockers.

As in younger patients, octogenarians with drug-resistant sustained ventricular tachycardia or ventricular fibrillation should be referred for nonpharmacological interventions. In such patients, Tresch et al demonstrated identical 80% 25-month survival in patients older versus younger than 65 years, treated with an automatic implantable cardioverter defibrillator (AICD).[38] Thus, an AICD appears to be the treatment of choice in such elderly patients. A large percentage of these patients will also require anti-arrhythmic drugs, most often amiodarone, to reduce the likelihood of AICD discharge.

Conduction disturbances: anatomical changes

Multiple anatomical changes in the cardiac conduction system occur with advancing age. Increases in collagenous and elastic fibers are observed throughout the conduction system. Fat deposits around and within the sinoatrial (SA) node may produce a partial or complete separation of the node from the atrial musculature. This separation, if extreme, may result in sick sinus syndrome. In addition, a marked reduction in the number of pacemaker cells in the SA node begins by 60 years; by age 75, less than 10% of the cell numbers found in young adults remains. Calcification of the left side of the cardiac skeleton, involving the aortic and mitral annuli, the central fibrous body and the summit of the interventricular septum, occurs to a variable extent. Because of their proximity to these structures, the atrioventricular (AV) node, His bundle, bifurcation and proximal left and right bundle branches may be infiltrated, causing major conduction disturbances.[39]

Sinoatrial node function

Although resting heart rate is not age-related in healthy subjects, the phasic variation in R–R interval known as respiratory sinus arrhythmia declines with age due to a reduction in cardiac parasympathetic activity.[40,41] In an institutionalized population aged 81 ± 8 years, Aronow et al[42] noted a 1.14-fold risk for new coronary events for each 5 beat/min increment of mean 24-hour heart rate, a finding similar to that in younger populations. Maximal sinus rate is reduced by approximately one beat per year due to the well-documented decrease in beta-adrenergic responsiveness seen with aging.[43] The formula $220 -$ age for predicting maximal exercise heart rate in younger individuals appears to be reasonably accurate beyond the age of 80 years as well.

On 24-hour ambulatory ECG recording in 50 apparently healthy octogenarians and nonagenarians, Kantelip et al observed no episodes of sinus bradycardia below 43 beats/min and no sinus pauses longer than 2.0 seconds,[6] findings parallel to those in BLSA volunteers 60–85 years.[1] Thus, sinus rates less than 40/min and pauses longer than 2.0 seconds are abnormal, even in octogenarians, and suggest the presence of sinus node disease. In 1372 subjects over 65 years in the CHS, bradycardia less than or equal to 40 beats/min was seen in 4.4% of men but only 1.4% of women.[8] Pauses longer than 3 seconds, however were equally rare in both sexes, 0.6% in men and 0.4% in women. Such pauses, although frequently considered to be diagnostic of sick sinus syndrome, do not automatically constitute a need for pacemakers in asymptomatic individuals. Hilgard et al[44] found pauses longer than 3.0 seconds in 53 (0.8%) of 6470 consecutive patients undergoing 24-hour ECG recordings; 42% of these were due to sinus arrest and the remainder to AV block. The 3-year survival probabilities were similarly high in the 26 patients who received pacemakers (78% survival) and the 26 who did not (85% survival). In Olmstead County, Minnesota, patients over 80 years old paced for isolated sick sinus syndrome enjoyed comparable survival to age- and sex-matched controls.[45] However, this study provided no follow-up information in unpaced individuals with this disorder.

Atrioventricular node function

The P–R interval undergoes a small but significant prolongation with age, increasing from 159 to 175 ms in men and from 156 to 165 ms in women between the fourth and eighth decades in healthy BLSA volunteers.[46] From high-resolution signal-averaged surface ECGs, the P–R prolongation was localized proximal to the His bundle deflection, presumably

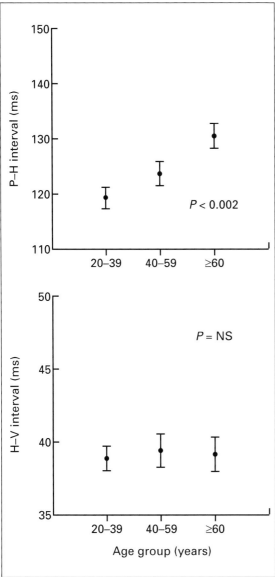

Figure 21.2
In 161 normal BLSA subjects ages 20–83 years who underwent noninvasive His bundle recording, an increase in the PR interval of 12 ms between Group 1 and Group 3 is explained entirely by a prolongation of conduction proximal to the His bundle (P–H interval, top panel), whereas conduction distal to the His bundle (H–V interval, bottom panel) is not age related. (From Fleg et al[46] with permission)

reflecting delay within the AV junction. In older men with first degree AV block, a similarly located but more pronounced delay was observed.[46] Given this age-associated slowing of AV conduction, the occurrence of first degree AV block rises markedly with age; in military air crewmen the incidence rose from 0.73/1000 person-years in the third decade to 6.0/1000 person-years in the eighth decade.[47] Isolated first degree AV block was found in 6.1% of 671 hospitalized subjects over 70 years old and occurred with similar frequency in healthy individuals and those with clinical heart disease.[48] The prevalence in octogenarians is also 6–8%, regardless of disease status.[3,4] In the 5150 subjects at least 65 years old in the CHS, first degree block was nearly three times as common in men (8.1%) as in women (3.2%).[49] First degree AV block has not been predictive of increased cardiac events in either apparently healthy older men[47] or nursing-home patients.[29]

Second and third degree AV block are uncommon even in older populations and usually indicate advanced disease of the conduction system. An exception is Mobitz type I AV block, in which a gradual prolongation of the P–R interval occurs until a ventricular complex is dropped. This type of AV block usually occurs in conjunction with enhanced vagal tone, myocardial ischemia or toxicity from digitalis and other anti-arrhythmic drugs. It is usually transient and rarely requires specific treatment. Mobitz type II AV block, in which ventricular complexes are dropped without progressive P–R interval prolongation was detected on 24-hour ECG recording in only 0.4% of women and 0.8% of men over 65 years old in the CHS.[8] In an institutionalized population 82 ± 8 years old, Aronow et al[29] detected type I second degree AV block in two of 960 patients and type II block in another six. Four of these latter six patients experienced coronary events over a 45-month mean follow-up.[29] Prior studies in younger populations have documented a poor prognosis in patients with chronic second degree AV block complicating organic heart disease. Symptomatic patients with type II block should receive a permanent pacemaker.

Third degree or complete AV block is the rarest form of AV block in older adults and indicates advanced conduction system disease. In the community-based CHS population, complete AV block was not seen in any of the 729 women and only twice in 643 men.[8] Many studies have documented the benefits of permanent pacemakers on life expectancy and recurrence of syncope in patients with complete AV block. The degree of survival benefit appears to vary with both age and the presence or absence of structural heart disease. In Olmstead County, Minnesota, survival in paced patients 65–79 years old with isolated AV block was similar to age- and gender-matched cohorts but in patients over 80 years, it was worse than for matched controls.[50] Not surprisingly, paced patients with AV block and associated heart disease had reduced survival compared with control subjects, both in 65–79 year old individuals and those over 80 years.

Ventricular conduction disturbances

Essentially all of the common ventricular conduction abnormalities increase with age. Because of the leftward shift of the QRS axis that accompanies normative aging, the prevalence of left-axis deviation of more than −30 degrees rises markedly with age, reaching as high as 20% by the 90s.[4] A prevalence of 7–8% is more typical for octogenarian cohorts.[3,29] The age-associated increase in left-axis deviation may be due in part to increased

left ventricular mass, superimposed upon intrinsic fibrosis of the left anterior fascicle. Institutionalized elderly patients 82 ± 8 years with left anterior fascicular block, defined by a QRS axis leftward of −45 degrees, experienced an incidence of new cardiac events similar to those with a normal QRS axis, parallel to findings in younger populations.[29]

Although both right and left bundle branch block (RBBB and LBBB) increase in prevalence with age,[51] these conduction disturbances should not automatically be attributed to the aging process. In younger populations RBBB is two to three times as common as LBBB, but this difference narrows with age.[51] RBBB was detected in 3% of clinically healthy subjects over 85 years old and 8–10% of those with heart disease.[3,4,29] In contrast to its left-sided counterpart, RBBB is often an isolated finding unassociated with organic heart disease.[51,52] Such individuals have no increased risk for cardiac events on long-term follow-up, but these data are derived from subjects in the fourth to seventh decades.[51,52] However, in 109 nursing home patients (mean age 82 years) with RBBB, Aronow et al also observed no significant increase in cardiac events over a 45 month average follow-up compared with control patients without ventricular conduction defects.[29] LBBB was observed in 3% of apparently healthy subjects over 85 years old,[3] 4% of nursing-home patients averaging 82 years[29] and 7% of 90–100 year old patients.[4] Because LBBB is usually accompanied by organic heart disease,[48,51,53] its prognosis primarily reflects that of the underlying cardiac disorder. For example, Aronow found a 71% incidence of new cardiac events in 42 institutionalized elderly patients with LBBB over a mean follow-up of 45 months compared with 31% in controls.[29] Thus, the presence of LBBB in an octogenarian should prompt a search for underlying cardiovascular disease if clinically warranted. A nonspecific intraventricular conduction defect exceeding 120 ms occurred in 2% of Framingham subjects over 70 years and, like LBBB, was strongly associated with organic heart disease.[54]

Summary

Nearly all of the major disturbances of cardiac rhythm, and atrioventricular or ventricular conduction increase with age. Although much of this increase is due to the presence of associated cardiac disease, intrinsic aging changes in cardiac electrophysiology and isolated sclerodegenerative changes in the conduction system also play important roles. Certain abnormalities such as atrial fibrillation or LBBB are uncommon in healthy octogenarians and are harbingers of subsequent cardiac morbidity and mortality. Treatment, however, should usually be based upon the presence and severity of underlying cardiovascular disease and not on the arrhythmia or conduction disturbance per se.

Acknowledgement

The secretarial assistance of Sharon Wright is gratefully acknowledged.

References

1. Fleg JL, Kennedy HL. Cardiac arrhythmias in a healthy elderly population. *Chest* (1982) **81**: 302–7.
2. Fleg JL. Electrocardiographic findings in older persons without clinical heart disease. In: Tresch DD, Aronow WS, eds, *Cardiovascular Disease in the Elderly Patient.* (Marcel Dekker: New York, 1994) 43–59.
3. Rajala SA, Geiger UKM, Haavisto MV et al. Electrocardiogram, clinical findings and chest X-ray in persons aged 85 years or older. *Am J Cardiol* (1985) **55**:1175–8.
4. Golden GS, Golden LH. The 'nona' electrocardiogram: findings in 100 patients of the 90+ age group. *J Am Geriatr Soc* (1974) **22**: 329–31.
5. Aronow WS, Epstein S, Schwartz KS, Koenigsberg M. Prevalence of arrhythmias detected by ambulatory electrocardiographic monitoring and of abnormal left ventricular ejection fraction in persons older than 62 years in a long-term health care facility. *Am J Cardiol* (1987) **59**:368–9.
6. Kantelip J-P, Sage E, Duchene-Marullaz P. Findings on ambulatory electrocardiologic monitoring in subjects older than 80 years. *Am J Cardiol* (1986) **57**:398–401.
7. Fleg JL, Kennedy HL. Long-term prognostic significance of ambulatory electrocardiographic findings in apparently healthy subjects ≥60 years of age. *Am J Cardiol* (1992) **70**:748–51.
8. Manolio TA, Furberg CD, Rautaharju PM et al. Cardiac arrhythmias on 24-hour ambulatory electrocardiography in older women and men: The Cardiovascular Health Study. *J Am Coll Cardiol* (1994) **23**:916–25.
9. Stemple DR, Fitzgerald JW, Winkel RA. Benign slow paroxysmal atrial tachycardia. *Ann Intern Med* (1977) **87**:44–8.
10. Drejarena LA, Vidaillet H Jr, Destefano F et al. Paroxysmal supraventricular tachycardia in the general population. *J Am Coll Cardiol* (1998) **31**:150–7.
11. Maurer MS, Shefrin EA, Fleg JL. Prevalence and prognostic significance of exercise-induced supraventricular tachycardia in apparently healthy volunteers. *Am J Cardiol* (1995) **75**: 788–92.
12. Epstein LM, Chiesa N, Wong MN et al. Radiofrequency catheter ablation in the treatment of supraventricular tachycardia in the elderly. *J Am Coll Cardiol* (1994) **23**:1356–62.
13. Kannel WB, Abbott RD, Savage DD, McNamara PM. Epidemiologic features of chronic atrial fibrillation. *N Engl J Med* (1982) **306**:1018–22.
14. Staffurth JS, Gibberd MC, Ng Tang Fui S. Arterial embolism in thyrotoxicosis with atrial fibrillation. *BMJ* (1977) **2**:688–90.
15. Brand FN, Abbott RD, Kannell WB, Wolf PA. Characteristics and prognosis of lone atrial fibrillation. 30-year follow-up in the Framingham Study. *JAMA* (1985) **254**:3449–53.
16. Kopecky SL, Gersh BJ, McGoon MD et al. The natural history of lone atrial fibrillation. A population-based study over three decades. *N Engl J Med* (1987) **317**:669–74.
17. Wolf PA, Abbott RD, Kannel WB. Atrial fibrillation: a major contributor to stroke in the elderly. The Framingham Study. *Arch Intern Med* (1987) **147**:1561–4.
18. Petersen P, Boysen G, Gottredsen J et al. Placebo-controlled randomized trial of warfarin and aspirin for prevention of thromboembolic complications in chronic atrial fibrillation. *Lancet* (1989) **i**:175–9.
19. Stroke Prevention in Atrial Fibrillation Study Group Investigators. Preliminary report of the Stroke Prevention in Atrial Fibrillation Study. *N Engl J Med* (1990) **322**:863–8.
20. The Boston Area Anticoagulation Trial for Atrial Fibrillation Investigators. The effect of low-dose warfarin on the risk of stroke in patients with non-rheumatic atrial fibrillation. *N Engl J Med* (1990) **323**:1505–11.
21. Ezekowitz MD, Bridgers SL, James KE et al for the Veterans Affairs Stroke Prevention in Non-rheumatic Atrial Fibrillation Investigators. Warfarin in the prevention of stroke associated

with nonrheumatic atrial fibrillation. *N Engl J Med* (1992) **327**:1406–12.

22. Camm AJ, Evans KE, Ward DE, Martin A. The rhythm of the heart in active elderly subjects. *Am Heart J* (1980) **99**:598–603.

23. Kostis JB, McCrone K, Moreyra AE et al. Premature ventricular complexes in the absence of identifiable heart disease. *Circulation* (1981) **63**:1351–6.

24. Busby MJ, Shefrin EA, Fleg JL. Significance of exercise-induced frequent or repetitive ventricular ectopic beats in apparently healthy volunteers. *J Am Coll Cardiol* (1989) **14**:1659–65.

25. Fleg JL. Ventricular arrhythmias in the elderly: prevalence, mechanisms and therapeutic implications. *Geriatrics* (1988) **43**:23–9.

26. Cullen KJ, Stenhouse NS, Wearne KL et al. Electrocardiograms and thirteen year cardiovascular mortality in Busselton study. *Br Heart J* (1982) **47**:209–12.

27. Kannel WB, Doyle JT, McNamara PM et al. Precursors of sudden death: factors related to the incidence of sudden death. *Circulation* (1975) **57**:606–13.

28. Abdalla ISH, Prineas RJ, Neaton JD et al. Relations between ventricular premature complexes and sudden cardiac death in apparently healthy men. *Am J Cardiol* (1987) **60**: 1036–42.

29. Aronow WS. Correlation of arrhythmias and conduction defects on the resting electrocardiogram with new cardiac events in 1153 elderly patients. *Am J Noninvas Cardiol* (1991) **5**: 88–90.

30. Kirkland JL, Lye M, Faragher EB, dos Santos AGR. A longitudinal study of the prognostic significance of ventricular ectopic beats in the elderly. *Gerontology* (1983) **29**:199–201.

31. Martin A, Benbow LJ, Burous GS et al. Five-year follow-up of 106 elderly subjects by means of long-term ambulatory cardiac monitoring. *Eur Heart J* (1984) **5**:592–6.

32. Aronow WE, Epstein S, Koenigsberg M, Schwartz KS. Usefulness of echocardiographic abnormal left ventricular ejection fraction, paroxysmal ventricular tachycardia, and complex ventricular arrhythmias in predicting new coronary events in patients over 62 years of age. *Am J Cardiol* (1988) **61**:1349–51.

33. The Cardiac Arrhythmia Suppression Trial (CAST) Investigators Preliminary Report.

Effect of encainide and flecainide on mortality in a randomized trial of arrhythmia suppression after myocardial infarction. *N Engl J Med* (1989) **321**:406–12.

34. The Cardiac Arrhythmia Suppression Trial II Investigators. Effect of the antiarrhythmic agent moricizine on survival after myocardial infarction. *N Engl J Med* (1992) **327**:227–33.

35. Aronow WS, Mercando AD, Epstein S, Kronzon I. Effect of quinidine or procainamide versus no antiarrhythmic drug on sudden cardiac death, total cardiac death, and total death in elderly patients with heart disease and complex ventricular arrhythmias. *Am J Cardiol* (1990) **66**:423–8.

36. Aronow WS, Ahn C, Mercando AD et al. Effect of propranolol versus no antiarrhythmic drug on sudden cardiac death, total cardiac death, and total death in patients ≥62 years of age with heart disease, complex ventricular arrhythmias, and left ventricular ejection fraction ≥40%. *Am J Cardiol* (1994) **74**: 267–70.

37. Aronow WS, Ahn C, Mercando AD et al. Decrease of mortality by propranolol in patients with heart disease and complex ventricular arrhythmias is more an antiischemic than an antiarrhythmic effect. *Am J Cardiol* (1994) **74**:613–15.

38. Tresch DD, Troup PJ, Thakur RK et al. Comparison of efficacy of automatic implantable cardioverter defibrillator in patients older and younger than 65 years of age. *Am J Med* (1991) **90**:717–24.

39. Lev M. The pathology of complete atrioventricular block. *Prog Cardiovasc Dis* (1964) **6**:409–44.

40. Schwartz J, Gibb WJ, Tran T. Aging effects on heart rate variation. *J Gerontol A Biol Med Sci* (1991) **46**:M99–106.

41. Byrne EA, Fleg JL, Vaitkevicius PV et al. Role of aerobic capacity and body mass index in the age-associated decline in heart rate variability. *J Appl Physiol* (1996) **81**:743–50.

42. Aronow WS, Ahn C, Mercando AD, Epstein S. Association of average heart rate on 24-hour ambulatory electrocardiograms with incidence of new coronary events at 48-month follow-up in 1311 patients (mean age 81 years) with heart disease and sinus rhythm. *Am J Cardiol* (1996) **78**:1175–6.

43. Fleg JL, Schulman S, O'Connor F et al. Effects of acute β-adrenergic receptor blockade on age-associated changes in cardiovascular performance during dynamic exercise. *Circulation* (1994) **90**:2333–41.

44. Hilgard J, Ezri MD, Denes P. Significance of ventricular pauses of three seconds or more detected on twenty-four-hour Holter recordings. *Am J Cardiol* (1985) **55**:1005–8.

45. Tung RT, Shen W-K, Hayes DL et al. Long-term survival after permanent pacemaker implantation for sick sinus syndrome. *Am J Cardiol* (1994) **74**:1016–20.

46. Fleg JL, Das DN, Wright J, Lakatta EG. Age-associated changes in the components of atrio-ventricular conduction in apparently healthy volunteers. *J Gerontol A Biol Med Sci* (1990) **45**:M95–100.

47. Mymin D, Mathewson FAL, Tate RB, Manfreda J. The natural history of primary first-degree atrioventricular heart block. *N Engl J Med* (1986) **315**:1183–7.

48. Mihalick MJ, Fisch C. Electrocardiographic findings in the aged. *Am Heart J* (1974) **87**:117–28.

49. Furberg CD, Manolio TA, Psaty BM et al. Major electrocardiographic abnormalities in persons aged 65 years and older (the Cardiovascular Health Study). *Am J Cardiol* (1992) **69**:1329–35.

50. Shen W-K, Hammill SC, Hayes DL et al. Long-term survival after pacemaker implantation for heart block in patient ≥65 years. *Am J Cardiol* (1994) **74**:560–4.

51. Fahy GJ, Pinski SL, Miller DP et al. Natural history of isolated bundle branch block. *Am J Cardiol* (1996) **77**:1185–90.

52. Fleg JL, Das DN, Lakatta EG. Right bundle block: long-term prognosis in apparently healthy men. *J Am Coll Cardiol* (1983) **1**:887–92.

53. Schneider JF, Thomas HE Jr, McNamara PM, Kannel WB. Clinical-electrocardiographic correlates of newly acquired left bundle branch block: the Framingham study. *Am J Cardiol* (1985) **55**:1332–8.

54. Kreger BE, Anderson KM, Kannel WB. Prevalence of intraventricular block in the general population: the Framingham study. *Am Heart J* (1989) **117**:903–10.

22

Cardiopulmonary resuscitation in the elderly: beneficial or an exercise in futility?

Donald D Tresch and Hossein Amirani

Introduction

Sudden cardiac death increases with age.[1,2] In some elderly persons sudden cardiac death will be the terminal event after a prolonged debilitating and painful illness, such as cancer, or it may occur following many years of symptoms related to a cardiac disorder. In many elderly persons, however, the cardiac arrest will be the first manifestation of cardiac disease in a supposedly healthy and physically active 75 or 80 year old. Depending upon the situation, plus the person's beliefs, sudden cardiac death will be viewed differently by various persons. In certain situations it may be an answer to a person's prayer, whereas in other situations it will be a tragedy. Certainly, the age of the person sustaining the cardiac arrest will influence the manner in which sudden cardiac arrest is perceived by both individuals and society in general.

Whether cardiopulmonary resuscitation (CPR) should be performed in elderly patients who sustain cardiac arrest is a significant issue confronting the medical profession, as well as the general public. The issue has both ethical and economic implications. What percentage of elderly patients will survive the CPR? Are elderly survivors, compared with younger survivors, more likely to have significant neurological impairment? Will they be able to live independently functional lives or will they spend their remaining years in a long-term care institution? What about the hospital course in elderly patients who are successfully resuscitated? Will the hospital stay be significantly longer in elderly survivors, and will medical costs be extremely expensive for this group of patients whose long-term survival is problematic? Such questions require answers in a society that is struggling with the ethical issues of providing meaningful life versus prolonging suffering in the current environment of medical care cost containment.

This chapter attempts to decide whether CPR is beneficial in elderly patients compared with younger patients who receive CPR following cardiac arrest. Emphasis will be on survival in reference to the site of the cardiac arrest, including in-hospital, out-of-hospital, and nursing home settings. The functional status of survivors and the duration of hospitalization and stays in intensive care units will be assessed. We will determine whether significant differences exist in the clinical characteristics between elderly and younger patients who sustain cardiac arrest and determine whether any prearrest or arrest characteristics are predictive of survival. Lastly, a possible difference in the mechanism of the cardiac arrest between the age groups will be investigated.

The specific age criterion for elderly varies depending upon the specific study discussed. In most studies, elderly are classified as 70 years or older. We are unaware of any study that specifically studied very elderly patients, although in all studies the elderly groups included some patients 80 years or older, and some studies included patients 100 years old or older.

In-hospital cardiac arrest

Findings of studies of CPR in hospitalized elderly patients following cardiac arrest have been variable (Table 22.1). Many early studies[3-6] of CPR in hospitalized patients, mainly of small numbers of patients, did not find patient age to be a significant determinant of survival. Gulati and associates,[4] in a prospective study of 52 patients age 64–91 years, found 27% of patients who sustained cardiac arrest in 1983 were initially resuscitated and 17% survived to be discharged. Age was not a determinant of survival, although the initial documented cardiac rhythm at the time of the arrest was highly predictive. Twenty-three percent of the patients survived if their initial rhythm was ventricular fibrillation (VF), compared to only 5% of patients whose rhythm was asystole. Similar findings were reported by Bedell and associates in one of the largest prospective studies of CPR performed in hospitalized patients.[5] Of 294 consecutive hospital patients who received CPR for a cardiac arrest during an 18-month period between 1981 and 1983, 42 (14%) survived to be discharged. Patients' ages ranged from 18 to 101 years (mean age 70) and age was not a significant predictor of survival. Pre-arrest determinants of survival included severity of illness and level of patient's functional activity. At the time of arrest, as in Gulati's study, the presence of VF was the most favorable deter-minant of survival: 27% of patients with VF survived compared with only 8% of those with other rhythms. Other adverse predictors of survival at the time of arrest included increased duration of CPR and whether intubation was necessary.

In contrast to the results of many early studies of CPR, other studies have reported less favorable survival rates in elderly hospitalized patients receiving CPR.[7-10] George and associates,[7] in a prospective study of 140 consecutive hospitalized patients (age range 18–92 years) in 1985, reported a 24% survival rate (hospital discharge) with CPR following cardiac arrest. The survival rate increased to 36% in the patients who demonstrated ventricular tachyarrhythmias. A statistical difference in survival was found when patients were partitioned at age 65 years, but 'chi-square' analysis revealed no association between mortality and age partitioned at 60, 63, 67, or 80 years. Of the patients older than 80 years, 11% survived to hospital discharge. In an attempt to determine the influence of specific pre-arrest clinical characteristics upon survival, hypotension and azotemia were the only significant adverse predictors of survival; however, the collective effect of various clinical characteristics that assessed the patient's pre-arrest comorbidity significantly correlated with survival. The higher the patient's pre-arrest comorbidity classification, the less chance the patient had of surviving the cardiac arrest with CPR. The authors concluded that increased comorbidity was a more important prognostic factor than patient age in determining success of CPR. Tortolani and associates[8] in a retrospective study of hospitalized patients (age range 18–99 years, mean age 69.5) published in 1989, reported a survival rate of 19% in hospitalized patients under 68 years of age who received CPR following cardiac arrest, compared to a 10% survival rate in patients

Study (location, year)	Survival to hospital discharge (%)		
	Younger* patients	Elderly* patients	Total patients
Gulati et al (Lancashire, UK, 1982)[4]			
All rhythms	18	17	17
VF	—	—	—
Bedell et al (Boston, USA, 1981–1982)[5]			
All rhythms	—	—	14†
VF	—	—	27†
Woog et al (Sydney, Aus, 1984)[6]			
All rhythms	15	17	16
VF	—	—	22
George et al (Nashville, USA, 1985)[7]			
All rhythms	—	—	24‡
VF	—	—	36‡
Tortolani et al (Manhasset, USA, 1990)[8]			
All rhythms	—	—	15‡
VF	—	—	21‡
Taffet et al (Houston, USA, 1984–1985)[9]			
All rhythms	16	0	—
VF	—	0	—
Murphy et al (Boston, USA, 1977–1987)[10]			
All rhythms	—	6.5	—
VF	—	21	—
Robinson and Hess (York, USA, 1989)[11]			
All rhythms	—	—	29†
VF	—	—	50†
Roberts et al (Winnipeg, Canada, 1985–1986)[12]			
All rhythms	—	—	10†
VF	—	—	19†
Rosenberg et al (Portland, USA, 1989–1990)[13]			
All rhythms	25	22	23
VF	—	—	—
Berger and Kelly (Lexington, USA, 1985–1989)[14]			
All rhythms	—	—	11†
VF	—	—	15†
Tresch et al (Milwaukee, USA, 1989–1990)[18]			
All rhythms	27	24	26
VF	35	39	37

* See text for specific ages in each study.
† Age not determinant of survival.
‡ Older age unfavorable determinant of survival.
VF, ventricular fibrillation.

Table 22.1
Survival rates after in-hospital cardiac arrest

68 years or older. The authors did not explain their reasoning for using age 68 years for dividing the age groups. Therefore, the possibility of post hoc selection must be considered.

Two other studies published in 1988 and 1989 reported very dismal results with CPR in hospitalized elderly patients; the findings of these studies received much attention from both the medical profession and the lay press. Taffet and associates[9] in a retrospective study of CPR in a Veterans Administration hospital found that although elderly patients (aged ≥70 years) who received CPR could be initially resuscitated as successfully as younger patients, none of the elderly patients survived hospitalization. In comparison, 16% of the patients under 70 years who received CPR survived to be discharged from the hospital. The authors did not assess the cardiac arrest rhythm, but found the presence of sepsis, cancer, increased number of pre-arrest drugs, absence of witnessed arrest and increased patient age all to be predictors of poor outcome. In the other study, Murphy and associates[10] retrospectively analyzed the success of CPR in 503 persons aged at least 70 years (range 70–103) who sustained cardiac arrest between 1977 and 1987. Of the 503 persons, 259 were hospitalized at the time of cardiac arrest and 244 were living in the community (out-of-hospital arrest). Of the 259 hospitalized patients, 36% were initially resuscitated, although only 6.5% survived to be discharged. Furthermore, at the time of discharge approximately 50% of survivors had significant neurological or functional impairments and over 50% of the patients were discharged to either a rehabilitation institution or a long-term care facility. Pre-arrest clinical characteristics which favored survival included lack of chronic and multiple acute illnesses. There was a trend, although the difference was not significant, that patients with functional or mental

impairments had worse outcomes than patients without such impairments. As in the other previous studies, the presence of VF at the time of the arrest was a significant favorable predictor of survival. Twenty-one percent of elderly survived if their cardiac arrest rhythm was VF or ventricular tachycardia (VT) compared with a survival rate of only 2.6% in those with other rhythms. Ventricular fibrillation or VT, however, were not common cardiac rhythms; they were demonstrated only in 27% of patients at the time of arrest. Electromechanical dissociation or asystole was the more common rhythm in these elderly patients. Other arrest characteristics that favored survival were a witnessed arrest and CPR duration less than 5 min. Based on these unfavorable results, both Taffet[9] (1988) and Murphy[10] (1989) concluded that CPR is rarely beneficial in hospitalized elderly patients who sustained cardiac arrest and questioned whether the procedure should be performed in this age group.

Contrary to the dismal findings of Taffet's and Murphys' studies, more recent published studies of CPR performed on hospitalized elderly patients reported more favorable results.[11–20] Robinson and associates[11] reported a 29% hospital discharge survival rate in hospitalized patients (age range 2–93 years) who received CPR following cardiac arrest. In this study, patient age was not a significant determinant of survival (mean age of survivors 68.8 years, range 2–83 and mean age of nonsurvivors 70.4 years, range 44–93; $P = 0.36$). As in many of the previous studies, patients demonstrating VT or VF had a significantly better chance of surviving compared to patients with other arrhythmias. None of the patients who demonstrated asystole survived and only 1% of patients with electrical mechanical dissociation survived. Duration of CPR was the other arrest determinant of survival; CPR of duration no more than 10 minutes was associated with favorable results, compared with CPR greater than 10 minutes. Pre-arrest functional status was not specifically assessed, although all but one of the survivors lived at home prior to the hospital CPR and none of the survivors had any limitations in their daily activities prior to the hospital admission. Follow-up evaluation of the patients at mean 31 months demonstrated that 54% were alive and the majority were living independently at home without any compromise in activities. In another retrospective study published in 1993, Rosenberg and associates[13] assessed success of CPR in two university affiliated community hospitals. The average age of 300 patients who received CPR was 70.4 years; 59% of the patients were over 70 years of age. Survival to hospital discharge was 23% in the total patient population. Patient age was not a significant determinant of survival, although, as in other studies, ventricular tachyarrhythmias and short CPR duration were favorable determinants of survival. Survival to hospital discharge was also significantly influenced by the patient's pre-arrest comorbidity. The specific comorbidities, however, differed in each of the two hospitals and combinations of comorbidities were much more predictive of survival than a specific comorbidity.

In a more recently published study (1994) comparing success of hospital CPR between patients 70 years or older (mean age 78 years, range 70–91) and patients under 70 years (mean age 58 years, range 22–69), Tresch and associates[18] found no significant difference in hospital or long-term survival between the age groups. Over 25% of all patients survived to be discharged, and if their initial cardiac rhythm was VF at the time of arrest, over 35% survived. At 2-year follow-up, over 70% of all patients were alive, and the majority

were functioning at their pre-arrest status, regardless of patient age. In assessing pre-arrest clinical characteristics, the only significant difference between elderly and younger patients was that the elderly more commonly demonstrated atrial fibrillation. Prior to hospitalization, the patients, including the elderly, were very active and functionally independent, with most patients free of significant chronic illnesses or disabilities. The majority of patients were hospitalized for acute coronary syndromes, including unstable angina and acute myocardial infarction, and over 80% had their rhythm monitored either in an intensive care unit or on telemetry at the time of arrest. The arrest was witnessed in over 50% of patients. Based upon the results of this study, the investigators concluded that hospitalized patients who received CPR in the 1990s are a highly selected group, compared to patients who received CPR in previous years. Regardless of age, the patients who receive CPR are usually highly functional, are commonly hospitalized for acute coronary syndromes, and the majority are closely monitored prior to a cardiac arrest. In these patients, CPR can be very gratifying and elderly patients will benefit from the procedure as well as younger patients. Other recent studies[19] have confirmed that elderly patients whose primary illness is a cardiac disorder have a much better chance of surviving with CPR than patients whose primary illness is noncardiac.

Out-of-hospital cardiac arrest

In general, most studies[20–26] of out-of-hospital cardiac arrest have reported that elderly victims benefit from CPR (Table 22.2). Tresch and associates,[20] in a study of paramedics published in 1988, reported that elderly patients ($\geq$70 years) could be initially resuscitated as successfully as younger patients under 70 years of age, although elderly patients were less likely to survive hospitalization. Nine percent of elderly patients survived to be discharged from the hospital compared with 16% of younger patients. As in studies of in-hospital CPR, the survival significantly improved in patients whose cardiac rhythm at the time of arrest was VF. Sixteen percent of elderly patients and 23% of younger patients survived if their cardiac rhythm was VF. Even in patients over 80 years of age, 14% survived if their initial documented arrhythmia was VF. Unfortunately, only 44% of elderly patients demonstrated VF, which was significantly less than that demonstrated by younger patients. Electromechanical dissociation and asystole were the more common rhythms in

Study (location, year)	Survival to hospital discharge (%)	
	Younger patients	Elderly patients
Murphy et al (Boston, USA, 1977–1987)[10]		
All rhythms		0.8
VF		2.0
Tresch et al (Milwaukee, USA, 1983–1985)[20]		
All rhythms	16	9
VF	23	16
Tresch et al (Milwaukee, USA, 1980–1985)†[38]		
All rhythms	24	10
VF	47	24
Bonnin et al (Houston, USA, 1987)[21]		
All rhythms	12	7
VF	20	14
Denes et al (Minneapolis, USA, 1987–1988)[22]		
All rhythms	—	—
VF	16	18
Eisenberg et al (King City, WA, USA, 1975–1989)[23]		
All rhythms	22	9
VF	32	20
Longstreth et al (Seattle, USA, 1983–1988)[24]		
All rhythms	14	10
VF	30	24
Juchems et al (Aschaffenburg, GDR, 1981–1991)[26]		
All rhythms	14	11
VF	—	—

* See text for specific ages in each study.
† Arrest witnessed by paramedics.
VF, ventricular fibrillation.

Table 22.2
Survival rates after out-of-hospital cardiac arrest

elderly patients. Besides rhythm differences, elderly patients' arrests were more commonly witnessed compared with younger patients. Even though the arrest was more likely to be witnessed, elderly patients were less likely to receive CPR by a bystander at arrival of paramedics.

Other recent studies have reported similar favorable findings to those of Tresch and associates. In two separate studies of paramedics, Bonnin et al[21] and Denes et al[22] reported survival rates of 14% and 18%, respectively, in elderly patients (≥70 years of age) who received CPR following out-of-hospital cardiac arrest if the initial arrest rhythm was VF. Eisenberg and associates,[23] in one of the largest patient series in the US, reported even more favorable results. Of 569 patients 20% aged 75 years and older who sustained out-of-hospital cardiac arrest between 1975 and 1989 survived following CPR if their arrest rhythm was VF. More recently, Longstreth and associates[24] reported a 24% survival in elderly patients age 70 years and over who received out-of-hospital CPR; this was not significantly different compared with patients younger than 70 years. Outcome was independent of patient age until the ninth decade. As in all studies, patients in Longstreth's study who demonstrated asystole or electromechanical dissociation at the time of cardiac arrest had little chance of surviving. Only 1% of patients 70 years and over and 2% of patients under 70 years of age survived the cardiac arrest if their rhythm was electromechanical dissociation or asystole at the initiation of CPR.

As in their study of elderly hospitalized patients, Murphy and associates[10] reported very poor survival rates in patients 70 years and older who sustained out-of-hospital cardiac arrest (1977–1987) and received CPR. Less than 1% of patients 70 years or older survived. The authors did not assess survival in patients under 70 years receiving CPR; thus we do not know if the poor results in the elderly patients were related to patient age, or merely reflected the poor success of CPR during this period. Two other recent studies[26,27] of out-of-hospital CPR in large metropolitan areas (Chicago and New York) also reported very poor success. In New York City, during a 6-month period in 1990–1991 only 1.4% of all persons who received out-of-hospital CPR by paramedics survived; even of those who demonstrated VF, only 5.3% survived.[27] Similar dismal results were noted in the Chicago study, and the findings of this study suggested that older age was an adverse determinant of survival.[28] Such poor survival rates are troublesome. The explanation for these poor results, compared to other studies, is unclear but such differences suggest variability in outcome according to community.

Nursing home cardiac arrest

Until recently, CPR in nursing homes has not received much interest from the medical profession. However, in the last decade, perhaps because of the increased emphasis on long-term care and the increased pressure from society for medical cost containment, the issue has attracted much attention from both the medical profession and from society in general. As expected, when dealing with such a complex topic involving both medical and ethical questions, the answers are controversial and emotional, as well as unresolved.

In general, CPR is infrequently used in this setting. Studies have reported that CPR is used in only 2–5% of all nursing homes with some nursing homes never performing CPR.[29] In reference to success of CPR in nursing homes, most studies[30–33] have reported very poor survival rates in the majority of patients who received CPR (Table 22.3). Applebaum and

Study (location, year)	No. of patients	Mean age (years)	Survival to hospital discharge
Kaiser et al (Rochester, USA, 1977–1985)[33]			
All rhythms	32	72	16*
Applebaum et al (Baltimore, USA, 1987)[30]			
All rhythms	117	82	2
Awoke et al (Washington DC, USA, 1987–1990)[31]			
All rhythms	57	75	0
Gordon and Cheung (Toronto, Canada, 1988–1991)[32]			
All rhythms	41	81	0
Tresch et al (Milwaukee, USA, 1986–1991)[34]			
All rhythms	196	79	5
VF	39	—	15
VF witnessed arrests	22	—	27
Ghusn (Houston, USA, 1986–1991)[35]			
All rhythms	114	81	11
VF	16	—	13
Witnessed arrests	—	—	0

* Alive at 30 days.

Table 22.3
Survival rates after nursing home cardiac arrest

associates[30] reported that only 2 of 117 (2%) nursing-home residents (mean age 82 years) who received CPR in 1987 by trained ambulance teams survived. In comparison, 11% of nonnursing-home residents 65 years or older (mean age 75 years) who received CPR survived. Similar dismal findings were reported in separate studies by Awoke[31] and Gordon.[32] In both studies, no residents in long-term care facilities who received CPR survived. Cardiopulmonary resuscitation in both studies was performed by trained on-site physicians and resuscitation teams. Mean age of residents in the two studies was 75 years and 81 years, respectively. On the basis of the results of these studies, the use of CPR in nursing homes has been questioned.

Two recent studies,[34,35] however, found success of CPR to be variable among nursing-home patients; in a subset of patients, the survival rate was not significantly different from that reported in elderly persons living in the community. In both studies, the success of CPR was highly dependent upon whether the arrest was witnessed and whether the initial documented cardiac arrest rhythm was VF. In Tresch's study[34] of 196 nursing home patients, mean age 78.5 years (range 31–107), 27% of the patients whose arrest was witnessed and who demonstrated VF survived with CPR. At follow-up, the majority of patients were without a significant functional change from their pre-arrest status. Without the presence of the two determinants (witnessed arrest and presence of VF), the survival rate was only 2.5%. Patients' pre-arrest clinical characteristics did not separate survivors from nonsurvivors. The mean length of hospital stay for all patients who were initially successfully resuscitated was 9.9 days and 63% of the patients who died in the hospital died within 24 hours. From the findings of these studies it appears that selected nursing-home patients sustaining cardiac arrest will survive with CPR. Therefore, some investigators have concluded that CPR should be offered to those nursing-home residents who desire it, but CPR should be initiated only if the arrest is witnessed, and continued only if the patient's initial documented rhythm is VT or VF.

Functional status of survivors of cardiac arrest

Most studies of elderly survivors of cardiac arrest show that the majority of survivors are without significant neurological or functional impairments and return to their pre-arrest activities. Tresch and associates[36] found that the deterioration of pre-arrest functional status to hospital discharge status was no different between elderly (≥70 years) and younger (< 70 years) survivors of out-of-hospital cardiac arrest; and the majority of survivors, regardless of age, were functionally independent at hospital discharge. Furthermore, duration of hospitalization and length of stay in an intensive care unit was not different between the age groups. Long-term survival and functional status was also similar with approximately 65% of elderly and younger survivors alive and functionally independent at 2-year follow-up.

In another study Tresch and associates[18] assessed the functional status of 39 survivors of in-hospital cardiac arrest. As in the study of out-of-hospital survivors of cardiac arrest, pre-arrest to postarrest functional deterioration was not different between elderly (≥ 70 years) and younger (< 70 years) survivors. Functional status was good in these survivors and most patients were completely independent at the time of hospital discharge. Moreover, at mean follow-up of 29 months, all living survivors were functioning independently.

The lack of significant neurological and functional impairment in elderly survivors of cardiac arrest has been further corroborated by the findings from recent studies of other investigators. As in the studies by Tresch and associates,[18,36] Longstreth and associates[24] found no significant difference between the number of survivors over 70 years and survivors under 70 who were discharged to nursing homes. And, in a prospective study of in-hospital CPR, Berger and associates[14] reported that the majority of survivors (mean age 68 years, range 53–94) discharged alive, regardless of age, had no significant neurological defects, and all but one returned to their pre-arrest environment.

In contrast to these favorable findings concerning functional status of elderly survivors of cardiac arrest, some studies[10,37] have found significant deterioration of pre-arrest functional status following CPR in survivors. Also, the deterioration was noted to be more severe in elderly compared to younger survivors. As previously noted, Murphy and associates[10] reported approximately 50% of survivors age 70 years or older of in-hospital cardiac arrest had significant neurological and functional impairment with some patients in a persistent vegetative state. Over 30% of the survivors required placement in nursing homes following hospital discharge. Fitzgerald and associates[37] also found significant deterioration in functional status in survivors (mean age 64 years) of in-hospital cardiac arrest and worse functional deterioration was associated with older age and longer hospital stay prior to the cardiac arrest. Multivariant logistic regression analysis demonstrated that survivors older than 75 years were 5.3 times as likely to have worse deterioration of function after CPR than patients 55 years or younger.

The explanation for the differences between the unfavorable findings of the Fitzgerald study and the previous studies that reported favorable findings concerning functional status of survivors of cardiac arrest is unclear. In the studies that reported favorable findings, only patients who survived to hospital discharge were analyzed, whereas some of the patients analyzed by Fitzgerald died in hospital. Thus, it is possible that the patients who died in hospital had severe neurological impairments, which may partially explain the increased number of patients with functional impairment in Fitzgerald's study, compared to other studies that analyzed only hospital survivors. Furthermore, the patients in Fitzgerald's study were patients enrolled in the Study to Understand Prognosis and Preferences for Outcomes and Risks of Treatment (SUPPORT), a group of patients who were seriously ill with an aggregate 6-month survival of only 47%. Some of the SUPPORT patients had metastatic cancer, nontrauma coma, severe heart failure or end-stage renal disease. Therefore, the patients in Fitzgerald's study had much worse pre-arrest comorbidities than those in other studies, which may be another reason for the worse postarrest functional status of their survivors. Elderly patients more commonly have increased comorbidity compared to younger patients, which may explain why the elderly survivors in Fitzgerald's study demonstrated severe functional deterioration following successful resuscitation; minor changes could produce significant functional deterioration in frail chronically ill patients.

Possible difference in characteristics of cardiac arrest between age groups

A difference in cardiac rhythm at the time of arrest and a difference in the mechanism of cardiac arrest between patients older and younger than 70 years of age has been proposed by some investigators. In some studies of CPR[18,20,21] VF was the most common initial documented arrhythmia in younger patients, whereas electromechanical dissociation or asystole were the more common initial documented arrhythmias in elderly patients. In addition, elderly patients who sustained cardiac arrest commonly had a history of heart failure and were taking digitalis at the time of the arrest. To assess whether the asystole and electromechanical dissociation arrhythmia in elderly patients were not merely degeneration of an initial ventricular tachyarrhythmia, Tresch and associates studied a subset of patients whose out-of-hospital arrest was witnessed by paramedics.[38] In this group of patients, the cardiac arrest occurred after the arrival of paramedics and the patient's cardiac rhythm was monitored at the time of the arrest. As noted in their previous studies, the investigators found a significant difference in cardiac rhythm between age groups. Only 22% of patients older than 70 years demonstrated VF as their initial cardiac rhythm at the time of the onset of arrest, compared with 42% of younger patients. In turn, elderly patients more commonly demonstrated electromechanical dissociation. Besides rhythm, symptoms preceding the arrest were age related. Younger patients were more likely to complain of chest pain, whereas elderly patients were short of breath. Regardless of age, patients with chest pain before the arrest were more likely to demonstrate VF at the time of arrest, whereas patients with dyspnea more commonly demonstrated electromechanical dissociation or asystole. Survival was dependent upon both the patient's cardiac rhythm at the time of arrest and the patient's symptoms preceding arrest. Approximately 60% of the younger and elderly patients survived if they complained of chest pain before the arrest and demonstrated VF at the time of arrest. Patients who complained of dyspnea were less likely to survive, as were patients who did not demonstrate VF at the time of arrest.

The explanation for the difference in the cardiac rhythm at the time of arrest and the difference in symptoms before the arrest between age groups is unclear. Tresch and associates, in some studies[36,38] found that more elderly patients who sustained out-of-hospital cardiac arrest had a history of heart failure and were receiving digoxin and diuretics compared with younger patients. The investigators hypothesized that cardiac arrest in many elderly patients may be related to abnormal left ventricular function with underlying heart failure, which would explain the dyspnea in the elderly patients preceding arrest, and might also explain the bradyasystole noted at the time of arrest. Compared with elderly patients, cardiac arrest in younger patients more commonly may be related to acute myocardial ischemia or infarction manifested as acute chest pain with the development of VF and cardiac arrest. Other investigators[39] have reported severe bradycardia or electromechanical dissociation to be common cardiac arrhythmias in patients with advanced heart failure who sustained cardiac arrest, compatible with the proposal of Tresch and associates. Also, other investigators also found VF to be less common in elderly patients who sustain cardiac arrest, compared with younger patients. A low prevalence of ventricular fibrillation associated with cardiac arrest has been found in nursing-home residents who sustain cardiac arrest and many nursing-home patients are elderly, have a history of heart failure, and are taking digitalis and diuretics. By contrast, not all investigators found a significant difference in rhythms between elderly and younger patients who experience cardiac arrest.

Conclusions and considerations

Age alone does not appear to be the most significant determinant of survival in patients who receive CPR following cardiac arrest; and CPR does not appear to be necessarily an 'exercise in futility' in elderly patients. Based upon the results of numerous studies, we now understand some factors that influence success of CPR. Patient's pre-arrest comorbidity is one of the most significant determinants. Patients with acute cardiac illness have more favorable success with CPR than do patients with such chronic illnesses as renal failure or cancer. Not only the specific comorbidity, but the number of chronic illnesses present appear to be an important determinant of survival; the more illnesses present and the more medications taken, the less chance of surviving with CPR. In addition to comorbidity, functional status is important. Patients with chronic disabilities, physical or mental, are less likely to do well with CPR. The influence of such variables may be the reason that hospitalized patients who sustain cardiac arrest do worse with CPR than do out-of-hospital persons who receive CPR. The presence of such variables may also partially explain the poor results with CPR in nursing homes.

Besides pre-arrest variables, certain arrest characteristics are important determinants of survival with CPR. The most important arrest variable is the specific cardiac rhythm initiating the cardiac arrest. All studies show that patients with VF or VT comprise the bulk of the patients in whom CPR is beneficial. Some investigators have found witnessed arrest another favorable variable for survival. Duration of CPR is also an important factor, as is whether intubation is necessary.

Recognizing that there are always exceptions, we are now better able to determine which patients are unlikely to survive with CPR. Physicians have to assume the responsibility for the selection of proper patients for CPR, as well as for developing guidelines for the duration and continuation of CPR. Too often the patient or the patient's family is not properly informed concerning the chance of surviving with CPR and decisions concerning CPR or DNR (do not resuscitate) are emotional responses, instead of rational reasoned decisions. At other times the decision concerning CPR reflects the physician's, or in some cases, the nurse's preferences, rather than the patient's.

Some recent studies show that patients receiving CPR are becoming a more 'selective group'; in these patients, results of CPR are rewarding in elderly, as well as younger patients. Such selection, however, occurs too infrequently. If physicians fail to accomplish the task of 'selecting' patients we most probably will lose the right to participate in CPR decision making. That would invite continued erosion of the clinical skill, art and judgment that results in appropriate individual care,[40] which is so important in caring for elderly patients.

References

1. Kannel WB, Thomas HE Jr. Sudden coronary death: the Framingham study. *Ann NY Acad Sci* (1982) **382**:3–21.

2. Kuller L, Lilienfeld A. Epidemiological study of sudden and unexpected deaths due to arteriosclerotic heart disease. *Circulation* (1966) **34**:1056–68.

3. Fusgen I, Summa JD. How much sense is there in an attempt to resuscitate an aged person? *Gerontology* (1978) **24**:37–45.

4. Gulati RS, Bhan GL, Horan MA. Cardiopulmonary resuscitation of old people. *Lancet* (1983) **ii**:267–9.

5. Bedell SE, Delbanco TL, Cook EF et al. Survival after cardiopulmonary resuscitation in the hospital. *N Engl J Med* (1983) **309**:569–75.

6. Woog RH, Torzillo PJ. In-hospital cardiopulmonary resuscitation: prospective survey of management and outcome. *Anaesth Intensive Care* (1987) **15**:193–8.

7. George AL Jr, Folk BP III, Crecelius PL, Campbell WB. Pre-arrest morbidity and other correlates of survival after in-hospital cardiopulmonary arrest. *Am J Med* (1989) **87**:28–34.

8. Tortolani AJ, Risucci DA, Rosati RJ, Dixon R. In-hospital cardiopulmonary resuscitation: patient, arrest and resuscitation factors associated with survival. *Resuscitation* (1990) **20**:115–28.

9. Taffet GI, Teasdale TA, Luchi RJ. In-hospital cardiopulmonary resuscitation. *JAMA* (1988) **260**:2069–72.

10. Murphy DI, Murry AM, Robinson BE et al. Outcomes of cardiopulmonary resuscitation in the elderly. *Ann Intern Med* (1989) **111**:199–205.

11. Robinson GR II, Hess D. Postdischarge survival and functional status following in-hospital cardiopulmonary resuscitation. *Chest* (1994) **105**:991–6.

12. Roberts D, Landolfo K, Light RB, Dobson K. Early predictors of mortality for hospitalized patients suffering cardiopulmonary arrest. *Chest* (1990) **97**:413–19.

13. Rosenberg M, Wang C, Hoffman-Wilde S, Hickham D. Results of cardiopulmonary resuscitation. *Arch Intern Med* (1993) **153**:1370–5.

14. Berger R, Kelley M. Survival after in-hospital cardiopulmonary arrest of noncritically ill patients. *Chest* (1994) **106**:872–9.

15. Ebell MH, Preston PS. The effect of the APACHE II score and selected clinical variables on survival following cardiopulmonary resuscitation. *Fam Med* (1993) **25**:191–6.

16. Varon J, Fromm RE Jr. In-hospital resuscitation among the elderly: substantial survival to hospital discharge. *Am J Emerg Med* (1996) **14**:130–2.

17. Peterson MW, Geist LJ, Schwarz DA et al. Outcome after cardiopulmonary resuscitation in a medical intensive care unit. *Chest* (1991) **100**:168–74.

18. Tresch DD, Heudebert G, Kutty K et al. Cardiopulmonary resuscitation in elderly patients hospitalized in the 1990s: a favorable outcome. *J Am Geriatr Soc* (1994) **42**:137–41.

19. Quill TE, Bennett NM. The effects of a hospital policy and state legislation on resuscitation orders for geriatric patients. *Arch Intern Med* (1992) **152**:569–72.

20. Tresch DD, Thakur R, Hoffman R et al. Comparison of outcome of resuscitation of out-of-hospital cardiac arrest in persons younger and older than 70 years of age. *Am J Cardiol* (1988) **61**:1120–2.

21. Bonnin MJ, Pepe PE, Clark PS. Survival in the elderly after out-of-hospital cardiac arrest. *Crit Care Med* (1993) **21**:1645–51.

22. Denes P, Long L, Madison C et al. Resuscitation from out-of-hospital ventricular tachycardia/fibrillation (VT/VF): the effect of age on outcome. *Circulation* (1990) **82**:III-81.

23. Eisenberg MS, Horwood BT, Larson MB. Cardiopulmonary resuscitation in the elderly. *Ann Intern Med* (1990) **113**:408–9.

24. Longstreth WT Jr, Cobb LA, Fahrenbruch CE et al. Does age affect outcomes of out-of-hospital cardiopulmonary resuscitation? *JAMA* (1990) **264**:2109–10.

25. Weston CFM, Wilson RJ, Jones SD. Predicting

survival from out-of-hospital cardiac arrest: a multivariate analysis. *Resuscitation* (1997) **34**:27–34.

26. Juchems R, Wahlig G, Frese W. Influence of age on the survival rate of out-of-hospital and in-hospital resuscitation. *Resuscitation* (1993) **26**:23–9.

27. Lombardi G, Gallagher EJ, Gennis P. Outcome of out-of-hospital cardiac arrest in New York City: the pre-hospital arrest survival evaluation (PHASE) study. *JAMA* (1994) **271**:678–83.

28. Becker LB, Han BH, Meyer PM. Racial differences in the incidence of cardiac arrest and subsequent survival. *N Engl J Med* (1993) **329**:600–6.

29. Duthie E, Mark D, Tresch D et al. Utilization of cardiopulmonary resuscitation on nursing homes in one community: rates and nursing home characteristics. *J Am Geriatr Soc* (1993) **41**:384–8.

30. Applebaum GE, King JE, Finucane TE. The outcome of CPR initiated in nursing homes. *J Am Geriatr Soc* (1990) **38**:197–200.

31. Awoke S, Mouton CP, Parrott M. Outcomes of skilled cardiopulmonary resuscitation in a long-term care facility: futile therapy? *J Am Geriatr Soc* (1992) **40**:593–5.

32. Gordon M, Cheung M. Poor outcome of on-site CPR in a multi-level geriatric facility: three and a half years experience at the Baycrest Center for Geriatric Care. *J Am Geriatr Soc* (1993) **41**:163–6.

33. Kaiser TE, Kayson EP, Campbell RG. Survival after cardiopulmonary resuscitation in a long-term care institution. *J Am Geriatr Soc* (1986) **34**:909.

34. Tresch DD, Neahring JM, Duthie EH et al. Outcomes of cardiopulmonary resuscitation in nursing homes: can we predict who will benefit? *Am J Med* (1993) **95**:123–30.

35. Ghusn HF, Teasdale TA, Pepe PE et al. Older nursing home residents have a cardiac arrest survival rate similar to that of older persons living in the community. *J Am Geriatr Soc* (1995) **43**:520–7.

36. Tresch DD, Thakur R, Hoffman R et al. Should the elderly be resuscitated following out-of-hospital cardiac arrest? *Am J Med* (1989) **86**:145–50.

37. FitzGerald JD, Wenger NS, Califf RM et al. Functional status among survivors of in-hospital cardiopulmonary resuscitation. *Arch Intern Med* (1997) **157**:72–6.

38. Tresch DD, Thakur R, Hoffman R et al. Comparison of outcome of paramedic witnessed cardiac arrest in patients younger and older than 70 years. *Am J Cardiol* (1990) **65**:453–7.

39. Luu M, Stevenson WG, Stevenson LW et al. Diverse mechanism of unexpected cardiac arrest in advanced heart failure. *Circulation* (1989) **80**:1675–80.

40. Combs AH. CPR: A plea for patient selection. *Hosp Prac* (1996) **31**:13–16.

23

Atrial fibrillation in the very old: incidence, mechanism and therapy

Joseph S Alpert and Lorraine L Mackstaller

Introduction

Atrial fibrillation (AF) is the cardiac arrhythmia most frequently encountered in clinical practice. The prevalence of AF increases with age, doubling in incidence for each decade above 60 years of age. Nearly 10% of persons older than age 80 have a history of atrial fibrillation.[1-3] With continuing growth of the elderly population in industrial nations, AF will have an ever larger impact on cardiovascular morbidity and mortality. Indeed, examination of discharge patterns from short-stay hospitals in the US reveals a steady and substantial increase in AF prevalence rates for patients discharged between 1982 and 1993.[4,5] In the population-based Framingham Study, AF increased in prevalence between 1968 and 1989; the prevalence of AF increased with rising age in the Framingham population.[1] Thus, in the period 1987–1989, men aged 65–74 had a 7.8% prevalence of AF while men aged 75–84 had an 11.7% prevalence. More modest increases were noted for women. Of particular interest was the observation that the *age-adjusted* prevalence of AF also increased between 1968 and 1989.[6] Therefore, an aging population cannot be the only explanation for the rise in AF prevalence.[1] Age-adjusted prevalence of AF rose strikingly in men with prior myocardial infarction (4.9% to 17.4%) suggesting that increased survival of patients with heart disease, for example myocardial infarc-

tion, might account for some of the overall, age-adjusted increase in AF prevalence.

Atrial fibrillation is more prevalent in men than in women. For the Framingham population during 1987–1989, men aged 75–84 and without a history of myocardial infarction had an 8.7% prevalence of AF while a similarly aged female cohort had a prevalence of 5.2%. When a history of myocardial infarction was present, the prevalence of AF in 75–84 year old men was 21.8% versus 9.5% for a similar cohort of women (1983–1989).[1]

Similar age- and gender-related prevalences were noted in the Cardiovascular Health Study, a population-based, longitudinal study of risk factors for coronary artery disease and stroke in more than 5000 men and women aged 65 years and over. The prevalence of AF increased from 2.8% in women aged 65–69 to 6.7% in women aged 80 years and above. The prevalence for men in these two age groups rose from 5.9% to 8%.[7]

Most elderly patients with AF have associated cardiovascular disease. The presence of any cardiovascular disease increases the risk for AF by three- to five-fold. Specifically, the presence of coronary heart disease doubles the risk for developing AF in men of all ages but not in women.[8] Rheumatic heart disease increases the risk of AF eight-fold in men and 27-fold in women, while heart failure increases AF risk eight times in men and 14 times in women. The marked increase in heart failure prevalence in elderly patients undoubtedly contributes to the frequency with which AF is observed in elderly populations. In the Cardiovascular Health Study, the prevalence of AF in men and women with neither clinical nor subclinical cardiovascular disease was 1.6%. The prevalence of AF rose to 4.6% in individuals with subclinical cardiovascular disease and 9.1% in patients with clinically overt cardiovascular conditions (Table 23.1).[7]

Pulmonary disease is also associated with atrial fibrillation; approximately 2–3% of patients with clinically important pulmonary disease develop AF.[8] Right atrial dilation, hypoxemia, acidosis and therapy with beta-1 sympathomimetic amines all undoubtedly contribute to the pathogenesis of the arrhythmia.

Important noncardiovascular conditions that predispose to atrial fibrillation are hyperthyroidism and the use/abuse of alcohol. Atrial fibrillation develops in 10–20% of patients with clinically evident hyperthyroidism.[7] A

low serum thyrotropin (TSH) level in the absence of symptomatic thyrotoxicosis is associated with a three-fold higher risk of AF during the next 10 years in patients 60 years of age or older.[9] In this population, the cumulative incidence of AF during a 10-year follow-up was 28% in patients with low serum TSH levels but no clinical evidence of hyperthyroidism.[9]

Atrial fibrillation may also develop in the setting of various infections, particularly in patients with pre-existing cardiovascular disease. Pneumonia and empyema are two of the most common infections during which AF develops. Other entities that may lead to the development of AF include smoke inhalation, toxic exposures, electrolyte abnormalities such as hypokalemia, hypocalcemia, hypomagnesemia, as well as hypothermia, hypoxemia and hypoglycemia.

Sympathomimetic amines such as bronchodilating beta-agonists, cold remedies, antihistamines, local anesthetics and caffeine-containing beverages can also precipitate AF.[8] Finally, surgery can lead to AF especially in patients with heart disease. Cardiac surgery of any type can also precipitate AF, particularly in elderly individuals. Atrial fibrillation occurs in 5–40% of such patients.[10,11] Thoracotomy for lung surgery also carries a significant risk for the development of AF.[12]

Feinberg et al[2] estimated that, based on the recent US census, there are 2.2 million people in the United States with AF, with a median age of 75 years. The prevalence of AF was estimated to be 2.3% in people over 40 years of age and 5.9% in those over 65 years of age. Of patients with AF, 70% were between the ages of 65 and 85 years.

Of the Veterans Administration's (VA) 2.9 million patients in 1995, 38% were over the age of 65, while 40% of the VA's outpatient clinic visits were for persons 65 years and older.[6] The VA estimates that by the year

History of heart failure
Valvular heart disease
Stroke
Enlarged left atrium (echocardiography)
Abnormal mitral or aortic valve function
Systemic hypertension, treated
Advancing age
Adapted from Furberg et al.[7]

Table 23.1
Factors independently associated with the prevalence of atrial fibrillation in the Cardiovascular Health Study[7]

2010 the number of patients who will be 85 years or older will increase by 400%. This aging population will automatically increase the prevalence of AF in VA hospitals and clinics.

Etiology of AF

Atrial fibrillation usually occurs in patients with pre-existing cardiovascular disease. Thus, Lok and Lau[13] noted that the conditions most frequently associated with AF were hypertension and hypertensive heart disease (28.9%), atherosclerotic cardiovascular disease (24.7%) and rheumatic heart disease (17.5%). Mitral valve disease and cardiomyopathy were also associated with AF. Enlarged left atrial (LA) diameter has also been said to play an important role in the etiology of AF as well as the physician's ability to cardiovert and maintain sinus rhythm (NSR). Brodsky et al[14] found that patients with moderate LA enlargement (45–60 mm) could be maintained in NSR with anti-arrhythmic medication after cardioversion, but patients with markedly dilated LA (>60 mm) were unlikely to maintain NSR.

In one study, the following noncardiac conditions were also associated with AF: pulmonary disease (18.6%), diabetes mellitus (12.7%) and thyrotoxicosis (5.2%).[13] Mandel[15] found major predisposing factors to AF in patients without overt heart disease to be hypertension, diabetes mellitus, left ventricular hypertrophy by EKG criteria, and nonspecific EKG repolarization abnormalities. Diabetes and hypertension carried the greatest risk for developing AF. High consumption of alcohol is a known cause of cardiomyopathy, but excessive alcohol ingestion by itself can result in isolated AF without evidence of myocardial disease.[16]

Mechanism of AF

Patients with AF do not belong to a homogeneous population. Many different factors contribute to this arrhythmia, producing direct clinical and therapeutic consequences. The currently accepted theory for the mechanism of AF involves random waves of intra-atrial re-entry with multiple macrore-entrant circuits moving from one area of the atrial muscle to another.[17] This mechanism produces an EKG pattern with an undulating baseline without discernible P-waves. The ventricular response to this atrial activity is irregularly irregular depending on the refractory period and conductivity of the AV node.

The chaotic atrial contractions of AF result in a 20–30% decline in stroke volume and cardiac output in normal individuals and a greater decrease of cardiac output in patients with heart disease.[3] The falls in stroke volume and cardiac output are the result of a decrease in the volume of blood arriving in the left ventricle during diastole due to the asynchronous atrial contractions and loss of the atrial booster function or 'kick'.

The onset of tachyarrhythmias such as AF is often related to the action of the autonomic nervous system. Coumel et al[18] observed that the parasympathetic (vagal) and sympathetic nerve terminals are anatomically close to each other in the myocardium, and thus are affected by each other. The functional response to cholinergic (vagal) stimulation occurs within milliseconds, while the response to adrenergic (sympathetic) stimulation takes seconds. According to Coumel, this temporal difference has important clinical implications for heart rate variability. Diseased atrial muscle may react differently from normal atrial muscle fibers with increased sensitivity to adrenergic stimulation. Coumel states that 'there is a predominance of vagal influence in the normal atria ... vagal withdrawal is an early characteristic of diseased hearts that even precedes the increase of sympathetic drive.'[18] Therefore, either the parasympathetic or the sympathetic portion of the autonomic nervous system may produce arrhythmias via vagal stimulation in normal atria and by sympathetic stimulation in diseased atria. In actual practice, patients with new onset AF and no organic heart disease are more likely to have been vagally induced, while patients with structural heart disease tend to have sustained attacks mediated by a sympathetic nervous mechanism.[18]

Multiple short episodes of paroxysmal AF commonly precede the onset of chronic or persistent AF. Allessie et al[19] reported experiments in chronically instrumented goats that revealed marked electrophysiological changes in the atrium during the first days after the onset of AF. These changes favored induction and perpetuation of AF. Allessie suggested that these electrophysiological changes may be due to chronic shortening of atrial refractoriness during atrial fibrillation based on changes in composition of the ion channels responsible for atrial repolarization. With new onset AF, these electrophysiological changes reverse within several days after conversion to NSR. Therefore, early treatment of acute AF with maintenance of NRS may prevent the onset of chronic AF due to electrophysiological remodeling. Furthermore, AF can be associated with reversible impairment of ventricular function, cardiac chamber enlargement, heart failure and thromboembolic events.[20]

Morbidity of untreated or sustained AF

Morbidity from AF is related to the sustained rapid, irregular heart rate, decreased ventricular preload and atrial thrombosis. Excessive ventricular rate may lead to hypotension, pulmonary congestion, angina pectoris and anxiety in susceptible individuals. Rapid ventricular rate in elderly patients with paroxysmal AF and sick sinus syndrome can result in syncopal episodes due to ventricular asystole or severe bradycardia following cessation of the tachyarrhythmia.[21,22] The loss of synchronized atrial contraction, the so-called 'atrial kick,' can compromise cardiac output and produce fatigue. Systemic embolization from atrial stasis is the most devastating complication and will be addressed separately (see below).

Complications are more common in patients with advanced age, prior history of congestive heart failure, a history of smoking, echocardiographic evidence of enlarged left atrial diameter (>40 mm) and recent myocardial infarction.[23]

Thromboembolic events and anticoagulation

AF is an important cause of stroke in the elderly. The Framingham Study found that the risk of stroke rose from 1.5% in the age group 50–59 to 23.5% in people over 80 years of age.[24] The risk of stroke varies depending on age and pre-existing structural heart disease. In a recent analysis, patients under age 60 and without hypertension or cardiovascular disease had a very low incidence of stroke.[25]

Patients over 75 years of age with at least one risk factor (diabetes, hypertension, prior TIA/stroke) have an annual stroke rate of 8.1%.[25] The European Atrial Fibrillation Trial noted an annual stroke rate of 12% in patients with AF and TIA.[26]

A major dilemma in treating AF and preventing stroke is deciding the balance between those individuals at greatest risk for stroke compared with those who are at greatest risk for hemorrhagic complications of anticoagulant therapy. The elderly have an increased rate of AF and stroke, as well as an increased risk of hemorrhage during chronic warfarin therapy. It seems reasonable therefore, to provide anticoagulation for elderly patients without an increased risk of intracranial hemorrhage from falls, dementia, or uncontrolled hypertension.[2] It is essential that the clinician monitor the intensity of anticoagulation and the blood pressure in all patients, especially the very elderly. Concomitant medications, for example over-the-counter drugs such as nonsteroidal anti-inflammatory agents, aspirin and cimetidine can have a marked effect on warfarin anticoagulation and thereby increase the risk for hemorrhage.

Avoiding the complication of thromboembolic events in patients with AF requires intervention by the physician based on risk stratification. In comparing treatment with the anticoagulant warfarin, or the antiplatelet agent, aspirin, the European Atrial Fibrillation Trial found that oral anticoagulation reduced the annual rate of primary events (major intracranial hemorrhage) from 17% to 8% and the risk of strokes from 12% to 4%.[26] In the same trial, aspirin decreased the risk of a primary event from 19% to 15% and the risk of stroke from 12% to 10%.

It is recommended that long-term anticoagulation with warfarin (International Normalized Ratio (INR) 2.0–3.0) be strongly considered for all patients older than age 65 years with AF, and for patients younger than 65 years with the following risk factors: previous TIA or stroke, hypertension, diabetes, heart failure, clinical coronary artery disease, mitral stenosis, prosthetic heart valves or thyrotoxicosis.[27] Patients who either decline anticoagulation or are poor candidates for any reason should be given aspirin 325 mg/day.[27] Patients

younger than 65 years without risk factors for stroke can probably be treated with aspirin alone or possibly no antithrombotic therapy.

In patients between the ages of 65 and 75 without risk factors, the use of antithrombotic therapy must be a negotiated decision, made between the patient and his/her physician based on risk assessment, side-effects and convenience.[27]

In patients older than 75 years of age, chronic, life-long anticoagulation with warfarin is recommended because of the high prevalence of stroke in the elderly; however, this fact must be weighed against the increased risk of cerebral hemorrhage. Anticoagulation at the lower end of the therapeutic range (INR 2.0–3.0) might be appropriate in the very elderly.[27] Because elderly individuals have an increased sensitivity to warfarin, therapy should be initiated at low dose, for example 2.5–5 mg of warfarin daily.

Goals of therapy for AF

The immediate cause of symptoms when AF develops is usually the rapid, irregular heart rate. The primary goal of therapy, therefore, is to control the ventricular response, prevent arterial embolism, and to convert the patient to NSR, if possible. Control of the ventricular response can be accomplished by three classes of medications used alone or in combination: beta-blockers such as propanolol, atenolol or metoprolol; the calcium channel blockers verapamil and diltiazem; and/or digoxin.[28] Restoration of sinus rhythm can be achieved by direct-current cardioversion or traditional anti-arrhythmic drug (classes IA, IC, III) therapy. Successful cardioversion is more likely to occur if AF has been present for less than 12 months with minimal left atrial enlargement.[29] A secondary goal of therapy is to prevent the recurrence of AF.

Managing the patient with new-onset, rapid AF

New-onset or acute AF can occur in the setting of acute myocardial infarction or following open-heart surgery. It may also develop de novo in a patient with previously recognized arteriosclerotic heart disease, valvular heart disease (especially mitral valve disease), cardio-myopathy or hypertensive heart disease. On occasion, atrial fibrillation results from primary cardiac electrical disease (so-called 'lone AF'). Lone AF is exceedingly rare in elderly patients.

Figure 23.1 depicts a schema that offers clinicians a number of choices for managing this common clinical problem. Certain strategies aim to restore sinus rhythm while others merely slow the rapid ventricular response. In many patients, the clinician should be satisfied initially with merely controlling the ventricular response. Thereafter, he/she can employ techniques aimed at restoring sinus rhythm. However, restoration of sinus rhythm is not

Clinically and/or hemodynamically <u>stable</u>	Clinically and/or hemodynamically <u>unstable</u>
(a) oral or intravenous beta-blockers	(a) cardioversion
or	or
(b) oral or intravenous verapamil or diltiazem	(b) intravenous procainamide (800–1000 mg/30 min)
or	or
(c) oral or intravenous digoxin (loading dose 0.75–1.0 mg over 12–24 hours; maintenance dose 0.25–0.50 mg/24 hours	(c) intravenous verapamil (5–10 mg/15–20 seconds) or an intravenous diltiazem infusion
or	or
(d) oral or intravenous type IA or IC anti-arrhythmic agents (procainamide, quinidine, disopyramide, propafenone)	(d) intravenous beta-blockers: propranolol (4–8 mg over 5–10 minutes); metoprolol (10–15 mg over 5–10 minutes); atenolol (5–10 mg over 5–10 minutes)
or	
(e) elective cardioversion	

Figure 23.1.
Managing rapid atrial fibrillation.

feasible or possible in all patients. In individuals who remain in atrial fibrillation, chronic control of the ventricular response is essential. Each of the choices listed in the two columns of Figure 23.1 can lead to excellent clinical results in a given patient. Which option one chooses depends on certain characteristics of the patient (e.g. known allergy to one of the drugs), the clinical setting (e.g. coronary care unit versus the office) and the experience of the physician (e.g. has the physician much experience with DC cardioversion?).

As seen in Figure 23.1, the clinician must first determine whether the patient is stable or unstable. An unstable patient with rapid AF might manifest one or more of the following characteristics: rest angina, left ventricular failure or hypotension. If any of these characteristics is present, then the patient is a candidate for one of the therapeutic options listed in the column labelled 'clinically and/or hemodynamically *unstable*'. Option (a), cardioversion, should be undertaken if the patient is very unstable (e.g. acute MI with hypotension) and if contraindications to cardioversion are absent (e.g. patient recently ate lunch). Sinus rhythm is usually restored. Another effective therapeutic option (b) is the administration of intravenous procainamide (800–1000 mg over 30 minutes). Many patients will return to sinus rhythm during infusion of this agent. The clinician has to monitor the patient closely to avoid hypotension, excessive QRS widening on the electrocardiogram (50% increase in QRS duration), and the development of ventricular arrhythmias (torsades de pointes). Procainamide is contraindicated in patients who are known to be allergic to this agent.

Intravenous verapamil or diltiazem (option c) are very effective in slowing the ventricular response in patients with rapid AF. Approximately 10% of patients with AF are restored to sinus rhythm by this technique, but all patients manifest a marked decrease in ventricular rate. A constant infusion of verapamil or diltiazem may be required to maintain adequate control of the ventricular response until sinus rhythm can be restored by other means (e.g. cardioversion or intravenous procainamide infusion). Intravenous beta-blockers are as efficacious as verapamil or diltiazem in slowing the ventricular response in patients with rapid AF. As noted earlier, sinus rhythm can be restored later by cardioversion or intravenous procainamide infusion. Repeated doses of beta-blockers may be administered if the ventricular response fails to slow sufficiently, and if adequate systemic blood pressure is maintained. Intravenous beta-blockers and intravenous verapamil should never be administered in close proximity since asystole may result.

Similar agents and procedures are employed in the patient who is 'clinically and hemodynamically *stable*' despite rapid AF (Figure 23.1). However, drugs are usually administered orally, and cardioversion for restoration of sinus rhythm is performed electively if the patient fails to revert with pharmacological therapy. Oral or intravenous digoxin followed by oral digoxin (option c) is the most widely employed therapeutic strategy for patients who are stable despite rapid AF. The initial dose of digoxin is 0.50–0.75 mg followed by 0.25–0.50 mg in 4–6 hours. The size of the second dose depends on the extent to which the ventricular rate slows in response to the first dose of digoxin. A maintenance dose of digoxin (often 0.25 mg/day) is often administered once adequate control of the heart rate has been obtained. Oral beta-blockers, verapamil or diltiazem (options a and b) are preferable to digoxin. On occasion, one of these three agents (digoxin, beta-blocker, verapamil) does not slow the heart rate sufficiently. In this situation, the clinician may choose to employ two of these agents together (e.g. digoxin plus a beta-blocker) to slow the heart rate. The physician should employ such combinations cautiously since excessive slowing of the ventricular response is possible. One should aim for a resting heart rate between 70–90 beats/min.

Once the ventricular rate has been adequately controlled, the clinician often attempts to restore sinus rhythm (options d, e) with an anti-arrhythmic agent (IA, IC or III) and/or elective DC cardioversion. If AF has been present for more than 2 days, a period of prophylactic anticoagulation (e.g. 30 days of oral warfarin) should be given before cardioversion to sinus rhythm is attempted. One hopes thereby to prevent episodes of arterial embolism.

A number of patients will be refractory to all attempts at restoration of sinus rhythm and will remain in AF even though the ventricular response is adequately controlled (e.g. 70–90 beats/min). For many such individuals, AF is an acceptable rhythm as long as the ventricular response is controlled. For other patients, however, particularly those with left ventricular hypertrophy or poor ventricular function, restoration of sinus rhythm is important since it leads to a 30–50% increase in cardiac output. For such patients, administration of amiodarone may be of considerable benefit since it usually enables the clinician to restore stable sinus rhythm despite failure of previous attempts. As already noted, patients who remain in AF should be anticoagulated with warfarin. Aspirin is a less acceptable second choice. Factors that should influence the clinician in deciding for restoration of NSR versus rate control in AF are listed in Table 23.2.

Maintenance of NSR after conversion of AF

Patients cardioverted from AF to NSR have a decreased likelihood of maintaining NSR unless they receive anti-arrhythmic drug therapy. In six studies comparing no drug therapy or placebo to active drug therapy after cardioversion, the overall percentage of patients in NSR after 1 year was 29% without anti-arrhythmic drug therapy;[17] treatment with quinidine, flecainide or disopyramide increased that percentage to 49%. Sotalol has been noted to have efficacy similar to that of quinidine.[17] Amiodarone has greater efficacy for maintaining NSR 1 year after conversion from AF. Seventy-one percent of patients were maintained in NSR after 1 year of amiodarone therapy.[17]

The maintenance of NSR with type I or type III anti-arrhythmic agents is not without risks. All of these drugs have pro-arrhythmic potential mediated by early after-depolarizations or by blockade of sodium channels, thereby allowing the development of electrical re-entry.[17,30,31] Multicenter randomized trials, for example the AFFIRM trial, are currently underway to compare the risk-benefit ratio of maintaining NSR versus controlling the ventricular rate and chronically anticoagulating patients in AF.[32]

As noted earlier, multiple factors have to be considered in deciding between rate control versus conversion of AF to NSR (Table 23.2). Factors that favor conversion of AF to NSR with anti-arrhythmic drug therapy include LA size less than 50 mm, duration of AF less than 1 year, increased symptoms of CHF or fatigue with AF, 'younger,' more active patients, and/or contraindications to chronic anticoagulation. Most patients deserve at least one attempt at conversion of AF to NSR with drug therapy to maintain NSR; however, multiple

Factors favoring conversion of AF to NSR and anti-arrhythmic drug therapy to maintain NSR
1. Symptoms of CHF or fatigue increase when NSR is not present
2. Left atrial size less than 50 mm
3. LVH or markedly decreased LV function: AF usually associated with increased symptoms
4. Duration of AF less than 1 year
5. 'Younger', more active patients
6. Presence of paroxysmal AF
7. Contraindication to chronic anticoagulation

Factors favoring maintenance of AF with pharmacological rate control and anticoagulation
1. No deterioration in symptomatic status with AF when heart rate is controlled
2. Left atrial size greater than 50 mm
3. Duration of AF greater than 1 year
4. Normal or near normal LV function
5. 'Older', less active patients
6. Sustained AF
7. No contraindications to anticoagulation
8. Failure to maintain NSR despite cardioversion and adequate anti-arrhythmic drug therapy

Table 23.2
Conversion of AF to NSR versus rate control: factors to be considered

clinical factors must be taken into account in deciding a course of action.

Rate control as a goal in place of conversion to NSR

Maintenance of sinus rhythm may not be possible despite medical therapy, or the risk of therapy may be too great, for example compromised left ventricular function increases the risk of pro-arrhythmia with anti-arrhythmic drug therapy, thereby favoring rate control as the treatment of choice. Factors that favor maintaining AF with pharmacological rate control include LA size greater than 50 mm, AF of more than 1 year in duration, 'older', less active patients, no contraindication to anticoagulation and/or prior failure to maintain NSR after conversion from AF (see Table 23.2). Adequate rate control can minimize both the hemodynamic consequences and the symptoms associated with excessive heart rate. Anticoagulation for thromboembolic prophylaxis and rate control medication are increasingly popular therapeutic strategies. Drugs that control rate include digoxin, calcium channel blockers and beta-blockers (Figure 23.1).

References

1. Wolf PA, Benjamin EJ, Belanger AJ et al. Secular trends in the prevalence of atrial fibrillation: the Framingham Study. *Am Heart J* (1996) **131**:790–5.

2. Feinberg WM, Blackshear JL, Laupacis A et al. Prevalence, age distribution, and gender of patients with atrial fibrillation: analysis and implications. *Arch Intern Med* (1995) **3**: 469–75.

3. Alpert JS, Peterson P, Godtfredsen J. Atrial fibrillation: natural history, complications, and management. *Ann Rev Med* (1988) **39**:41–52.

4. Haupt BJ, Graves EJ. Detailed diagnosis and procedures for patients discharged from short-stay hospitals. United States, 1979. Dept. of Health and Human Services publication no. (PHS) 82-1274-1. (National Center for Health Statistics: Hyattsville, MD 1982.)

5. Graves EJ. Detailed diagnoses and procedures, National Hospital Discharge Survey, 1992, Vital Health Statistics (13). (National Center for Health Statistics: Hyattsville, Maryland, 1994) 118.

6. Kizer KW. Geriatrics in the VA: providing experience for the nation. *JAMA* (1996) **275**:1303–7.

7. Furberg CD, Psaty BM, Manolio TA et al. Prevalence of atrial fibrillation in elderly subjects (the Cardiovascular Health Study). *Am J Cardiol* (1994) **74**:236–41.

8. Readon M, Camm AJ. Atrial fibrillation in the elderly. *Clin Cardiol* (1996) **19**:765–75.

9. Sawin CT, Geller A, Wolf PA et al. Low serum thyrotropin concentrations as a risk factor for atrial fibrillation in older persons. *N Engl J Med* (1994) **331**:1249–52.

10. Fuller JA, Adams GC, Buxton B. Atrial fibrillation after coronary artery bypass surgery: is it a disorder of the elderly? *J Thorac Cardiovasc Surg* (1989) **97**:821–5.

11. Hochberg MS, Levine FH, Daggett WM et al. Isolated coronary artery bypass grafting in patients seventy years and older. *J Thorac Cardiovasc Surg* (1982) **84**:219–23.

12. Von Knorring J, Lepantalo M, Lindgren L, Lindfors O. Cardiac arrhythmias and myocardial ischaemia after thoracotomy for lung cancer. *Ann Thorac Surg* (1992) **53**:642–7.

13. Lok NS, Lau CP. Presentation and management of patients admitted with atrial fibrillation: a review of 291 cases in a regional hospital. *Int J Cardiol* (1995) **48**:271–8.

14. Brodsky MA, Allen BJ, Capparelli EV et al. Factors determining maintenance of sinus rhythm after chronic atrial fibrillation with left atrial dilation. *Am J Cardiol* (1989) **63**: 1065–8.

15. Mandel WJ. Should every patient with atrial fibrillation have the rhythm converted to sinus rhythm? *Clin Cardiol* (1994) **17**:II-16–20.

16. Karlson BW, Herlitz J, Edvaedsson N, Olsson SB. Prophylactic treatment after electroconversion of atrial fibrillation. *Clin Cardiol* (1990) **13**:279–86.

17. Repique LJ, Shah SN, Marais GE. Atrial fibrillation 1992: management strategies in flux. *Chest* (1992) **101**:1095–1103.

18. Coumel P, Thomas O, Leenhardt A. Drug therapy for prevention of atrial fibrillation. *Am J Cardiol* (1996) **77**:3–9A.

19. Allessie MA, Konings K, Kirchhof CJHJ, Wijffels M. Electrophysiologic mechanisms of perpetuation of atrial fibrillation. *Am J Cardiol* (1996) **77**:10–23A.

20. Sopher SM, Camm AJ. Atrial fibrillation: maintenance of sinus rhythm versus rate control. *Am J Cardiol* (1996) **77**:24–37A.

21. Aroesty JM, Cohen SI, Morkin E. Bradycardia–tachycardia syndrome: results in twenty-eight patients treated by combined pharmacologic therapy and pacemaker implantation. *Chest* (1974) **66**:257–63.

22. Ferrer MI. Sick sinus syndrome. *J Cardiovasc Med* (1981) **8**:743–51.

23. Friedman HZ, Goldberg SF, Bonema JD et al. Acute complications associated with new-onset atrial fibrillation. *Am J Cardiol* (1991) **67**: 437–9.

24. Wolf PA, Abbott RD, Kannel WB. Atrial fibrillation as an independent risk factor for stroke:

the Framingham study. *Stroke* (1991) **22**:983–8.

25. Atrial Fibrillation Investigators: Risk factors for stroke and efficacy of anti-thrombotic therapy in atrial fibrillation: analysis of pooled data from five randomized controlled trials. *Arch Intern Med* (1994) **154**:1449–57.

26. EAFT Study Group. European Atrial Fibrillation Trial: secondary prevention of vascular events in patients with nonrheumatic atrial fibrillation and a recent transient ischaemic attack or minor ischaemic stroke. *Lancet* (1993) **342**:1255–62.

27. Laupacis A, Albers G, Dalen J et al. Antithrombotic therapy in atrial fibrillation. *Chest* (1995) **108**:352S–9S.

28. Atrial fibrillation: new approaches to old problem. *Harvard Heart Letter* (1995) **6**:3–4.

29. Pritchett ELC. Management of atrial fibrillation. *N Engl J Med* (1992) **326**:1264–70.

30. Nguyen PT, Scheinman MM, Seger J. Polymorphous ventricular tachycardia: clinical characterization, therapy, and the QT interval. *Circulation* (1986) **74**:340–9.

31. Echt DS, Liebson PR, Mitchell LB et al and the CAST Investigators. Mortality and morbidity in patients receiving encainide, flecainide, or placebo: the Cardiac Arrhythmia Suppression Trial. *N Engl J Med* (1991) **324**:781–8.

32. Antman EM. Atrial fibrillation and flutter: maintaining stability of sinus rhythm versus ventricular rate control. *J Cardiovasc Electrophysiol* (1995) **6**:962–71.

24

Pacemaker and ICD indications in the elderly

Philippe Delfaut, Sanjeev Saksena, Atul Prakash, Ryszard B Krol and Betty Wang

Introduction

Pacemaker and implantable cardioverter-defibrillator (ICD) therapies are important advances in the treatment of cardiac rhythm disorders. In specific populations, improvement of patient survival by such implantable devices has been shown in clinical studies.[1–4] Although clinical decisions for ICD or pacemaker implantation are usually based on symptoms, the patient's brady- or tachy-arrhythmia and the presence of heart disease, indications for these therapies may vary to some extent according to individual situations or in particular subgroups of patients. The elderly patient presents one such subgroup. With progressively increasing medical expenditures, the patient benefit versus risk and the cost–benefit ratios of therapies are becoming major concerns for all health-care systems. The paucity of scientific data in any group leads to the obvious question as to whether the elderly patient population obtains the full advantages of pacemaker and ICD therapies, since advanced age or multiple concomitant illnesses may reduce life expectancy. Even physicians, based on subjective evaluations, are often reluctant to initiate aggressive or expensive interventions in elderly patients. Implantable cardiac rhythm management devices fit into this category. The psychological impact of device therapy, the often more complicated organization of device follow-up and challenges in patient education are some issues that may influence the physician's decision before device insertion. The choice of the device is also affected. It may be guided by the physician's assessment of individual patient benefit, the associated cardiac or other diseases and the general status of the patient. It is the purpose of this chapter to review the recently approved ACC/AHA guidelines for pacemaker and defibrillator therapy and evaluate available scientific data in the elderly population.

Indications for cardiac pacemaker therapy
Standard indications

With increasing age, the probability of developing cardiac conduction disturbances becomes more likely. Abnormalities in the atrial or ventricular substrate resulting from frequent concomitant heart disease in the elderly may lead to severe bradyarrhythmias. Even in the absence of heart disease, in many cases, idiopathic or isolated conduction system disease may appear in the elderly patient. Over 85% of patients receiving pacemaker therapy are over 64 years old.[4] Prospective and retrospective studies have shown that elderly patients also benefit from the use of sophisticated pacemakers with dual-chamber pacing and rate-response function.[5–6] These pacemakers improve survival and quality of life compared with ventricular pacing and nonrate-responsive devices.

Tables 24.1 and 24.2 outline the recently approved and published ACC/AHA practice guidelines and address indications for cardiac pacing in 1998.[4] Table 24.1 enumerates indications in atrioventricular (AV) block and Table 24.2 in sinus node dysfunction. Class I indications are the conditions for which there is evidence and/or agreement that a given procedure or treatment is beneficial, useful and effective. Class II indications are conditions for which there is conflicting evidence and/or a divergence of opinion about the usefulness/efficacy of a procedure or treatment. Class II is divided into two subclasses: class IIa for which there is a weight of evidence/opinion in favor of usefulness and efficacy and class IIb for which there is less

---

Class I
Third degree AV block and
    Bradycardia with symptoms *or*
    Arrhythmias and symptomatic bradycardia (drugs) *or*
    Asystole >3.0 s or rate <40 bpm in symptom-free patients *or*
    AV node ablation *or*
    Postoperative AV block *or*
    Neuromuscular diseases
Second degree AV block and symptomatic bradycardia

Class IIa
Asymptomatic third degree AV block
Asymptomatic type II second degree AV block
Asymptomatic type I second degree AV block (intra- or infra-His levels)
First degree AV block with 'pacemaker syndrome'

Class IIb
First degree AV block with LV dysfunction and symptoms of CHF

Class III
Asymptomatic first degree AV block
Asymptomatic type I second degree AV block (supra-His level)
AV block expected to resolve

From Gregoratos et al.[4]

Table 24.1
ACC/AHA 1998 guidelines for permanent pacing in the AV block

Class I
Sinus node dysfunction with symptomatic bradycardia
Symptomatic chronotropic incompetence

Class IIa
Spontaneous or drug-induced sinus node dysfunction

Class IIb
Chronic heart rates <30 bpm in minimally symptomatic patient

Class III
Sinus node dysfunction in asymptomatic patients
Sinus node dysfunction with symptoms not related to bradycardia
Sinus node dysfunction with symptomatic bradycardia due to nonessential drug therapy

From Gregoratos et al.[4]

Table 24.2
ACC/AHA 1998 guidelines for permanent pacing in sinus node dysfunction

well-established usefulness and efficacy by evidence and opinion. The conditions for which there is evidence and/or general agreement that a procedure and treatment is not useful and effective and potentially harmful are represented in class III. Based on available data, there is no evidence for increased risk of pacemaker implantation in the elderly patient.

AV block

It is now recognized that pacemaker therapy can improve survival especially in patients with high-degree AV block, with underlying heart disease and using dual-chamber pacemakers. While device implantation is faster, easier and often less expensive with single-chamber ventricular demand pacemakers, ventricular demand (VVI) pacing as a primary therapy is becoming less and less frequent.[5,7] Resolution of AV block-related symptoms is also observed with cardiac pacing in general and dual chamber demand (DDD) pacing in particular.[8,9] However, the existence of a pre-existing heart disease undoubtedly worsens the prognosis of the elderly patient with AV block after pacemaker implantation.[1] Advanced ventricular dysfunction and the presence of prior coronary artery disease are two predictors of poorer outcome of permanent pacing for this indication. After acute myocardial infarction in the elderly patient, persistent second and third degree AV blocks are important indications for demand pacing especially if associated with symptoms.

Bifascicular and trifascicular blocks are also frequently associated with transient high-degree AV block and sudden death in the elderly patient. Symptomatic patients with such electrocardiographic abnormalities and without other causes explaining the symptoms are candidates for permanent pacing. In the absence of symptoms, prolongation of H–V interval beyond 80ms is, for some investigators, an index of potential high-degree AV block and an indication for prophylactic permanent pacing.[10,11] Other investigators consider prolongation of H–V interval to be due to the underlying heart disease and a marker for sudden death.[12,13]

Sinus node dysfunction

Sinus node dysfunction is the major indication for pacemaker implantation in elderly patients in the USA. Sinus node dysfunction is frequently associated with symptoms (syncope, dizziness, dyspnea) related to inappropriate sinus bradycardia, sinus pauses and chronotropic incompetence. Furthermore, patients with this abnormality often experience other complications such as tachyarrhythmias, for example atrial fibrillation with a risk of thromboembolism and precipitating congestive heart failure. Due to the frequent association of sinus node dysfunction with paroxysmal or chronic atrial fibrillation, VVI or VVIR pacing was preferred by many as the primary pacing mode. However, during the last decade, retrospective and prospective studies[14–18] showed the superiority of DDD and DDDR pacing in terms of mortality and morbidity. Atrial pacing not only improves survival but reduces the incidence of atrial fibrillation and reduces thromboembolic events and NYHA functional class. Moreover, new pacemaker technology now allows mode switching from DDD to VVI or DDI in case of paroxysmal atrial fibrillation episodes avoiding ventricular tracking by fast atrial rates. Some groups[19,20] advocate AAI or AAIR pacing as the best pacing modes in such

patients, arguing that these pacing modes provide a more physiological ventricular activation and ease of implantation. Nevertheless, the risk of subsequent AV block, which may be up to 1–10% during long-term follow-up, tempers this approach. Pacemakers allowing automatic mode conversion from AAI to DDD pacing, in case of prolongation of AV delay may be an interesting compromise. In active patients with chronotropic incompetence, rate-responsive pacemakers increase heart rate during physical activity and show clinical benefits for the elderly patient.[21] The recent results of the THEOPACE study combining theophylline and dual-chamber pacing also suggest benefit.[22]

Supraventricular tachyarrhythmias

Atrial fibrillation incidence increases with age and affects 2% of the population over 65 years and 4% of the population over 80 years. The presence of pre-existent paroxysmal or chronic atrial fibrillation at the time of pacemaker implantation strongly discourages many physicians from choosing a dual-chamber pacemaker for atrial pacing. However, permanent atrial pacing in patients with or without pre-existing atrial fibrillation is now recognized to decrease atrial fibrillation recurrences. Single- and dual-site atrial pacing is included as a standard indication in 1998 ACC/AHA guidelines for prevention of symptomatic supraventricular tachycardia that is drug or catheter-ablation resistant.[4] Furthermore, as reported by us and others,[23,24] atrial multisite pacing can prevent and reduce supraventricular tachyarrhythmia recurrences. We obtained, in our prospective sequential crossover pilot study comparing dual-site right atrial pacing and single-site right atrial pacing, promising results with a combination of simultaneous pacing from the high right atrium and the coronary sinus ostium and atrial overdrive pacing. In our series of 30 patients with drug-refractory frequent atrial fibrillation,[25] 67% being older than 65 years, with bradycardia and symptomatic drug-refractory atrial fibrillation, 78% were atrial arrhythmia-free at 1 year, 63% at 2 years and 56% at 3 years. These data improve results obtained with antiarrhythmic drug therapy alone in other studies.[26–28] In patients without atrial fibrillation recurrences for 1 year, one may stop the antithrombotic treatment. This was seen in one-third of our population and thromboembolic complications have not been observed. This is a major advantage for elderly patients who are at higher risk for complications from warfarin. This study was also designed to compare the efficacy of dual-site right atrial pacing and single pacing site (i.e. high right atrium and coronary sinus ostium). Arrhythmia-free intervals significantly increased from 9 ± 10 days before pacing, to 143 ± 110 days in single-site right atrial pacing ($P < 0.0001$), and to 195 ± 96 days (range 25–270 days) in dual-site right atrial pacing ($P < 0.005$ versus single site right atrial pacing and $P < 0.0001$ versus control). This study shows a beneficial effect of dual-site atrial pacing compared with single-site pacing modes and no pacing. In this study, there was no difference in terms of atrial fibrillation prevention efficacy between the two single sites of pacing from the high right atrium and the coronary sinus ostium.

Syncope due to other causes

Hypersensitive carotid sinus syndrome affects predominantly the older patients. Cardioinhibitory and/or vasodepressor reflexes from carotid sinus stimulation may induce syncope and severe injuries. Regression of symptoms is usually obtained with cardiac pacing.[29,30] However, about 10% of implanted patients have recurrent syncope probably due to the vasopressor component of this disease. DDD or DDI pacing with hysteresis and automatic mode conversion is considered as the best choice for these patients. Efficacy of new algorithms like 'rate-drop response' accelerating the heart rate when the device detects an episode has been shown.[31,32] Association of dual-chamber pacing with drugs like midodrin, anticholinergenic agents, beta-blockers or fludrocortisone may provide symptomatic improvement also.

Even if pharmacological therapy improves symptoms in most patients with vasovagal syncope, some of them still break through and remain severely symptomatic with asystole or severe bradycardias during tilt testing. Initial studies of cardiac pacing in vasovagal syncope show disappointing results even in patients with a mainly bradycardiac mechanism.[33] The hypotensive component of the syncope is incompletely controlled by the pacemaker therapy, and this may explain the recurrence of symptoms. This is in contrast to the efficacy of pacing in carotid sinus syndrome. However, rate-drop response algorithms, allowing faster pacing rate when a vasovagal episode is suspected by the device, give encouraging results. Benditt et al[32] observed that 59% of patients with vasovagal syncope were recurrence-free with dual-chamber pacing during a mean follow-up of 7 months. In this condition, the challenge is to find the method for appropriate recognition of the onset of the vasovagal episode by the implanted pacemaker device. Hybrid therapies combining pacemaker and drug therapy will most likely give better results in the future. Our studies also provide evidence for benefit of association between dual-chamber pacemaker and drug therapy.[34]

Particular indications

Hypertrophic obstructive cardiomyopathy

Hypertrophic obstructive cardiomyopathy causes severe symptoms (dyspnea, syncope, angina pectoris) and is associated with a poor prognosis (sudden death) if untreated. A beneficial effect of cardiac pacing has been suggested in selected drug-refractory patients.[35,36] Combination of right ventricular apex pacing and short AV delay decreases the left ventricular outflow tract gradient by as much as 50% in selected patients and improves the patient's symptomatology on long-term follow-up. This seems to result in functional and symptomatic patient benefit but probably does not remodel the ventricular myopathy. Symptoms and outflow tract gradient reappear after discontinuation of pacing, even after long-term periods of pacing. The atrial contraction for optimal ventricular filling is essential in this condition and dual-chamber pacemaker with DDD pacing is the preferred mode. However, to date, survival benefits with cardiac pacing and alteration of the course of the primary myocardial disease have not been clearly demonstrated. In the elderly patient with hypertrophic cardiomyopathy, cardiac pacing may alleviate symptoms and avoid surgical intervention.

Idiopathic dilated cardiomyopathy
Heart transplantation is the definitive therapy for end-stage dilated or ischemic cardiomyopathy. Some patients, especially in the elderly subgroup, are not eligible for this therapy. Standard dual-chamber pacing in severe idiopathic dilated cardiomyopathy was proposed almost 20 years ago based on encouraging results in a limited nonrandomized study of 16 patients.[37] Nevertheless, these preliminary results were not confirmed by other studies.[38,39] Moreover, DDD pacing does not seem to improve survival compared with VVI pacing.[40] Interesting results were obtained with individually optimized AV delays for some patients in order to re-establish left AV synchrony and improve left ventricular filling time.[41] However, even if acute improvements

in measured physiological parameters such as cardiac output and left ventricular diastolic filling were noted, no long-term data are available about functional improvement, mortality and morbidity. Bakker[42] introduced in 1994 biventricular pacing with a standard right ventricular lead and an epicardial left ventricular lead in a small group of five patients in NYHA class III or IV. At 3 months, he noticed improvements in NYHA functional class in four of the five patients. This was correlated with improvement in stroke volume, left ventricular ejection fraction and diastolic filling time. Another group[43] utilizing a transvenous lead for left ventricular pacing confirmed these data in a randomized acute study. The benefit of this pacing configuration seemed to persist with permanent pacing in three out of eight patients. Larger studies are, however, necessary to evaluate the real benefit in terms of survival and symptom relief with this pacing mode. At the present time, this is considered highly selected therapy for specific patients.

ICD therapy in the elderly
ICD therapy has been increasingly used in elderly patients. Most clinical series have almost 65% of patients older than 65 years of age. Sudden cardiac death due to ventricular fibrillation or sustained ventricular tachycardia is a common complication of coronary and other heart diseases in the elderly. Table 24.3 lists the recently approved practice guidelines detailing indications for ICD therapy in these patients. Note that no indication excludes or alludes to special considerations in the elderly patient.

Prior to ICD implant, the patient's clinical status assessment is of major importance. Existence of cardiac disease and altered left ventricular ejection fraction are the main

Class I
Cardiac arrest due to VF or VT without transient or reversible cause
Spontaneous sustained VT
Syncope of undetermined origin and inducible sustained VT or VF
Nonsustained VT with coronary disease, prior MI, LV dysfunction, and inducible VF or sustained
  VT not suppressible by class I anti-arrhythmic drugs

Class IIa
None

Class IIb
Cardiac arrest presumed to be due to VF with EPS precluded
Severe symptoms due to sustained VT or VF while awaiting cardiac transplantation
Familial or inherited conditions with high risk of VT or VF (long QT syndrome, hypertrophic
  cardiomyopathy)
Nonsustained VT with coronary artery disease, prior MI, LV dysfunction and inducible sustained
  VT or VF at EPS
Recurrent syncope of undetermined cause with LV dysfunction and inducible VT or VF at EPS
  when other causes of syncope are excluded

Class III
Syncope of undetermined cause in a patient without inducible VT or VF
Incessant VT or VF
VF or VT secondary to atrial arrhythmias amenable to ablation
VF or VT due to transient or reversible disorder
Significant psychiatric disorder that may be aggravated by device implant or preclude
  systematic follow-up
Terminal illnesses with projected life expectancy of <6 months
Coronary disease LV dysfunction, prolonged QRS duration in the absence of VT and undergoing
  coronary bypass surgery
NYHA class IV drug refractory congestive heart failure in patients who are not candidates for
  cardiac transplant

From Gregoratos et al.[4]

Table 24.3
ACC/AHA 1998 guidelines for ICD implantation

parameters influencing the patient's life expectancy. Severe coronary artery disease with uncontrolled ischemia as well as a very low ejection fraction will probably result in increased risk during defibrillation threshold testing. The benefits and risks of ICD insertion in the elderly must be also evaluated according to eventual concomitant disease. ICD insertion is not recommended for patients with life expectancy less than 6 months. To date, few

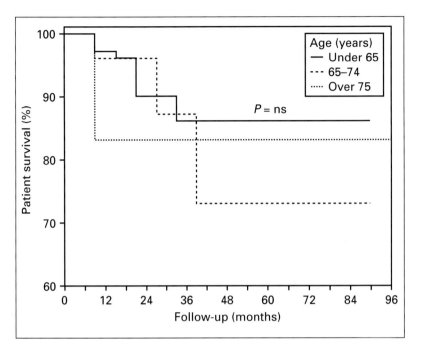

Figure 24.1
Survival in younger and older patients with ICDs.

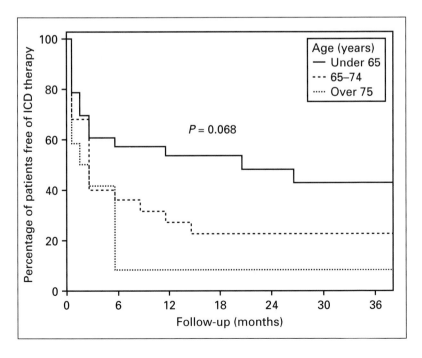

Figure 24.2
Freedom from ICD therapy in younger and older patients with ICDs.

studies[44–46] have compared the outcome of ICD insertion in the elderly with younger patients. In these reports, it appears that prevention of sudden cardiac death by ICD therapy is as effective in the elderly as in the younger patient. Panotopoulos et al[47] noticed 100% survival at 4 years in over 75 year old patients and 97% in under 75 year old patients (*P*: not significant). In this particular study, cardiac mortality and noncardiac mortality were increased in the elderly resulting in a lower survival in this group. Factors associated with mortality were age over 75 years, ejection fraction less than 30%, NYHA class III and appropriate shocks. This study, like others, included both epicardial and transvenous ICD insertions and several device generations without distinction in the analysis. That may explain why other studies show different results. Tresch et al[44] compared patient characteristics, surgical complications and long-term survival rates in elderly and younger patients. The two populations were not different in terms of cardiac disease, ejection fraction, myocardial revascularization frequency and peri-operative mortality. Long-term survival at 3 years was similar in both groups. In a similar comparison study, Manolis et al[46] noted more frequent coronary artery disease and less frequent concomitant cardiac surgical procedures such as subendocardial resection at the time of epicardial ICD insertion in the elderly group. There was, however, no difference in defibrillation thresholds.

We have recently reported the survival and need for device therapy in consecutive patients implanted with transvenous ICD during the period 1989–1996 at our center.[45] Remarkably, there was no peri-operative mortality with this ICD implant method in the elderly or very elderly patient. There was no significant difference in survival between the age groups. The survival from all-cause mortality was 96% at 1 year, 87% at 3 years and 73% at 5 years (Figure 24.1). Survival was not significantly different between the subgroups of age (Figure 24.1). In this analysis the very elderly aged over 75 years did not have impairment of survival compared with younger patients, but used the device more frequently and earlier (Figure 24.2).

Conclusions

With increasing experience with cardiac pacemaker and ICD therapy, it is apparent that both can be implemented safely without evidence of increased implant risk or reduced benefit to the elderly patient. Thus, standard indication and clinical consideration would be applicable to this group. No evidence suggests that the elderly or very elderly should be limited in their access to these valuable cardiac therapies.

References

1. Moss AJ, Hall WJ, Cannom DS et al and the MADIT Investigators. Improved survival with an implanted defibrillator in patients with coronary artery disease at high risk for ventricular arrythmia. *N Engl J Med* (1996) **335:** 1933–40.

2. Shen WK, Hammil SC, Hayes DL et al. Long-term survival after pacemaker implantation for heart block in patients >65 years. *Am J Cardiol* (1994) **74:**560–4.

3. Amikam S, Lemer J, Roguin N et al. Long-term survival of elderly patients after pacemaker implantation. *Am Heart J* (1976) **91:** 445–9.

4. Gregoratos G, Cheitlin MD, Conill A et al. ACC/AHA guidelines for implantation of cardiac pacemakers and antiarrhythmia devices. A report of the American College of Cardiology/American Heart Association Task Force on practice guidelines. *J Am Coll Cardiol* (1998) **31:**1175–209.

5. Lamas GA, Pashos CL, Normand SLT, McNeil B. Permanent pacemaker selection and subsequent survival in elderly medicare pacemaker recipients. *Circulation* (1995) **91:**1063–9.

6. Hargreaves MR, Channon KM, Cripps TR et al. Comparison of dual chamber and ventricular rate responsive pacing in patients over 75 with complete heart block. *Br Heart J* (1995) **74:**397–402.

7. Bernstein AD, Parsonnet V. Survey of cardiac pacing in the United States. *Am J Cardiol* (1992) **69:**331–8.

8. Zion MM, Marchand PE, Obel IWP. Long term prognosis after cardiac pacing in atrioventricular block. *Br Heart J* (1973) **35:** 359–64.

9. Alpert MA, Katti SK. The natural history of high-degree atrioventricular block following permanent pacemaker implantation. *J Chronic Dis* (1982) **35:**341–4.

10. Scheinman MM, Peters RW, Sauve MJ et al. Value of the H–Q interval in patients with bundle branch block and the role of prophylactic permanent pacing. *Am J Cardiol* (1982) **50:**1316–22.

11. Petrac D, Radic B, Birtic K, Gjurovic J. Prospective evaluation of intrahisiar second-degree AV block induced by atrial pacing in the presence of chronic bundle branch block. *Pacing Clin Electrophysiol* (1996) **19:**784–92.

12. McAnulty JH, Rahimtoola SH, Murphy E et al. Natural history of 'high risk' bundle branch block: final report of a retrospective study. *N Engl J Med* (1982) **307:**137–43.

13. Denes P, Dhingra RC, Wu D et al. Sudden death in patients with chronic bifascicular block. *Arch Intern Med* (1977) **137:**1005–10.

14. Andersen HR, Nielsen JC, Thomsen PEB et al. Long-term follow-up of patients from a randomised trial of atrial versus ventricular pacing for sick-sinus syndrome. *Lancet* (1997) **305:** 1210–16.

15. Stangl K, Seitz K, Wirtzfeld A et al. Differences between atrial single chamber pacing and ventricular single chamber pacing with respect to prognosis and antiarrhythmic effect in patients with sick sinus syndrome. *Pacing Clin Electrophysiol* (1990) **13:**2080–85.

16. Sgarbossa EB, Pinski SL, Maloney JD et al. Chronic atrial fibrillation and stroke in paced patients with sick sinus syndrome: relevance of clinical characteristics and pacing modalities. *Circulation* (1993) **88:**1045–53.

17. Rosenqvist M, Brandt J, Schuller H. Long-term pacing in sinus node disease: effect of stimulation mode on cardiovascular mortality and morbidity. *Am Heart J* (1988) **116:**16–22.

18. Lamas GA, Ellenbogen KA, Griffin JJ et al for the PASE Investigators. Quality of life and clinical events in DDDR versus VVIR paced patients: design and preliminary results of a randomized trial. *Circulation* (1992) **92**(Supplement):I-533 (abst).

19. Santini M, Ansalone G, Cacciatore G et al. Status of single chamber atrial pacing. In: Barold SS, Mujica J, eds, *New Perspectives in Cardiac Pacing* (Futura Publishing: Mount Kisco, NY, 1991) 273–301.

20. Rosenqvist M, Aren C, Kristensson BE et al. Atrial rate-responsive pacing in sinus syndrome disease. *Eur Heart J* (1990) **11:**537–42.

21. Gammage M, Schofield S, Rankin I et al. Benefit of single setting rate responsive ventricular pacing compared with fixed rate demand pacing in elderly patients. *Pacing Clin Electrophysiol* (1991) **14**:174–80.

22. Alboni P, Menozzi C, Brignole M et al. Effects of permanent pacemaker and oral theophylline in sick sinus syndrome the THEOPACE study: a randomized controlled trial. *Circulation* (1997) **96**:260–6.

23. Saksena S, Prakash A, Hill M et al. Prevention of recurrent atrial fibrillation with chronic dual-site right atrial pacing. *J Am Coll Cardiol* (1996) **28**:687–94.

24. Daubert C, Mabo PH, Berder V et al. Atrial tachyarrhythmias associated with high degree interatrial conduction block: prevention by permanent atrial resynchronisation. *Eur JCPE* (1994) **1**:35–44.

25. Delfaut P, Saksena S, Prakash A, Krol RB. Long-term outcome of patients with drug-refractory atrial fibrillation after single and dual site right atrial pacing for arrhythmia prevention. *J Am Coll Cardiol* (in press).

26. Coplen SE, Antman FM, Berlin JA et al. Efficacy and safety of quinidine therapy for maintenance of sinus rhythm after cardioversion. *Circulation* (1990) **82**:1106–16.

27. Juul-Moller S, Edvardsson N, Rehnqvist-Ahlberg N. Sotalol versus quinidine for the maintenance of sinus rhythm after direct current conversion of atrial fibrillation. *Circulation* (1990) **82**:1932–9.

28. Gosselink ATM, Crijns HJGM, Van Gilst WH et al. Low-dose amiodarone for maintenance of sinus rhythm after cardioversion of atrial fibrillation or flutter. *JAMA* (1992) **267**:3289–96.

29. Sutton R, Ahmed R, Ingram A. 12-year pacing experience in carotid sinus syndrome. *Pacing Clin Electrophysiol* (1989) **11**:1253 (abst).

30. Brignole M, Oddone D, Cogorno S et al. Long-term outcome in symptomatic carotid sinus hypersensitivity. *Am Heart J* (1992) **123**:687–92.

31. Bexton RS, Davies A, Kenny RA. The rate-drop response in carotid sinus syndrome. *Pacing Clin Electrophysiol* (1997) **20**:840–6.

32. Benditt DG, Sutton R, Gammage MD et al and the International Rate-drop Investigators Group. Clinical experience with Thera DR rate-drop response pacing algorithm in carotid sinus syndrome and vasovagal syncope. *Pacing Clin Electrophysiol* (1997) **20**:832–9.

33. Fitzpatrick AP, Travill CM, Cardas PE et al. Recurrent symptoms after ventricular pacing in unexplained syncope. *Pacing Clin Electrophysiol* (1990) **13**:619–24.

34. Krol R, Prakash A, Delfaut P et al. Head up tilt table testing in patients with carotid sinus syndrome modifies response to carotid sinus stimulation and influences selection of therapy. *J Am Coll Cardiol* (1998) **31**:37A.

35. Jeanrenaud X, Goy JJ, Kappenberger L. Effects of dual-chamber pacing in hypertrophic obstructive cardiomyopathy. *Lancet* (1992) **339**:1318–23.

36. Fananapazir L, Cannon RO III, Tripodi D, Panza JA. Impact of dual-chamber pacing in patients with obstructive hypertrophic cardiomyopathy with symptoms refractory to verapamil and beta-adrenergic-blocker therapy. *Circulation* (1992) **85**:2149–61.

37. Hochleitner M, Hortnagl H, Ng CK et al. Usefulness of physiologic dual-chamber pacing in drug-resistant idiopathic dilated cardiomyopathy. *Am J Cardiol* (1990) **66**:198–202.

38. Brecker SJ, Xiao HB, Sparrow J, Gibson DG. Effects of dual-chamber pacing with short atrioventricular delay in dilated cardiomyopathy. *Lancet* (1992) **340**:1308–11.

39. Gold MR, Feliciano Z, Gottlieb SS, Fisher ML. Dual-chamber pacing with a short atrioventricular delay in congestive heart failure: a randomized study. *J Am Coll Cardiol* (1995) **26**:967–73.

40. Brady PA, Shen WK, Neubauer SA et al. Pacing mode and long-term survival in elderly patients with congestive heart failure. *J Intervent Cardiol Electrophysiol* (1997) **1**:1980–5.

41. Nishimura RA, Hayes DL, Holmes DR, Tajik AJ. Mechanism of hemodynamic improvement by dual-chamber pacing for severe left ventricular dysfunction: an acute Doppler and catheterization study. *J Am Coll Cardiol* (1995) **25**:281–88.

42. Bakker PF, Meijburg H, De Jonge N et al. Beneficial effect of biventricular pacing in congestive heart failure. *Pacing Clin Electrophysiol* (1994) **17**:820 (abst).

43. Cazeau S, Ritter P, Lazzarus A et al. Multisite pacing for congestive heart failure. *Pacing Clin*

Electrophysiol (1996) **19**:568 (abst).

44. Tresch DD, Troup PJ, Thakur RK et al. Comparison of efficacy of automatic implantable cardioverter defibrillator in patients older and younger than 65 years of age. *Am J Med* (1991) **90**:717–24.

45. Saksena S, Mathew P, Giorgeberidze I et al. Implantable defibrillator therapy for the elderly. *Am J Geriatr Cardiol* (1998) **7**:11–14.

46. Manolis AS, Rastegar H, Wang PJ et al. Implantation of the automatic defibrillator system in elderly and younger patients: comparative results. *J Am Coll Cardiol* (1993) **21**:212A (abst).

47. Panotopoulos PT, Axtell K, Anderson AJ et al. Efficacy of the implantable cardioverter-defibrillator in the elderly. *J Am Coll Cardiol* (1997) **29**:556–60.

25

Major pericardial disease
David H Spodick

Introduction

Pericardial anatomy and physiology are inseparable.[1] The pericardium is a complex membrane: an inner sac of monocellular epithelium lying on the heart like a latex glove with projections along all the great vessels clasped by an outer tough fibrous sac. Together they are the *parietal pericardium* and the mesothelial layer on the heart surface is the *visceral pericardium* separated by 15–35 ml of fluid, an ultrafiltrate of plasma. The parietal pericardium prevents sudden cardiac dilation during hypervolemia and exercise and resists penetration of infection from neighboring structures.[2] However, congenital or surgical absence of the entire pericardium does not produce recognizable disease.[3] Table 25.1 outlines the diseases of the pericardium. *All must be anticipated at all ages.*[3] Although there are no formal investigations of age predilection, like other diseases, viral infection is more frequent in younger patients and most systemic diseases, neoplasms and chronic infections such as tuberculosis, in older patients.[4]

Pericarditis can be acute, subacute or chronic, the latter two preceded by an acute phase which sometimes escapes detection. Table 25.2 summarizes the principal etiologies.[3]

Acute pericarditis

The most common clinically recognized form of pericardial disease, acute pericarditis has cardinal manifestations that include a pericardial rub, typical electrocardiographic changes, pain and frequently pericardial effusion with or without cardiac compression (tamponade).[5–8] Chest pain is not invariable; it is expected in acute infectious pericarditis and many traumatic and immunopathic types, but is most often absent in neoplastic, rheumatoid, postradiation and subacute or chronic tuberculous pericarditis.[3,9] Most types, even purulent pericarditis, can be 'silent' in elderly patients, sometimes due to cognitive impairment. Typically, pain is left precordial and retrosternal and usually pleuritic (aggravated by inspiration, coughing, recumbency and body movements), although sometimes steady, 'pressing' and radiating to one or both arms or even the jaw, resembling pain of myocardial ischemia; *radiation to or perception in one or both trapezius ridges is almost pathognomonic*.[3,10] Also pathognomonic are pericardial rubs (friction sounds) with one, two or (usually) three components.[8] Rises in white blood cell counts and serum enzymes reflect superficial myocardial involvement and are usually small. In *myopericarditis*, with strong myocardial involvement, they tend to be higher and longer lasting.[3]

Classically, electrocardiograms show J–ST

Congenital pericardial abnormalities
   Congenital pericardial abnormalities
      Partial (usually left)
         Incidental
         With herniation of portions of the heart
      Total
   Congenital pericardial cysts and diverticula

Acute and subacute inflammatory pericardial disease
   Acute pericarditis and myopericarditis
      Noneffusive
      Effusive
         Without cardiac compression
         With tamponade of the heart
      Pneumohydropericardium
   Recurrent acute pericarditis
   'Subacute pericarditis'
   Pericardial fat necrosis

Noninflammatory excess pericardial contents
   Hydropericardium
   Hemopericardium
      Traumatic
      In association with pathologic bleeding
         Hemorrhagic states
         Rupture of contiguous organs
   Chylopericardium
   Pneumopericardium
   Intrapericardial herniation of other organs

Chronic and constrictive pericardial disease
   Granulomatous
   Pericardial scarring
      Pericardial fibrosis/adhesions
      Pericardial calcification/ossification
      Inflammatory cysts and diverticula
   Chronic pericardial effusion
   Amyloidosis of pericardium

Table 25.1
Categories of pericardial disease

and T-wave changes due to an accompanying epimyocarditis which is usually mild.[6,7] However, PR-segment depression occurs first in electrocardiograms soon after onset: sometimes this is the only change. *Stage 1, the key ECG finding, is pathognomonic*: widespread J-point elevation with normally configured T-waves (concave upward) in almost all leads.[6] In elderly patients, Stage 1 may be absent or missed in those with 'painless' lesions. In *Stage 2*, J-points return to the baseline after which the T-waves become inverted. (In contrast, acute myocardial infarction features reciprocal J-point depressions, T-waves convex upward and few if any PR-segment deviations, along with QRS changes and T-wave inversions that occur before ST-segments become isoelectric).[3,11] In *Stage 3*, T-wave inversion occurs in almost all leads. *Stage 4* is a return to normal or baseline. In elderly patients with marked pre-existing ECG abnormalities pericarditic J–ST and T changes may be minimal or absent.

Tachycardia is the rule except in many uremics and many elderly patients with altered cardiac pacemaking, conduction and autonomic function. Febrile responses may also be blunted in the elderly.

Pericardial effusion and cardiac tamponade

Acute pericarditis may be 'clinically dry' (without significant effusion) or frankly effusive with variable pericardial fluid volume that may contain fibrin, cellular debris and often hemorrhagic components. Rapidly developing effusion, particularly with bleeding, however, will not permit the parietal pericardium to stretch so that it compresses the heart (cardiac tamponade).[2,12] Heart sounds may become faint and the pericardial rub sometimes disappears. The apex impulse may or may not become impalpable. Chest X-rays may show enlargement of the cardiac silhouette which can be normal or flask-shaped. Lateral films often show pericardial fat lines. Echo-Doppler cardiography is the most efficient diagnostic technique.[3] Large effusions (and some small effusions with a noncompliant parietal pericardium), permit the heart to swing freely with each cardiac cycle; during tamponade there may be one swing for every two cycles producing ECG electric alternation.[13]

In frank tamponade the right heart increases markedly in size at the expense of the left during inspiration with reversal on expiration—the main cause of *pulsus paradoxus* (often palpable, an inspiratory blood pressure drop of 10 mmHg or more), reflected in reciprocal Doppler flow velocities and other respiratory reciprocation.[10] Usually early diastolic collapse of the right ventricular free wall and late diastolic collapse of the right atrium signifies some degree of tamponade. Computed tomography (CT) and magnetic resonance imaging (MRI) or transesophageal echocardiograms (TEE) may be needed to detect loculated pericardial fluid, especially when transthoracic echocardiograms (TTE) are equivocal.[3] While hemorrhagic fluid is most common in severe pericarditis and in neoplastic involvement, the *presence of blood in the pericardial effusion is nonspecific for etiology*. Pure blood (hemopericardium) occurs acutely in some patients receiving anticoagulants or thrombolytic agents and in cardiac or pericardial trauma.[14,15]

Almost any etiological type of pericarditis may cause tamponade. Most common causes (depending on the patient population) are idiopathic (presumably usually viral) pericarditis, malignancy (usually metastatic) and trauma. *In the elderly, malignancy and vasculitic disorders must always be ruled in or out*. Postmyocardial infarction syndrome after a silent myocardial infarction may present as

Idiopathic pericarditis (syndrome)
Infectious pericarditis
    Bacterial
        Suppurative
        Tuberculous
    Viral
        Coxsackie
        Influenza
        Other
    Mycotic (fungus)
    Rickettsial
    Parasitic
    Other
        Spirochetal
        Spirillum infection
        Mycoplasma pneumoniae
        Leptospira
        Listeria
        Lymphogranuloma venereum
        Psittacosis (chlamydiaceae)
        AIDS (probably viral; HIV-4; other)
Pericarditis in diseases of contiguous structures
    Myocardial infarction
        Acute myocardial infarction
        Postmyocardial infarction syndrome
        Postpericardiotomy syndrome
        Ventricular aneurysm
    Dissecting aortic aneurysm; intramural aortic hematoma (IAH)
    Pleural and pulmonary diseases
        Pneumonia
        Pulmonary embolism
        Pleuritis (pleuropericarditis)
Pericarditis in the vasculitis–connective tissue disease group
    Rheumatoid arthritis
    Systemic lupus erythematosus (SLE); drug-induced SLE
    Scleroderma
    Sjögren's syndrome
    Whipple's disease (bacterial)
    Mixed connective tissue disease (MCTD)
    Reiter's syndrome
    Ankylosing spondylitis
    Inflammatory bowel disease
    Serum sickness
    Wegener's granulomatosis
    Vasculitis
    Polymyositis (dermatomyositis)
    Behcet's syndrome
    Familial Mediterranean fever
    Dermatomyositis
    Panmesenchymal reaction of steroid hormone withdrawal
    Polyarteritis
    Thrombohemolytic thrombocytopenic purpura
    Other
Pericarditis in immunopathies and 'hypersensitivity' states
    Drug reactions

Table 25.2
Etiology of acute pericarditis and myopericarditis

Serum sickness
Allergic granulomatosis
Giant urticaria
Other sensitivity reactions (see under Pericarditis in diseases of contiguous structures: dissecting aortic aneurysm; pleural and pulmonary diseases)

Neoplastic percarditis
Secondary (metastatic, hematogenous or by direct extension): carcinoma, sarcoma, lymphoma, leukemia, other)
Primary: mesothelioma, sarcoma, fibroma, lipoma

Pericarditis in disorders of metabolism
Renal failure
Uremic (chronic/acute renal failure)
'Dialysis' pericarditis
Myxedema
Cholesterol pericarditis
Gout

Traumatic Pericarditis
Direct
Pericardial perforation
Penetrating chest injury
Esophageal perforation
Gastric perforation
Cardiac injury
Cardiac surgery
During catheterization
Pacemaker insertion
Diagnostic
'Foreign body' pericarditis
Indirect
Radiation pericarditis
Nonpenetrating chest injury

Pericarditis of uncertain pathogenesis
Postmyocardial and pericardial injury syndromes (? immune disorders)
Inflammatory bowel disease
Colitis (ulcerative, granulomatous)
Segmental enteritis
Löffler's syndrome
Thalassemia (and other congenital anemias)
'Specific' drug reactions (Psicofuranine, Minoxidil)
Pancreatitis
Sarcoidosis
Fat embolism
Bile fistula (to pericardium)
Wissler's syndrome
Stevens–Johnson syndrome
Gaucher's disease
Diaphragmatic hernia
? Atrial septal defect
Giant cell aortitis
Takayasu's syndrome
Mucocutaneous lymph node syndrome
Fabry's disease
Kawasaki's disease
Degos' disease
Other

Table 25.2
Continued

'idiopathic' pericarditis.[9,16] Elderly patients are especially prone to traumatic complications of cardiac catheterization, pacemaker installation and cardiac surgery which induce hemopericardium. Unless the patient is hypovolemic (e.g. taking diuretics) catheterization shows cardiac diastolic pressures to be significantly elevated and nearly equal (within 5 mmHg) in all chambers, usually equilibrating at between 15 and 30 mmHg, with variable reduction in systolic pressures.[2,10,12] The time needed for critical tamponade depends on the rate of fluid accumulation, the degree of pericardial 'give' and the absolute amount of fluid. Myocardial abnormalities, especially hypertrophy and aortic valve disease, may resist cardiac compression, and damp critical signs such as pulsus paradoxus. Moreover, coronary and other heart disease may interfere with dynamic compensation by impairing contractility.[11,15]

Rapidly developing tamponade resembles cardiogenic shock, but with venous hypertension and engorgement, excepting with brisk bleeding where intravascular volume may not have sufficient time to expand and to be transferred to the venous circulation.[2] *Slow tamponade* resembles heart failure because of systemic congestion, dyspnea and even orthopnea. Treatment is by drainage of fluid.[15] Before drainage, the size and distribution of effusions should have been determined by imaging cardiography, especially echo-Doppler.[3] Pericardial fluid drainage is safest by subxiphoid surgical incision[17] with or without thoracoscopic guidance; with large effusions and in emergencies pericardial paracentesis is justified and pericardiocentesis is quite safe in almost any situation under transesophageal echocardiographic guidance.[3]

General treatment of pericarditis

Treatment aims to relieve symptoms and destroy etiological agents as well as to relieve tamponade. In acute pericarditis the cornerstones are rest, analgesics (usually non-steroidal anti-inflammatory agents), and antipyretics. Specific infections require demonstrably effective antibiotics. Tuberculosis should have at least triple drug therapy. Colchicine may be added.[18] *Corticosteroids should be avoided* unless they are for treatment of a systemic etiological form (e.g. a vasculitis) or if all other means fail to deal with the patient's discomfort. [2,15]

Principal etiological forms of acute pericarditis (Table 25.2)
Idiopathic/viral pericarditis

Idiopathic/viral pericarditis is a frequent form and is only 'idiopathic' because no etiology can be discovered (there is general agreement, usually without direct proof, that in its acute form it is usually viral).[3] It may occur in the course of or following recognized viral illness, or viral elements may be shown by serological tests. ('Idiopathic' pericarditis, of course, may be due to *any* disease that first appears in the pericardium). Unmistakably viral forms occur mainly in younger patients. They present the epitome of the symptoms and signs of acute pericarditis mentioned earlier.[10,15] Pericardial effusions are frequent, but tamponade is not (although it must always be anticipated); constrictive evolution is not rare. Pneumonia and pleurisy are frequent and, as in most forms of pericarditis, left pleural effusion is not rare.[2] C-reactive protein, erythrocyte sedimentation rate and white blood cell counts are usually elevated, but in some elderly patients these acute phase reactants may not respond.

Bacterial and other infections

Bacterial and other infections are likely to be more dramatic than idiopathic, presumed viral, pericarditis, and much more likely to result in constriction.[15,19,20] Traditionally, tuberculous pericarditis was the most feared of these and may still be found especially in elderly residents of nursing homes. Infections can be deceptively 'quiet', particularly in the elderly in whom pneumonia is frequently a precursor or concomitant. Treatment is as above along with specific antibiotics (NB most antibiotics given orally achieve good levels within the pericardium). Corticosteroids appear to reduce the morbidity and complication rate of acute tuberculous pericarditis as long as adequate multiple antibiotic treatment is also provided. However, as in all forms of pericarditis, corticosteroids do not prevent eventual constriction.[3]

Immunopathies (presumptive mechanism)

Acute pericarditis may appear after injury to the heart such as surgery (postpericardiotomy syndrome: PPS) and myocardial infarction (postmyocardial infarction syndrome: PMIS).[9,16] All probably have the same pathogenesis: anti-heart antibodies (exact role uncertain) and, at least for the PPS, presence of community-prevalent viruses. These syndromes often resemble acute idiopathic pericarditis, but develop in days to weeks after myocardial injury. They are prone to recurrences,[18] although if the initial illness was missed or remote they present as a form of 'idiopathic' pericarditis. Frequent signs of immune involvement include arthralgis, recurring fever and sometimes rashes. ECG changes of acute pericarditis may or may not occur although they usually become rare after the index recur-

rence. General treatment is as mentioned above, although a corticosteroid agent such as prednisone may be required when all else fails. Colchicine, if tolerated, should be included.[15,18]

Vasculitis–connective tissue disease group

This group is one of the largest generators of pericarditis due to the prevalence of rheumatoid arthritis in which pericardial lesions and pericardial effusions, usually subclinical, occur in about 50% of patients. Almost the whole group is involved, particularly lupus erythematosus, both the 'natural' kind and that due to drugs (e.g. procainamide); it is identified by increased antinuclear antibodies (ANA). (NB all women with apparent 'idiopathic' pericarditis should have ANA tests.)

Selected other etiologies

Uremic pericarditis, which can be severe, fibrinous and hemorrhagic, occurs typically in nondialyzed patients. It usually has the loudest pericardial rubs, varies from severely painful to painless, and responds to intense hemodialysis and anti-inflammatory medication. Unless there is an intercurrent infection, in purely uremic pericarditis the ECG does not change. *Dialysis pericarditis* is much more difficult to treat and is often painless; effusion and constriction may occur. Treatment is to increase hemodialysis or switch to peritoneal dialysis. *Neoplastic pericarditis*, usually due to metastasis or extension from nearby tumors and rarely to primary pericardial tumors, portends a prognosis for life of a few weeks to months. *Epistenocardiac pericarditis*: this pericarditis, usually subclinical and self-limited, accompanies and is localized over transmural myocardial infarctions. Occasionally, its pain is severe enough to require treatment. Generalized pericarditis, even during an acute myocardial infarction, (although usually 2 weeks to 4 months later) represents the PMIS (Dressler's syndrome) and is a contraindication for antithrombotic therapy.[11,16]

Recurrent and incessant pericarditis

Any etiological form may recur if the etiological agent or process is not destroyed. Autoimmune types, particularly recurrent 'idiopathic' pericarditis, tend to relapse either with a symptom-free interval (*recurrent pericarditis*) or flare repeatedly on reducing medication (*incessant pericarditis*). Many cases represent corticosteroid dependency. These patients are treated with reduction of physical activity, anti-inflammatory agents and colchicine if tolerated. Corticosteroids should be tapered very slowly, with other medications maintained for at least one or two months longer and then tapered.[15,18,20]

Chronic pericardial effusion

Chronic pericardial effusion, occurring mainly in middle-aged and older patients, sometimes with some degree of tamponade, may be an incidental finding on imaging or the residuum of a known bout of pericarditis. Most are idiopathic although some appear to be tuberculous.[3,20] Clinically significant chronic effusions usually are fairly large and sometimes massive. Among them conditions like *cholesterol pericarditis* are more threatening because of the danger of constrictive disease, which can occur rapidly after drainage if there is inflammatory activity. *Myxedema*, relatively rare today, may cause large to massive effusions, especially in elderly women. These usually have the greatest reduction of electrocardiographic QRST voltage: they usually respond promptly to thyroid therapy.

Since long-standing large effusions, particularly those that are increasing, may cause tamponade (especially after hemorrhage—always a danger following chest trauma) treatment must be individualized, but drainage, probably followed by pericardectomy, should be a main option. While needle and catheter drainage are quite feasible, surgical drainage permits biopsies of both the parietal and visceral pericardium. The latter is more likely to yield diagnostic material.[3,4]

Constrictive pericarditis

Constriction occurs in *acute, subacute, chronic and effusive-constrictive* forms. Acute constriction appears from a week to 2–3 months after an acute pericarditis usually with tamponade. Subacute constriction most often occurs as an element of effusive-constrictive pericarditis and produces variably mixed signs of each. The epitome of constrictive pericarditis is chronic constriction, which is increasingly rare in advanced countries because of the rapidity of diagnosis and frequent monitoring of patients who have had an acute attack. Usually, in chronic constriction there is little or no fluid and the scarred pericardium, largely or totally, obliterates the cavity, although effusive-constrictive cases are not rare. Most common current etiologies include surgical trauma, bacterial infection, mediastinal irradiation and viral or 'idiopathic' pericarditis.[3] With chronicity, the pericardium may calcify totally or, much more commonly, partly, sometimes producing confusing images (lateral chest films, CT and MRI are best to analyze calcification). Occasionally the heart can be constricted by chronic or, more often, subacute clotted hemopericardium or by encircling malignant tumors. More acute clotted hemopericardium produces *elastic constriction*.

Constriction reduces the ability of the heart to fill and to this extent resembles tamponade. However, tamponade impedes filling throughout diastole while constriction features a brief very rapid filling period after which there is a plateau of pressure and cessation of filling. These result from the 'rubber bulb' effect when the myocardium contracts, pulling in the stiff pericardium which thereafter springs back in diastole. (Diastolic suction may be present.) As in tamponade, there is diastolic pressure equilibration throughout the heart unless the constrictive tissue is variable or unequal. Atrial and venous pressure curves show both x and y descents with the y descent usually exaggerated. In effusive-constrictive pericarditis x and y may be equal (or even $x>y$) which produces mixed hemodynamic pictures. Ventricular pressure curves in both ventricles show the characteristic 'square root' sign during diastole (as in some patients with congestive failure and especially *in restrictive cardiomyopathies which are often very difficult to distinguish from constriction*).

Patients appear to have a form of heart failure although the myocardium need not fail (indeed, as in tamponade, it may have excellent systolic function excepting in some cases of chronic constriction)—it is 'prevented from succeeding', producing systemic congestion.[2] As in tamponade, the pulmonary alveoli show no edema although the lung interstitium may. The most common sign is dyspnea, particularly on exertion, and sometimes orthopnea. Jugular veins are dilated and during inspiration they may not collapse or even become more distended (*Kussmaul's sign*). Occasional patients have pulsus paradoxus but this is usually due to residual pericardial fluid, additional lung disease or because those parts of the heart that are not constricted—the atrial and ventricular septa—have excessive respiratory movement (right to left in inspiration).

The pulsus paradoxus in pure constriction is never large, that is, it is only slightly above the normal limit of 10 mmHg for respiratory change in brachial blood pressure. First and second heart sounds may be normal or of reduced intensity.[5] The hallmark is an early diastolic sound (EDS) with the exact mechanism of the abnormal early third sounds of cardiac failure excepting that it occurs sooner after the second sound due to the greatly abbreviated isovolumic relaxation and rapid filling periods. It is most common in chronic constriction and occasionally is striking (earning the sobriquet 'pericardial knock'). The EDS coincides with the sudden arrest of ventricular filling as the heart expands to the limit of its pericardial shell. Externally the EDS often coincides with an abnormal movement of the apex outward in diastole that follows abnormal apical inward movement in systole.[2] The abdominal organs, particularly the liver and spleen, are congested. Ascites and peripheral edema are common: occasionally ascites occurs with no pedal edema. Reduced serum proteins, particularly albumin, may be due to visceral congestion causing liver impairment and protein-losing enteropathy.[3]

The ECG often shows low voltage. Inter-atrial block resembling a low P-mitrale is frequent and, with chronicity, is often succeeded by atrial fibrillation. T-waves are nonspecifically changed. They may be inverted, especially if the patient never recovered from Stage 3 of the acute pericarditis ECG.[10] Imaging, particularly echocardiography, often shows compressed, tubular ventricles, sometimes with one or both atria enlarged.[15] The transthoracic echocardiogram alone is not reliable for pericardial thickening unless a careful damping maneuver is performed on the M-mode recording. CT and MRI are much better. MRI is best to gauge the condition of the myocardium before surgery since *there might be myocardial scarring, atrophy or invasion by calcium.* In many recent cases, especially constriction due to cardiac surgery, the pericardium can imprison the heart like a steel coat and yet be thin, negating thickness criteria (>4 mm) on imaging.[3]

While constriction may appear like early congestive failure, particularly in older patients with known heart disease, only *restrictive cardiomyopathy sometimes causes diagnostic difficulties since the hemodynamics of both may be identical* (rarely, both may be present simultaneously, e.g. due to thoracic radiation therapy). Usually, Doppler studies and advanced imaging techniques can distinguish the two, although diagnosis occasionally requires thoracotomy and biopsy.[3] Other patients, particularly with ascites, are thought to have hepatic cirrhosis (*Pick's disease*). Cirrhosis should not coexist with jugular venous distention. Conspicuous x and y collapses, pericardial thickening and calcification help the diagnosis, but none is specific. Tricuspid regurgitation is not rare, but significant murmurs do not occur in constriction unless there is additional heart disease or unless constriction or calcification over certain chambers and vessels (e.g. in the AV groove) causes external stenosis of underlying structures, such as valves.[5] Diastolic pressure equilibration within the heart is typical only of constriction, tamponade, and some cases of restrictive cardiomyopathy.

Like low pressure tamponade, constriction may be latent with relatively low cardiac diastolic pressures, particularly in patients treated for 'heart failure' with vigorous diuresis. Rapid intravenous infusion of 1 l of saline usually induces diastolic equilibration.

Treatment

Pericardiectomy is definitive and feasible in all but patients with severe myocardial damage and atrophy. Pre-operatively, sodium should be restricted and diuretics used as needed. Digitalis may prevent myocardial failure which sometimes follows resection of the pericardium. This is due to the unaccustomed hemodynamic burden of free inflow into a heart with a myocardium that often has disuse atrophy, especially in chronic cases. Operative risk thus depends on the condition of the myocardium, and also the metabolic impairment of long-standing systemic congestion and the technical problems faced by the surgeon when there is pericardial calcification, invasion of the myocardium by the constrictive tissue, or adhesions from previous surgery.[3,15] If tuberculosis is suspected, antituberculous therapy should be instituted before operation and continued thereafter.[20]

References

1. Spodick DH. Macro- and microphysiology and anatomy of the pericardium. *Am Heart J* (1992) **124**:1046–51.

2. Spodick DH. The normal and diseased pericardium: current concepts of pericardial physiology, diagnosis and treatment. *J Am Coll Cardiol* (1983) **1**:240–51.

3. Spodick DH. *The Pericardium: A comprehensive Textbook.* (Marcel Dekker: New York, 1997).

4. Spodick DH. Pericarditis in systemic diseases. *Cardiol Clin* (1990) **8**:709–16.

5. Spodick DH. Acoustic phenomena in pericardial disease. *Am Heart J* (1971) **81**:114–24.

6. Spodick DH. Diagnostic electrocardiographic sequences in acute pericarditis: significance of PR segment and PR vector changes. *Circulation* (1973) **48**:575–80.

7. Spodick DH. The electrocardiogram in acute pericarditis: distributions of morphologic and axial changes by stages. *Am J Cardiol* (1974) **33**:470–4.

8. Spodick DH. The pericardial rub: a prospective, multiple observer investigation of pericardial friction in 100 patients. *Am J Cardiol* (1975) **35**:357–62.

9. Khan AH. Review: the postcardiac injury syndromes. *Clin Cardiol* (1992) **15**:67–72.

10. Spodick DH. Pericarditis, pericardial effusion, cardiac tamponade and constriction. *Crit Care Clin* (1989) **5**:455–76.

11. Spodick DH. Pericardial complications of acute myocardial infarction. In: Francis GS, Alpert JS, eds, *Modern Coronary Care* (Little Brown: Boston, 1990) 331–9.

12. Spodick DH. Threshold of pericardial constraint: the pericardial reserve volume and auxiliary pericardial functions. *J Am Coll Cardiol* (1985) **6**:296–7.

13. Spodick DH. Electric alternation of the heart: its relation to the kinetics and physiology of the heart during cardiac tamponade. *Am J Cardiol* (1962) **10**:155–65.

14. Giles PJ, D'Cruz IA, Killam HAW. Tamponade due to hemopericardium after streptokinase therapy for pulmonary embolism. *South Med J* (1988) **81**:912–14.

15. Spodick DH. Critical care of pericardial disease. In: Rippe JM, Irwin RS, Alpert JS, Fink MP, eds, *Intensive Care Medicine*, 3rd edn (Little Brown: Boston, 1995) 282–95.

16. Spodick DH. Postmyocardial infarction syndrome (Dressler's syndrome). *ACC Curr J Rev* (1995) **4**:35–7.

17. Isselbacher EM, Cigarroa JE, Eagle KA. Cardiac tamponade complicating proximal aortic dissection: is pericardiocentesis harmful? *Circulation* (1995) **90**:2375–8.

18. Guindo J, Rodriguez de la serna A, Ramio J et al. Recurrent pericarditis: relief with colchicine. *Circulation* (1990) **82**:1117–20.

19. Mocchegiani R, Capestro F, Grancesconi M et al. Idiopathic acute pericarditis: a 10 year follow-up. *Eur Heart J* (1990) **11**(Supplement):404.

20. Permanyer-Miralda G, Sagrista-Sauleda J, Soler-Soler J. Primary acute pericardial disease: a prospective series of 231 consecutive patients. *Am J Cardiol* (1985) **56**:623–30.

21. Zayas R, Anguita M, Torres F et al. Incidence of specific etiology and role of methods for specific etiologic diagnosis of primary acute pericarditis. *Am J Cardiol* (1995) **75**:378–82.

26

Infective endocarditis

Gabriel Gregoratos and Kathryn A Glatter

Introduction

Infective endocarditis is a microbial infection of the cardiac valves, the endocardium or the endothelium adjacent to a cardiac or vascular malformation. It is caused by a large variety of micro-organisms, and the infection may pursue either a prolonged (subacute) or a fulminant (acute) course. Although much overlap exists, it is clinically useful to classify endocarditis as acute (generally caused by invasive pathogens such as *Staphylococcus aureus*, *Streptococcus pyogenes*, or *Neisseria*) or subacute (caused by more indolent organisms such as *Streptococcus viridans* or *Staphylococcus epidermidis*). Diagnosis and therapy differ considerably in these two forms of the disease.

Epidemiology

Incidence and age distribution

Despite conflicting reports in the literature, the incidence of infective endocarditis has not changed significantly since the advent of antibiotics. In 1936, the incidence of endocarditis in the United States was reported to be 4.2 per 100 000 person-years.[1] Reports from the Olmstead County, Minnesota Epidemiologic Survey indicate that the incidence of endocarditis in this area was 4.3 per 100 000 person-years in the 1950–1959 period and 3.9 per 100 000 person-years in the 1970–1981 era.[2] It is currently estimated that infective endocarditis accounts for 0.15 to 5.4 cases per 100 000 admissions to hospitals. The disease has undergone considerable change over the past 50 years with respect to age distribution. In the pre-antibiotic era, endocarditis involved primarily young adults. The mean age of patients with subacute endocarditis was reported to be 32 years in the 1930s and 1940s, 46 years in the 1950s, and 50 to 56 years in the 1960s. More recent studies suggest that the average age of patients with endocarditis is 57 years. Prior to 1923, fewer than 2% of patients with endocarditis were older than 60 years. It is now estimated that 55% of these patients are 60 or more years of age.[5–9]

The increasing age of patients with infective endocarditis poses a serious problem for older individuals because the clinical presentation may be atypical and may not suggest the diagnosis of endocarditis. Furthermore, even with appropriate therapy, the prognosis is generally poorer than in younger patients, for the following reasons. (1) An increase in the elderly population which has led to an increased number of persons with risk factors for endocarditis (e.g. calcific valvular disease). (2) A decline in new cases of rheumatic heart disease and increased survival in patients with prior rheumatic valvular lesions. (3) An increase in the use of prosthetic devices (e.g. prosthetic valves and pacemakers) which provide a substrate for endocarditis. (4) Increased survival of patients with congenital cardiac defects.[10,11]

(5) Increased incidence of manipulations of the genitourinary and gastrointestinal tracts of elderly patients, which may lead to bacteremia. (6) Increased incidence of line-related nosocomial bacteremias which develop frequently in elderly patients. It has been estimated that two-thirds of nosocomial staphylococcal bacteremias occur in elderly patients.[10] Studies of gender distribution in infective endocarditis indicate that the disease occurs much more frequently in men than in women. The male to female ratio has been reported as 2:1 in patients under age 50 and rises to at least 6.5:1 in patients over that age.[12,13]

Predisposing events

The source of bacteremia responsible for endocarditis in the elderly patient is often similar to that for patients under the age of 65 years. History of antecedent dental procedures is found in 15–20% of all patients with endocarditis due to nonenterococcal streptococcus. In one study, 25% of elderly patients with *Streptococcus viridans* endocarditis gave a prior history of dental manipulation. However, streptococcal endocarditis has also been reported in the edentulous patient.[14] Certain predisposing events occur more frequently in the elderly. These events include genitourinary tract infections and instrumentation such as cystoscopy, debridement of decubitus ulcers, gastrointestinal surgery with postoperative wound infection and biliary tract surgery.[15] Approximately half of all cases of nosocomial endocarditis in the elderly are associated with the use of intravascular catheters or other devices.[16]

Predisposing cardiovascular disease

Infective endocarditis develops most commonly in patients with underlying cardiac disease. In reported series, approximately 70% of patients with endocarditis had evidence of pre-existing structural cardiac abnormalities.[17] Rheumatic valvular and congenital structural defects each account for approximately one-quarter of the infective endocarditis cases while the remainder are degenerative-type structural defects. In patients with valvular disease, the mitral valve is involved most commonly, followed by aortic valve endocarditis and combined mitral and aortic valve infection. These various predisposing lesions have been classified into high-, moderate- and negligible-risk categories in the American Heart Association Scientific Statement on Prevention of Bacterial Endocarditis (Table 26.1).

Underlying rheumatic heart disease occurs less frequently in the elderly compared to younger patients. Rheumatic heart disease was found in only 20% of elderly patients with endocarditis.[18] In another study, underlying heart disease was absent in 40% of endocarditis patients over the age of 60 years.[19] Additionally, the importance of atheromatous deposits as a predisposing factor in endocarditis in the elderly has been emphasized.[20,21] In a recently reported study comparing underlying heart disease in two groups of patients with endocarditis, in patients over the age of 70 years, prosthetic devices were responsible for 52% of cases, 28% of patients had native valve disease and in 20% there was no evidence of pre-existing structural cardiac deformity.[20] Finally, endocarditis on transvenous pacemaker leads is an uncommon but increasingly frequent occurrence.[20,22]

Mitral annular calcification (MAC) is an important risk factor for endocarditis in the aging population. In patients with infective endocarditis associated with mitral annular calcification, the prognosis appears to be worse than in those without MAC due to the avascular nature of the mitral annulus that leads to the development of periannular and

Endocarditis prophylaxis recommended

High-risk category

> Prosthetic cardiac valves, including bioprosthetic and homograft valves
> Previous bacterial endocarditis
> Complex cyanotic congenital heart disease (e.g. single ventricle states, transposition of the great arteries, tetralogy of Fallot)
> Surgically constructed systemic–pulmonary shunts or conduits

Moderate-risk category

> Most other congenital cardiac malformations (other than above and below)
> Acquired valvular dysfunction (e.g. rheumatic heart disease)
> Hypertrophic cardiomyopathy
> Mitral valve prolapse with valvular regurgitation and/or thickened leaflets

Endocarditis prophylaxis not recommended

Negligible-risk category (no greater risk than the general population)

> Isolated secundum atrial septal defect
> Surgical repair of atrial septal defect, ventricular septal defect, or patent ductus arteriosus (without residua beyond 6 months)
> Previous coronary artery bypass graft surgery
> Mitral valve prolapse without valvular regurgitation
> Physiological, functional or innocent heart murmurs
> Previous Kawasaki disease without valvular dysfunction
> Previous rheumatic fever without valvular dysfunction
> Cardiac pacemakers (intravascular and epicardial) and implanted defibrillators

From Dajani et al[57] with permission.

Table 26.1
Cardiac conditions associated with endocarditis

myocardial abscesses.[21] In a prospective study of 976 elderly patients, including 526 with mitral annular calcification, Aronow reported a higher incidence of infective endocarditis in patients with MAC compared to patients without this abnormality.[22]

Microbiological features

Streptococci and staphylococci account for the majority of cases of endocarditis in both young and elderly patients. Streptococci have been reported to account for 25–80% of cases in the elderly.[19] However, enterococci may be responsible for up to 40% of streptococcal cases.[7] In a recently reported series of infective endocarditis in patients over the age of 70, Group D streptococci and enterococci were responsible for 48% of the cases, *S. viridans* accounted for 14%, staphylococci for 24% and miscellaneous other micro-organisms for 14%.[20] In patients with prosthetic valve endocarditis, *Staphylococcus epidermidis* is a common pathogen. The polymicrobial infections seen frequently in intravenous drug users are uncommon in the elderly.

An increasing number of infective endocarditis cases in the elderly are nosocomial in origin.[13,24,25] This finding is due mainly to an increased use of invasive procedures and prosthetic implants in this group of patients.[26] In a group of 56 patients with infective endocarditis aged 65 and older, fifteen acquired the infection in the hospital; 10 of these had intravenous lines and three genitourinary procedures.[7] An episode of infective endocarditis is considered nosocomial in origin when it appears 48 hours or more following hospitalization or when it follows a hospital-based procedure within 4 weeks.[27] The organisms responsible for nosocomial endocarditis vary depending upon the site of origin. Percutaneous invasive procedures are most often the source of staphylococcal infection whereas urinary tract manipulation predisposes to the development of enterococcal endocarditis.

Fundamental differences exist between nosocomial and community-acquired bacteremia caused by *Staphylococcus aureus*. In one study, community-acquired disease was not commonly associated with an extra-cardiac focus of infection and was more likely to lead to infective endocarditis and metastatic infections. In contrast, staphylococcal bacteremia that developed in a nosocomial setting was less likely to result in infective endocarditis and a portal of entry was frequently identified.[28] Several series have reported that nosocomially acquired infective endocarditis involved women more often than men.[6] Other investigators have emphasized that when Gram-negative micro-organisms are responsible for infective endocarditis in the elderly, the infecting organisms were frequently acquired in a hospital or in a chronic institutional setting.[27]

Clinical manifestations

Although the clinical manifestations of infective endocarditis are well described, they are frequently insidious and nonspecific, particularly in the elderly. Therefore, delays in diagnosis and treatment may occur and contribute to its mortality. Because comorbid illnesses are common among the elderly, these nonspecific symptoms of endocarditis may be incorrectly attributed to other underlying medical problems.[7,20,29] In reports from the older literature, Thell and colleagues described 42 patients over the age of 60 years with endocarditis confirmed either at autopsy or by surgical resection of the infected valve.[19] In 60% of these patients, the diagnosis of endocarditis was never suspected. In the largest comparative study by age group to date, Terpenning et al compared 52 patients under age 40 years and 49 patients over age 64 years with endocarditis.[16] The elderly patients in this cohort described fewer symptoms on admission to the hospital than did those under 40 years including a lower incidence of fever, chills, arthralgias, dyspnea or headache. Additional studies have also noted that the elderly patient with endocarditis may simply complain of 'not feeling well' due to vague or nonspecific symptoms of fatigue, malaise, and anorexia which are incorrectly attributed to other causes.[30–32] Patients over age 60 are more likely to present with hypotension and less likely with tachycardia than those under age 40 in Terpenning's study.[16] Finally, the classic peripheral stigmata of Osler's nodes, Roth spots or petechiae are present in only 1–14% of the elderly and are seen with a lower frequency than in younger patients.[16,20,29]

Signs and symptoms of endocarditis which involve the central nervous system are common among the elderly. Approximately one-third manifest neurological symptoms such as mental confusion, depression and paranoia which may be misdiagnosed as organic brain disorders attributed to the aging process. Hemiplegia, aphasia or focal cranial nerve palsies may be manifestations of septic cerebral emboli. One study found that the presence of neurological symptoms during the clinical course of endocarditis was an unfavorable prognostic factor and was associated with a 75% long-term mortality.[7] Meningitis may occur from direct extension from tissue infected by septic emboli. Additionally, mycotic aneurysms of the cerebral arteries occur in up to 10% of patients with endocarditis and may rupture several years after the initial infection.

The combination of fever and new or changing cardiac murmurs is an obvious clue to the diagnosis of endocarditis, yet both may be absent. Although fever greater than 100°F was present in over 80% of elderly patients in Terpenning's study at some point during their hospitalization, the height of the febrile response was lower than in younger patients.[16] The typical presentation of *acute* endocarditis with a marked toxic course, rigors and high-grade fevers is distinctly uncommon in this population. This poor febrile response to infection has been noted in previous studies and has been attributed to both the lower basal metabolic temperature of the elderly and diminished humoral response to infection.[29] The incidence of 'innocent' cardiac murmurs also increases in this population, particularly due to degenerative calcification of the aortic or mitral valve. One survey found that 58% of elderly patients in a veterans' hospital had some type of a cardiac murmur, the majority of which were of a low intensity and easily overlooked on physical examination.[33] Much of the emphasis in the older endocarditis literature placed on a changing cardiac murmur as an important diagnostic tool must be viewed

in this context. Conversely, it has been reported that 15–25% of patients with endocarditis have no murmur at presentation.[31] Therefore, the presence of a cardiac murmur in a febrile patient may not alone make the diagnosis of endocarditis and requires adjunctive data to correctly interpret this finding.

The cardiac complications of endocarditis can have serious hemodynamic consequences and contribute significantly to its morbidity. Refractory congestive heart failure is the most common cause of death in the elderly with this disease.[29] Heart failure occurs most frequently with acute aortic regurgitation through destruction of the aortic cusps, although severe mitral regurgitation may also be responsible. Valvular ring abscess can lead to conduction abnormalities by extension of the infection into the septum and adjacent conduction system, and may require surgical intervention for definitive therapy.[16] Embolization of vegetations to the coronary arteries may result in myocardial infarction in the absence of atherosclerotic disease. Finally, pyogenic bacteria such as *Staphylococcus aureus* can erode into the septum to create septal defects and shunts or into the pericardium with resultant cardiac tamponade.

Significant thromboembolic phenomena occur in about one-third of elderly patients with endocarditis.[7,16,29] Mesenteric embolic episodes may cause melena, ischemic bowel and acute abdominal pain. Septic pulmonary emboli from right-sided valvular lesions may lead to pneumonia, empyema and pulmonary infarction. Splenic emboli are generally clinically inapparent but are present in up to 44% of cases at autopsy. However, the late development of splenic abscess has been reported to carry a high mortality if emergent splenectomy is not performed.[34] Finally, septic embolization to the kidneys can induce hematuria, proteinuria or worsen the marginal renal function often present in the elderly.

Diagnosis

Laboratory data

The leukocyte count in endocarditis can be normal or markedly elevated, depending on the pathogen and acuity of illness. Normocytic, normochromic anemia is commonly present and may provide an important diagnostic clue. Because an elevated erythrocyte sedimentation rate (ESR) is present in up to 90% of cases, a normal ESR helps eliminate endocarditis from the differential diagnosis.[7,16,29] Immunoglobulin abnormalities occur commonly in endocarditis. A positive rheumatoid factor can be seen in up to 50% of cases of prolonged duration and may disappear after treatment.[7,29] Circulating immune complexes can be demonstrated and may play a role in the disease process. Since most patients with endocarditis have proteinuria and microscopic hematuria, examination of the urine sediment is generally helpful.

Blood cultures

Blood cultures must be obtained before the initiation of antibiotic therapy. Isolation of the pathogen is critical to guide appropriate treatment and to definitively diagnose infective endocarditis. Three sets of blood cultures (aerobic and anaerobic sets) within a 24-hour period are generally recommended with blood draws at least 15 minutes apart.[16,26,29] Although a minimum of 10 ml blood is required per set to identify the pathogen, 30 ml blood should be obtained to maximize the diagnostic yield.[16,26,29] The yield increases with each set of blood cultures drawn within 24 hours of bacteremia, and is reported to be 80% with the first set, 89% with the second set and 99% with the third set of blood cultures.[26] The most common cause of culture-negative endocarditis is failure to draw blood cultures prior to antibiotic treatment, although

the HACEK group (Hemophilus, Actinobacillus, Cardiobacterium, Eikenella and Klingella) of fastidious organisms can also lead to failures in diagnosis of the pathogen.[16,29]

Echocardiography

Echocardiography is used to confirm the presence of vegetations and to make a definite diagnosis of endocarditis, to define the anatomic location of the vegetations, and to determine the presence of complications such as annular abscess which might require surgical intervention. In patients with mitral regurgitation, vegetations commonly occur on the atrial wall or on the atrial side of the mitral valve leaflets. With aortic valvular disease, vegetations occur on the ventricular surface of the aortic valve or on the anterior mitral valve leaflet.[35,36]

Transesophageal echocardiography (TEE) has a specific role in the evaluation of endocarditis, particularly in the detection of prosthetic valve infection and paravalvular abscess. It can detect vegetations as small as 2–5 mm in diameter and has superior sensitivity and specificity compared to transthoracic echocardiography. The safety of TEE in patients over age 65 years was assessed by Zabalgoitia et al. No adverse outcomes related to the TEE were observed in this elderly group.[37] The authors noted that TEE may provide additional information in those elderly patients in whom the diagnosis of endocarditis was not strongly suspected. Werner et al observed that transthoracic echocardiography correctly identified vegetations in only 45% of patients over 70 years compared to 75% under age 40 years with endocarditis.[38] TEE increased the sensitivity of detection to over 90% in both groups. Thus, TEE may give critical information regarding the presence and size of endocarditis vegetations in the elderly, given the high incidence of pre-existing valvular abnormalities

Definite infective endocarditis
Pathological criteria
    Microorganisms: demonstrated by culture or histology in a vegetation, or in a vegetation that
    has embolized, or in an intracardiac abscess; or
    Pathological lesions: vegetation or intracardiac abscess present, confirmed by histology
    showing active endocarditis

Clinical criteria, using specific definitions listed in Table 26.3
    Two major criteria; or
    One major and three minor criteria; or
    Five minor criteria

Possible infective endocarditis
    Findings consistent with infective endocarditis that fall short of 'definite' but not 'rejected.'

Rejected
    Firm alternative diagnosis for manifestations of endocarditis; or
    Resolution of manifestations of endocarditis, with antibiotic therapy for 4 days or less; or
    No pathological evidence of infective endocarditis at surgery or autopsy, after antibiotic
    therapy for 4 days or less

From Durack et al[40] with permission

Table 26.2
Proposed new criteria for diagnosis of infective endocarditis

which may give false positive findings by transthoracic echocardiography.

Diagnostic criteria

The Beth Israel criteria put forth by von Reyn et al in 1981 were used for many years to confirm the diagnosis of endocarditis.[23] These criteria combined clinical signs and symptoms including the presence of new murmurs, positive blood cultures, fever, embolic phenomena and underlying heart disease to stratify patients into 'definite', 'probable', 'possible,' or 'rejected' categories of endocarditis. Although these commonly used sets of criteria are helpful to objectively evaluate the data, they fail in certain cases to accurately diagnose endocarditis when it is otherwise clinically obvious.[39,40] More recently, the Duke classification system has replaced the von Reyn criteria for diagnosis of endocarditis (Tables 26.2 and 26.3). The Duke classification proposes major and minor criteria similar to the Jones criteria for rheumatic fever. The major criteria include pathological diagnosis of valvular vegetations, positive blood cultures or echocardiographic findings consistent with endocarditis, while the minor criteria include fever, embolic phenomena or underlying valvular disease. Durack et al[40] compared the von Reyn with the Duke criteria to diagnose 405 suspected episodes of endocarditis with pathological confirmation. The authors found that

Major Criteria
Positive blood culture for infective endocarditis

Typical microorganism for infective endocarditis from two separate blood cultures
Viridans streptococci, *Streptococcus bovis*, HACEK group; or
Community-acquired *Staphylococcus aureus* or enterococci, in the absence of a primary focus; or
Persistently positive blood culture, defined as recovery of a microorganism consistent with infective endocarditis from:
(i) Blood cultures drawn more than 12 hours apart; or
(ii) All of three or a majority of four or more separate blood cultures, with first and last drawn more than 12 hours apart

Evidence of endocardial involvement
Positive echocardiogram for infective endocarditis
(i) Oscillating intracardiac mass, on valve or supporting structures, or in the path of regurgitant jets, or on implanted material, in the absence of an alternative anatomical explanation; or
(ii) Abscess; or
(iii) New partial dehiscence of prosthetic valve; or
New valvular regurgitation (increase or change in pre-existing murmur not sufficient)

Minor Criteria
Predisposition: predisposing heart condition or intravenous drug use

Fever: $\geq 38.0°C$ (100.4°F)
Vascular phenomena: major arterial emboli, septic pulmonary infarcts, mycotic aneurysm, intracranial hemorrhage, conjunctival hemorrhages, Janeway lesions

Immunological phenomena: glomerulonephritis, Osler's nodes, Roth spots, rheumatoid factor

Microbiological evidence: positive blood culture but not meeting major criterion as noted previously or serological evidence of active infection with organism consistent with infective endocarditis

Echocardiogram: consistent with infective endocarditis but not meeting major criterion as noted previously

---

* Including nutritional variant strains
From Durack et al[40] with permission.

Table 26.3
Definitions of terminology used in the proposed new criteria

80% were correctly classified as 'definite' for endocarditis by the Duke criteria compared to only 51% by the von Reyn.[40] The improved sensitivity of the Duke criteria has been confirmed by other investigators.[39] It is evident from the above that the diagnosis of infective endocarditis, particularly in the elderly, is frequently a complex and difficult process. The combination of clinical, microbiological and echocardiographic findings as proposed by the Duke investigators should minimize uncertainty.

Treatment

It is important to categorize elderly patients with infective endocarditis into complicated or uncomplicated groups. Patients with infection due to *Streptococcus viridans* and *Streptococcus bovis* can be placed in the uncomplicated group if there is no evidence of hemodynamically significant valve dysfunction because these organisms are all relatively penicillin-sensitive. Prognosis in this group is generally good, and a 90–97% cure rate is achieved with 4 weeks of antibiotic therapy.[41–43] These organisms rarely become resistant during therapy. Disk-diffusion studies are adequate guides of therapy for this patient group.

Patients should be classified in the complicated group if the causative organism is a staphylococcus, a fungus, or a Gram-negative organism. Similarly, patients with intracardiac prosthetic devices and patients allergic to penicillin also belong in the complicated group. Additionally, elderly patients presenting with heart failure due to valvular dysfunction, renal failure, extensive distal embolization or cerebral or other extravalvular cardiac complications must also be considered to have complicated disease. Prognosis in this group is uncertain, with a bacteriological cure reported in only 20–80% of cases.[3,12,17,44,45] Organisms involved in this patient group frequently become resistant during therapy, and the specific regimens are not well standardized. Quantitative tube dilution sensitivity studies are often necessary for bacteriological characterization and cardiovascular surgical support is often required to achieve a cure or to reduce complications. Whereas patients with uncomplicated endocarditis may be effectively treated in almost any well-staffed facility with an adequate microbiology laboratory, patients with complicated disease are best treated in a tertiary referral center with full support staff. The treatment of complicated infective endocarditis requires a team effort by cardiologists, infectious disease and renal specialists, and cardiac surgeons.

General principles of therapy

Microbiological diagnosis and accurate studies of the sensitivity of the isolated organism to antibiotic agents must be established as early as possible. This diagnosis is particularly important in the elderly since mortality is estimated to be 30%, about twice that of younger patients.[46] Patients with acute fulminant infective endocarditis must be treated with an empirical antimicrobial regimen as soon as possible after blood cultures have been obtained. Early cardiovascular surgical consultation should be obtained in all patients with endocarditis of a native aortic valve and in those with prosthetic valve infection even if hemodynamically stable. Blood cultures should be repeated 2 and 5 days after initiation of antibiotic therapy to document clearing and should be repeated 1–3 weeks after completion of therapy because of the possibility of relapse. Careful serial physical examinations should be performed because subtle changes, particularly in the elderly, may precede abrupt hemodynamic changes. Every patient should be examined to determine the portal of entry, particularly the oral cavity. Necessary dental therapy should be carried out along with antibiotic treatment. Patients with *Streptococcus bovis* endocarditis should undergo complete examination of the colon to exclude neoplasia.

Antibiotic therapy

A complete discussion of antimicrobial regimens employed in the treatment of infective endocarditis is beyond the scope of this chapter. The American Heart Association (AHA) has recently published revised recommendations for treating infective endocarditis.[47] Included in the revision is a regimen suitable for outpatient treatment of patients with endocarditis due to streptococci that are highly susceptible to penicillin: ceftriaxone 2 g administered intravenously or intramuscularly once daily for 4 weeks. This regimen allows for outpatient therapy which can be given by a visiting nurse or in an emergency department. Additional revisions are related to the recognition that enterococci are becoming increasingly resistant to penicillin G, vancomycin and aminoglycosides[48,49] and include guidelines for the appropriate therapy of endocarditis due to the HACEK group. These organisms are responsible for as many as 10% of endocarditis cases and are best treated with ceftriaxone.

Culture-negative endocarditis

The most common cause of culture-negative endocarditis is failure to obtain blood cultures prior to initiating antibiotic therapy. In the typical elderly patient with suspected endocarditis and negative blood cultures, it is recommended that empirical therapy with a regimen of ampicillin and gentamicin to cover *Enterococcus faecaelis* be initiated. Exceptions to this general rule include postoperative cardiosurgical patients and those with an acute fulminant course of endocarditis in whom the treatment regimen should include an aminoglycoside and a semisynthetic penicillin until the microorganism is positively identified. In cases of nosocomially acquired endocarditis with a fulminant septic course, vancomycin should be included in the therapeutic regimen. The clinical response to the various antibiotic regimens should be followed carefully and therapy should be continued for 4–6 weeks with a combination antibiotic regimen that produces symptomatic improvement and defervescence.

Prosthetic valve endocarditis

Treatment of an infected prosthetic valve, regardless of the infective organism, requires prolonged, aggressive antibiotic therapy and a combined team approach that includes specialists in infectious diseases, cardiology, nephrology and cardiovascular surgery. Aggressive bacteriocidal antimicrobial therapy alone or in combination with early surgery can successfully cure a substantial number of such patients. Surgical removal of the prosthesis is frequently necessary when the infective organism is a fungus, the infection relapses despite adequate antimicrobial therapy or there is a major embolic event or evidence of prosthetic valve dysfunction.

Surgical management

Congestive heart failure due to development of acute aortic regurgitation continues to be the leading cause of death from infective endocarditis.[44–46,50] Elderly patients who develop pulmonary edema during the active phase of left-sided endocarditis have a particularly poor prognosis on medical therapy alone; the mortality associated with this complication has been reported to range from 50 to 80%.[51] For these reasons early operative treatment with replacement of the incompetent valve has been advocated and extensively studied. Marked reductions in mortality have been reported to between 8 and 28% when valve replacement was undertaken during the active phase of the infection[52–53] and as low as 0% for valve replacement during the inactive phase of endocarditis. Other indications for early surgery include recurrent embolization, uncontrolled sepsis despite adequate antimicrobial chemotherapy, fungal infection, the development of extravalvular complications (conduction defects or pericarditis) and recurrence of the infection despite adequate antimicrobial chemotherapy.

In many cases of prosthetic valve endocarditis, surgery is the mainstay of treatment. New techniques have been described dealing with extracardiac extension of the infection and development of annular absesses. Operative mortality in one study was 17% in patients with annular abscess and 9% in patients with prosthetic valve endocarditis without an abscess.[54] Some patients may require complicated procedures that include valve conduits. Better detection of annular abscesses with transesophageal echocardiography and earlier surgical intervention might reduce further operative mortality.

Overall, valve replacement surgery is now being performed with lower rates of mortality and morbidity even in the very elderly. However elderly patients who are reoperated and those with active infective endocarditis fall into high risk categories.[55] Impaired left ventricular systolic function, low cardiac output, sepsis, endotoxemia, gut permeability and impaired hemostasis represent some of the pathophysiological mechanisms responsible for the increased surgical mortality in this patient group. Currently, measures to modify these mechanisms and improve surgical outcome in high-risk patients are being investigated. Such measures include pulsatile perfusion during cardiopulmonary bypass and aprotinin therapy to modify the inflammatory response and prevent hemostatic disorders. Similarly, the issue of bioprosthetic valve durability is of critical importance to elderly patients undergoing valve replacement surgery for infective endocarditis. Recent studies document excellent longevity of porcine bioprostheses in older patients. In one study of patients 70 years of age and older undergoing valve surgery and insertion of a porcine bioprosthesis, the actuarial freedom from valve failure at 9 years was 94% and at 18 years 84%.[56]

Prophylactic antibiotic therapy

Prophylactic antibiotic therapy to prevent the development of infective endocarditis following certain procedures remains a controversial topic. There are no randomized controlled human trials in patients with cardiac defects to establish definitively that antibiotic prophylaxis provides protection against the development of endocarditis during bacteremia-inducing procedures. Nevertheless, clinical consensus is that prophylactic antibiotics are useful and such prophylactic therapy has been standardized by the publication of the American Heart Association's scientific statement on prevention of bacterial endocarditis.[57] Various antibiotic chemoprophylaxis regimens are recommended depending on the source of bacteremia, the presence or absence of allergy to a particular antibiotic and the risk level of the patient. The reader is referred to the current AHA Guideline on Prevention of Bacterial Endocarditis for a full discussion of the antibacterial regimen recommendations.

References

1. Hedley OF. Rheumatic heart disease in Philadelphia hospitals. III. Fatal rheumatic heart disease and subacute bacterial endocarditis. *Pub Health Rep* (1940) **55**:1707–19.
2. Griffin M, Wilson W, Edwards E. Infective endocarditis. Olmstead County Minnesota, 1950 throughout 1981. *JAMA* (1985) **254**:1199–207.
3. Watanakunakorn C. Changing epidemiology and newer aspects of infective endocarditis. *Adv Intern Med* (1977) **22**:21–47.
4. Oakley C. Infective endocarditis. *Br J Hosp Med* (1980) **24**:239–43.
5. Kim E, Ching D, Pien F. Bacterial endocarditis at a small community hospital. *Am J Med Sci* (1990) **299**:487–93.
6. Kay D. Definitions and demographic characteristics. In: Kaye D, ed., *Infective Endocarditis*. (University Park Press: Baltimore, 1976) 1–10.
7. Robbins N, De Maria A, Miller MH. Infective endocarditis in the elderly. *South Med J* (1980) **73**:1335–8.
8. Rabinovich S, Evans J, Smith I et al. A long term view of endocarditis. *Ann Intern Med* (1965) **63**:185–98.
9. Venezio F, Westenfelder G, Gook F. Infective endocarditis in a community hospital. *Arch Intern Med* (1982) **142**:789–92.
10. Terpenning M, Buggy B, Kaufman C. Infective endocarditis: clinical features in young and elderly patients. *Am J Med* (1987) **83**:626–34.
11. Land M, Bisno A. Acute rheumatic fever: a vanishing disease in suburbia. *JAMA* (1983) **249**:895–8.
12. Lerner PI, Weinstein L. Infective endocarditis in the antibiotic era. *N Engl J Med* (1966) **274**:199–206, 259–66, 383–93.
13. Hayward GW. Infective endocarditis: a changing disease. *Br Med J* (1973) **ii**:706–9.
14. Berk SL, Smith JK. Infectious diseases in the elderly. *Med Clin North Am* (1983) **77**:273–93.
15. Gantz NM. Geriatric endocarditis: avoiding the trend toward mismanagement. *Geriatrics* (1991) **46**:66–8.
16. Terpenning MS, Buggy BP, Kauffman CA. Hospital acquired infective endocarditis. *Arch Intern Med* (1988) **148**:1601–3.
17. Pelletier LL Jr, Petersdorf RG. Infective endocarditis: a review of 125 cases from the University of Washington Hospitals 1963–72. *Medicine* (1977) **56**:287–313.
18. Applefield MM, Hornick RB. Infective endocarditis in patients over 60. *Am Heart J* (1974) **88**:90–4.
19. Thell R, Martin FH, Edwards JE. Bacterial endocarditis in subjects 60 years of age and older. *Circulation* (1975) **51**:174–82.
20. Selton-Suty C, Heon B, Grentzinger A et al. Clinical and bacteriological characteristics of infective endocarditis in the elderly. *Heart* (1997) **77**:260–3.
21. Aronow WS. Mitral annular calcification: significant and worth acting upon. *Geriatrics* (1991) **46**:73–86.
22. Klug D, Lacroix D, Savoye C et al. Systemic infection related to endocarditis on pacemaker leads. *Circulation* (1997) **95**:2098–107.
23. Aronow WS, Koenigsberg M, Kronzon I et al. Association of mitral annular calcification with new thromboembolic stroke and cardiac events at 39-month followup in elderly patients. *Am J Cardiol* (1990) **65**:1511–12.
24. Maki DG. Nosocomial bacteremia: an epidemiologic overview. *Am J Med* (1981) **70**:719–32.
25. Schlessinger LS, Ross SC, Schaberg DR. *Staphylococcus aureus* meningitis: a broad-based epidemiologic study. *Medicine* (1987) **66**:148–56.
26. Terpenning MS. Infective endocarditis. *Clin Geriatr Med* (1992) **8**:903–12.
27. Von Reyn C, Levy B, Arbeit R. Infective endocarditis: analysis based on strict case definitions. *Ann Intern Med* (1981) **94**:505–18.
28. Finklestein R, Sobel JD, Nagler A et al. *Staphylococcus aureus* bacteremia and endocarditis: comparison of nosocomial and community-acquired infection. *J Med* (1984) **15**:193–211.
29. Cantrell M, Yoshikawa TT. Infective endocarditis in the aging patient. *Gerontology* (1984) **30**:316–26.

30. Bayles TB, Lewis WH. Subacute bacterial endocarditis in older people. *Ann Intern Med* (1940) **13**:2154–63.

31. Tenenbaum MJ, Kaplan MH. Infective endocarditis in the elderly: an update. *Geriatrics* (1984) **39**:121–7.

32. Owen RE, Allen DM. Infections in the elderly. *Singapore Med J* (1991) **32**:179–82.

33. Wong M, Chuwa T, Shah P. Degenerative calcific valvular disease and systolic murmurs in the elderly. *J Am Geriatr Soc* (1983) **31**: 156–63.

34. Johnson JD, Raff MJ, Barnwell PA et al. Splenic abscess complicating infectious endocarditis. *Arch Intern Med* (1983) **143**:906–10.

35. Dillon JC, Feigenbaum H, Konecke LL et al. Echocardiographic manifestations of valvular vegetation. *Am Heart J* (1973) **86**:698–704.

36. Kim JH, Wiseman A, Kisslo J et al. Echocardiographic detection and clinical significance of left atrial vegetation in active infective endocarditis. *Am J Cardiol* (1989) **64**:950–2.

37. Zabalgoitia M, Gandhi DK, Evans J et al. Transesophageal echocardiography in the awake elderly patient: its role in the clinical decision-making process. *Am Heart J* (1990) **120**:1147–53.

38. Werner GS, Schulz R, Fuchs JB et al. Infective endocarditis in the elderly in the era of transesophageal echocardiography: clinical features and prognosis compared with younger patients. *Am J Med* (1996) **100**:90–7.

39. Hoen B, Selton-Suty C, Danchin N et al. Evaluation of the Duke criteria versus the Beth Israel criteria for the diagnosis of infective endocarditis. *Clin Infect Dis* (1995) **21**:905–9.

40. Durack DT, Lukes AS, Bright DK et al. New criteria for diagnosis of infective endocarditis: utilization of specific echocardiographic findings. *Am J Med* (1994) **96**:200–9.

41. Watanakunakorn D, Burkert T. Infective endocarditis at a large community teaching hospital, 1980–1990: a review of 210 episodes. *Medicine* (1993) **72**:90–102.

42. Steckelberg JM, Melton LJ III, Ilstrup DM et al. Influence of referral bias on the apparent clinical spectrum of infective endocarditis. *Am J Med* (1990) **88**:582–8.

43. Van der Meer JTM, Thompson J, Valkerburg HA et al. Epidemiology of bacterial endocarditis in the Netherlands. I. Patient characteristics. *Arch Intern Med* (1992) **152**:1863–8.

44. Weinstein L, Rubin RH. Infective endocarditis 1973. *Prog Cardiovasc Dis* (1973) **16**:239–74.

45. Rubenstein E, Lang R. Fungal endocarditis. *Eur Heart J* (1995) **16**(Suppl B):84–9.

46. Berman ND. Valvular heart disease in the elderly. *Mt. Sinai J Med* (1985) **52**:594–600.

47. Wilson WR, Karchmer AW, Dajani AS et al. Antibiotic treatment of adults with infective endocarditis due to streptococci, enterococci, staphylococci and HACEK microorganisms. *JAMA* (1995) **274**:1706–13.

48. Eliopoulos GM. Aminoglycoside resistant enterococcal endocarditis. *Infect Dis Clin North Am* (1993) **17**:117–33.

49. Eliopoulos GM. Enterococcal endocarditis. In: Kaye D, ed., *Infective Endocarditis*, 2nd edn. (Raven: New York, 1992) 209–29.

50. Stinson EB. Surgical treatment of infective endocarditis. *Prog Cardiovasc Dis* (1979) **22**: 145–68.

51. Richardson JV, Karp RB, Kirklin JW et al. Treatment of infective endocarditis: a 10 year comparative analysis. *Circulation* (1978) **58**: 589–97.

52. Kay PH, Oldershaw PJ, Dawkins K et al. The results of surgery for active endocarditis of the native aortic valve. *J Cardiovasc Surg* (1984) **25**:321–7.

53. Nelson RJ, Harley DP, French WJ et al. Favorable 10 year experience with valve procedures for active infective endocarditis. *J Thorac Cardiovasc Surg* (1984) **87**:493–502.

54. Jault F, Gandjbakhck I, Chastre JC et al. Prosthetic valve endocarditis with abscess: surgical management and long term results. *J Thorac Cardiovasc Surg* (1993) **105**:1106–13.

55. Taylor KM. Improved outcome for seriously ill open heart surgery patients: focus on reoperation and endocarditis. *Heart Lung Transplantation* (1993) **12**:S14–S18.

56. Pupello DF, Bessone LN, Hiro SP et al. Bioprosthetic valve longevity in the elderly: an 18-year longitudinal study. *Ann Thorac Surg* (1995) **60**:S270–S275.

57. Dajani AS, Taubert KA, Wilson W et al. Prevention of bacterial endocarditis. Recommendations by the American Heart Association. *JAMA* (1997) **277**:1794–1801.

27

Peripheral vascular disease
John A Spittell Jr

Introduction

Peripheral vascular disorders are common causes of significant morbidity in the octogenarian. The principal problems caused by the peripheral vascular disease(s) are pain in the extremities or digits, edema, and/or ulceration in the extremities or digits. Since the medical history may not be straightforward and/or difficult to elicit in the elderly, the clinical approach to peripheral vascular disorders in the elderly often is based more heavily on physical findings than on the historical details and this will be the format of this chapter. Furthermore, even when peripheral vascular disorders are asymptomatic, valuable therapeutic or prophylactic opportunities may be missed if they are not detected or recognized on physical exam.

Pain in the extremities or digits: occlusive peripheral arterial disease

The most common cause of occlusive peripheral arterial disease is arteriosclerosis obliterans. Arteriosclerosis obliterans is seen predominantly in men after the age of 60; from that age on, the prevalence in women increases, particularly when the risk factors of smoking and diabetes mellitus are present, so that arteriosclerosis obliterans in octogenarians is common in both sexes.[1]

The hallmark of symptomatic occlusive peripheral arterial disease is pain with walking but the octogenarian may consider it unimportant and not mention it unless specifically asked about it. Developing a classic story of intermittent claudication—lower extremity discomfort with walking and relief with standing still—is frequently difficult for several reasons. First, the elderly patient may not have the interest or need to walk far enough to produce intermittent claudication. Secondly, because atherosclerosis is the usual cause of occlusive peripheral arterial disease in the elderly patient, coronary artery disease is a common comorbid condition and if the patient has angina pectoris, it may limit walking to a level beneath the threshold for the intermittent claudication to occur. Thirdly, in persons of advanced age osteoarthritis of the knees and hips and/or spinal stenosis, when present, may limit walking. Fortunately, the diagnosis of occlusive peripheral arterial disease is not difficult if the extremities are carefully examined. It is useful to have some method of grading each of the arterial pulses (e.g. 0—pulse is absent, 4—pulse present and normal, 2—pulse present but reduced) in both the upper and lower extremities.

In the lower extremity the pulsations of the femoral artery in the groin and in the lower medial thigh (a common location for femoropopliteal aneurysm in elderly men), the popliteal artery, the dorsal pedis and posterior tibial artery should be evaluated. While one or both dorsalis pedis arteries may be congenitally absent in about 12% of persons, the posterior tibial artery is virtually never absent congenitally, so absence of the posterior tibial pulse is one of the best noninvasive indicators of occlusive arterial disease upstream.[2]

Occlusive arterial disease in the upper extremities, while less common than in the lower extremities, is not rare, particularly in the elderly. In addition to evaluating the radial and ulnar artery pulsations, their patency and the circulation in the hand can be readily confirmed by the Allen test (Figure 27.1). Another useful maneuver is palpation of both radial arteries to check for their pulsations being simultaneous; a delay in one or the other indicates subclavian artery occlusion on the ipsilateral side or innominate artery occlusion on the right; atherosclerotic occlusion of these branches of the aortic arch is common in smokers, while inflammatory occlusion may be seen in giant cell (cranial arteritis; temporal arteritis) arteritis, an arteritis seen only in the elderly.[3] Detection of subclavian or innominate artery occlusion can be an important finding in the patient with severe angina pectoris due to coronary disease since a favorite vessel for coronary artery bypass surgery is the internal mammary artery, a branch of the subclavian artery. Furthermore, in the patient who has had an internal mammary to left anterior descending bypass procedure to relieve angina, a recurrence of the angina may be due to development of occlusion of the subclavian artery rather than occlusion of the graft, and may be amenable to percutaneous angioplasty.[4]

Auscultation over peripheral arteries—the carotids, subclavians, abdominal aorta, the renal arteries and the femoral artery in the groin—should be a part of the vascular examination of the octogenarian. The presence of a bruit usually indicates turbulence of flow due to stenosis upstream; usually bruits are systolic only, but at times a bruit will continue into diastole indicating a stenosis severe enough (in the range of 80% of the lumen) to produce a gradient and therefore flow in diastole.

When occlusive arterial disease is present in the lower extremities, a rough estimate of the degree of ischemia can be obtained in the office or at the bedside by performance of elevation-dependency tests. Observing the skin color of the soles of the feet with the extremity raised 60° above the level for 1 minute will identify significant occlusive arterial disease if any pallor of the skin develops. By then observing the return of skin color to the skin of the foot and the filling of the superficial veins with dependency of the feet, the adequacy of circulation to the foot can be confirmed (Table 27.1).

Noninvasive testing using a hand-held Doppler and a standard blood pressure cuff can be used to take systolic blood pressures at the brachial and ankle levels in the supine position. Normally the ankle systolic pressure exceeds that at the brachial level, but with occlusive arterial disease in the lower extremity the ankle systolic pressure is lower than the brachial.

Even minor trauma to an ischemic limb can result in ischemic ulceration (Figure 27.2), which is characteristically extremely painful. The four common types of leg and foot ulcers have distinctive features that allow for differentiation on clinical features in most cases (Table 27.2). Because trauma can lead to poor or nonhealing ischemic ulceration, the patient with occlusive peripheral arterial disease should be instructed in proper foot care and protection of the ischemic limb from all types of trauma—mechanical, chemical and thermal. Proper footwear is essential and nail trimming is best carried out by a podiatrist or a trained

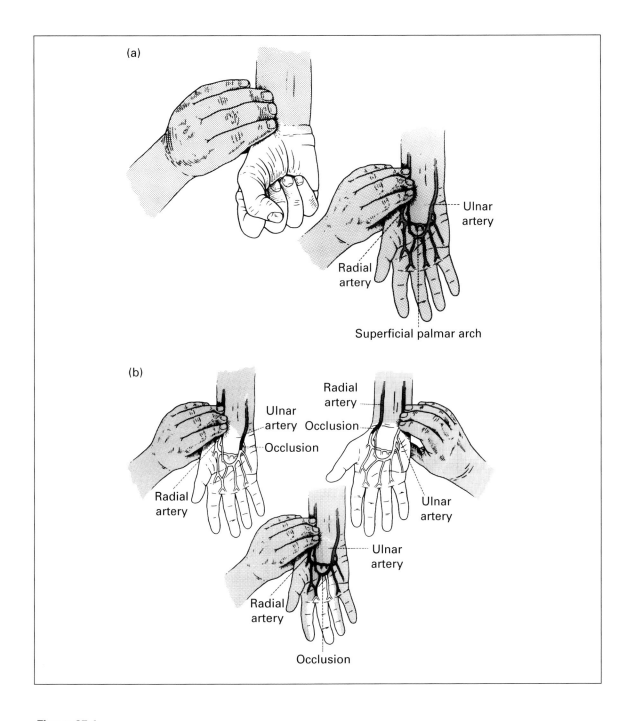

Figure 27.1
The Allen test. (a) Normal (negative) result, indicating patency of ulnar artery and superficial palmar arch. (b) Abnormal (positive) results due to occlusion of ulnar artery (left), radial artery (right), and superficial palmar arch (center). (Reproduced from Spittell[16] with permission from the Mayo Clinic)

Elevation pallor* grade	Appearance time (s)
0	No pallor in 60
1	Definite pallor in 60
2	Definite pallor in <60
3	Definite pallor in <30
4	Pallor on level

Dependency (time to:) Ischemia	Color return (s)	Venous filling (s)
None	10	15
Moderate	15–20	20–30
Severe	>40	>40

*Elevation of extremity at angle of 60° above level.
From Spittell[1] with permission.

Table 27.1
Elevation-dependency testing

	Arterial ischemic	Venous stasis	Neurotrophic	Arteriolar ischemic
Pain	+	+ with infection	0	+
Location	Toes, heel, foot	Medial leg	Weight bearing part of limb	Lateral and posterior or distal leg
Skin	Normal/atrophic	Stasis pigment	Callus	Normal/livedo
Ulcer margin	Discrete	Shaggy	Discrete	Serpiginous
Ulcer base	Pale, eschar	Healthy	Varies	Pale, eschar

Table 27.2
Differential features of common leg ulcers

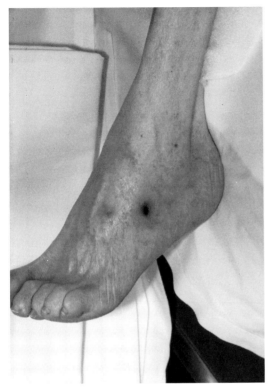

Figure 27.2
Ischemic ulceration on dorsum of foot produced by strap of lady's shoe.

should be avoided because of their tendency to cause cutaneous vasoconstriction. Likewise, if the patient has migraine, the ergot preparations should be avoided. Modifiable risk factors for atherosclerosis should be managed to try to lessen progression of the atherosclerosis.

For the patient with intermittent claudication there are three therapeutic options: a walking program; pharmacological therapy; and restoration of pulsatile flow. Natural history data are useful in deciding about the management of atherosclerotic occlusive arterial disease. In the nondiabetic person whose only complaint is intermittent claudication, the outlook for limb survival is rather favorable; only about 5% of such patients will lose a limb in the ensuing 5 years and about half of such patients will be able to walk as far or farther in 5 years.[5] Thus, the restoration of pulsatile flow for the nondiabetic person whose only symptom is intermittent claudication is elective, that is it is available for the patient who feels that his or her claudication is disabling. If restoration of pulsatile flow is not elected, a regular walking program—35 minutes a day, 5 days per week—should be followed and may, over a few months, as much as double the walking distance.[6] The addition of pentoxifylline 400 mg three times daily with meals may provide additional symptomatic relief.

For the patient with an ischemic ulcer or ischemic rest pain and for the diabetic person with symptomatic occlusive arterial disease, the prognosis for limb loss is unfavorable[7,8] and justifies an aggressive approach to restoring pulsatile flow to the ischemic extremity(ies) if possible.

When restoration of pulsatile flow is planned, careful consideration of comorbid conditions (coronary disease in particular) that may influence anesthetic and surgical risk is necessary. After the patient is deemed a

health-care professional rather than by the octogenarian (or spouse).

Decisions about management of peripheral occlusive arterial disease in the octogenarian or older patient are based on the same principles used in younger patients. Regardless of severity of the occlusive arterial disease, all patients should stop tobacco and avoid other things that may cause vasoconstriction, in addition to exercising fastidious foot care. For the treatment of coronary artery disease and hypertension, if feasible, beta-blocking agents

suitable risk for restoration of pulsatile flow, an arteriogram is needed to plan the appropriate procedure: interventional percutaneous procedure or vascular surgery. Until this point, arteriography is not necessary since the diagnosis can be made on physical examination and confirmed by noninvasive study (ankle–brachial systolic pressure). If the patient is allergic to contrast media or has renal failure, magnetic resonance (MR) angiography (Figure 27.3) can provide images of excellent quality.

Acute peripheral arterial occlusion can be embolic or thrombotic, but whatever the cause, can be dramatic with the 5 Ps—pain, pallor, paralysis, paresthesia, pulseless—or in the elderly can be much more subtle in onset with the patient or health-care provider merely commenting on the cold extremity, a painful digit or extremity, or pain in the extremity with walking. The initial management is heparinization while the general and cardiac status are being evaluated. The involved ischemic part should be protected from trauma, heat and cold and never be elevated. Arteriography is required to localize the occlusion and either thrombolytic therapy or thromboembolectomy is the treatment of choice. If the arterial occlusion is deemed to be embolic, the source—cardiac or proximal arterial aneurysm or atherosclerotic plaque—should be sought and if it cannot be removed, long-term oral anticoagulant therapy to prevent further embolization should be instituted if there is no contraindication to it. Any residual occlusive disease should be managed like other chronic occlusive peripheral arterial disease.

Aneurysmal disease[9]

In the octogenarian and even older persons, aneurysms of the aorta and peripheral arteries are atherosclerotic in origin except for aneurysms of the common femoral artery which are often false aneurysms occurring after transfemoral interventional procedures or aortofemoral bypass grafts. Infection may result in a mycotic aneurysm, usually in the aorta or visceral arteries and less often in extremity arteries.

The rate of enlargement of aneurysms is variable, but progressive enlargement may lead to pressure on surrounding structures or to rupture. Enlargement, coupled with slowing of flow within the aneurysm, contributes to the formation of laminated clot within the aneurysm creating the potential source for thromboembolic complications. Infection of an established aneurysm is the least common complication of aneurysms.

The size of an aneurysm generally influ-

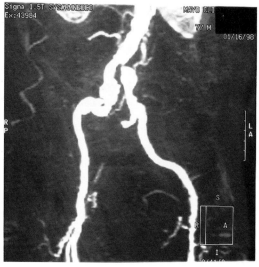

Figure 27.3
Iliac artery occlusion and aneurysms demonstrated by magnetic resonance angiography.

ences the frequency of complications and symptoms. Since aneurysms are so often asymptomatic, careful evaluation of the abdominal aortic pulsation and of the femoral and popliteal arteries, particularly in elderly men, is necessary if these potentially serious lesions are to be detected before complications occur. Thoracic aortic aneurysms are usually asymptomatic until complications—pressure on surrounding structures or chest pain—occur. Usually first noted on chest roentgenogram, they are best further evaluated and followed by CT scan. When suspected, aneurysms of the abdominal aorta and femoral and popliteal arteries can be confirmed by ultrasound. If aneurysm of the iliac artery is suspected from symptoms such as unexplained groin pain or proximal occlusion of an extremity vein, CT scan with contrast enhancement or MR angiography (Figure 27.3) can be used to confirm the diagnosis.

In good risk patients, the indications for surgical treatment of thoracic aortic aneurysms are an aneurysm 6.0 cm in diameter, an aneurysm enlarging under observation (particularly if the patient is hypertensive) or an aneurysm that is symptomatic. If the patient is not an acceptable anesthetic or surgical risk, careful control of hypertension is important, ideally with a beta-blocking drug.

The complications of abdominal aortic aneurysms in order of frequency are rupture, thromboembolism (atheroembolism) and pressure on surrounding structures, mainly the adjacent ureters. Rupture is rare in aneurysms less than 4.0 cm in diameter but the risk of rupture becomes significant when an aneurysm reaches 5.0 cm in diameter. Atheroembolism which presents with livedo reticularis of the lower extremities, blue toes, (Figure 27.4) hypertension and renal insufficiency may be either spontaneous or precipitated by the institution of anticoagulant therapy; it is best

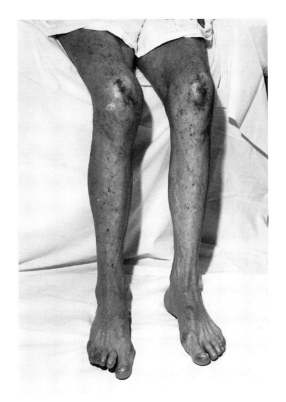

Figure 27.4
Livedo reticularis and blue toes due to atheroembolism (From Spittell[17] with permission).

treated by resection of the aneurysm to prevent progressive renal failure. Asymptomatic abdominal aortic aneurysms larger than 4.5 cm in diameter in good risk patients are best resected. In the poor risk patient with an abdominal aortic aneurysm 5.0 cm in diameter or larger, a percutaneous placement of a stented graft is an option, particularly for enlarging or symptomatic aneurysms.[10]

Iliac artery aneurysms, though less frequent than abdominal aortic aneurysms, are seen most often in men older than 60. Because they may rupture or cause obstructive uropathy, elective surgical resection with graft replacement is advisable in good risk patients.

Aneurysms of the femoral artery are most often atherosclerotic in origin but the frequency with which the femoral artery is used for access for diagnostic and interventional procedures has increased the incidence of false aneurysms. Likewise, the usual anastomoses of aortofemoral grafts have increased the occurrence of false aneurysms of the femoral artery in the groin. These aneurysms are easy to diagnose on physical examination and if confirmation is needed, ultrasound is excellent. Femoral aneurysms may cause obstruction of the companion vein or be the source of distal emboli from the laminated thrombus in the aneurysm; femoral artery aneurysms rarely rupture.

Popliteal artery aneurysms are seen almost exclusively in men, usually more than 60 years of age. These aneurysms may occur in three sites: in the lower medial thigh where the superficial artery exits the adductor canal; at the level of the knee joint in the popliteal space; and/or in the upper calf at the level of the trifurcation of the popliteal artery. Popliteal artery aneurysms are frequently bilateral. The most frequent complication is thromboembolic, but because of the confined space behind the knee, popliteal aneurysms can obstruct the popliteal vein and cause edema of the left leg. Popliteal artery aneurysms rupture rarely. Ideally popliteal aneurysms and femoral artery aneurysms should be resected and arterial continuity restored before complications occur.

Aneurysms of upper extremity arteries are rare; they are usually atherosclerotic. Complications are principally thromboembolic.

Ulceration in the extremity[11,12]

As indicated earlier, most ulcerations of the lower extremity are one of four common types (Table 27.2). Attention to the characteristics listed in the Table usually allows differentiation of the type or identifies the ulceration as a less common type. In the elderly, neoplastic lesions have to be kept in mind and, with any suspicion of neoplasm, should be biopsied promptly.

For ischemic ulceration due to occlusive arterial disease (Figure 27.5), restoration of pulsatile flow if at all possible, is indicated.

For venous stasis ulcerations (Figure 27.6), after healing, regular use of adequate (30–40 mmHg compression) elastic support (if no occlusive arterial disease coexists) to control the elevated ambulatory venous pressure is indicated. If occlusive arterial disease coexists, lighter-weight elastic support hose (20–30 mmHg compression at the ankle) should be used.

For the patient with neurotrophic ulceration (Figure 27.7) (usually a diabetic with diabetic neuropathy) local removal of the callus and rest are indicated; when the ulceration has healed, the footwear should be modified to have the patient bear weight on a different part of the foot.

The ulcerations due to arteriolar disease (Figure 27.8), being ischemic, are extremely painful. As noted in Table 27.2, these ulcerations occur on the lateral and/or posterior distal leg. These are seen in persons with long-standing rather benign hypertension or connective tissue disorders. Since the ischemia is in the skin, vasodilation is needed to effect healing. In many patients, bed rest, saline compresses for 30 minutes four to six times a day, with a sterile dry dressing between and an alpha-adrenergic blocking agent will relieve

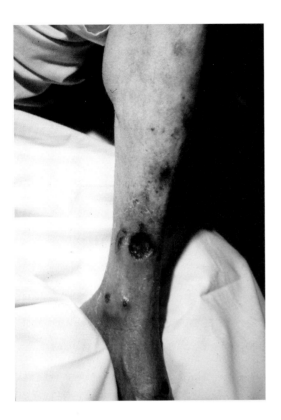

Figure 27.5
Ischemic ulcerations of the leg.

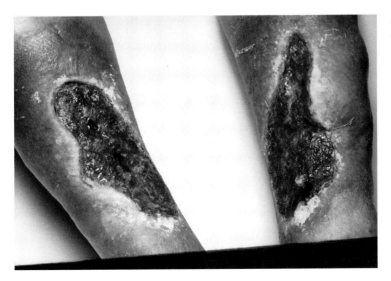

Figure 27.6
Bilateral venous stasis ulcerations.

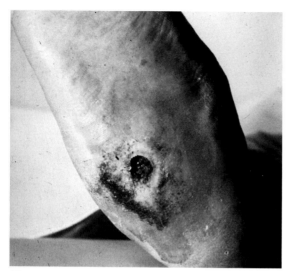

Figure 27.7
Neurotrophic ulceration of sole of foot.

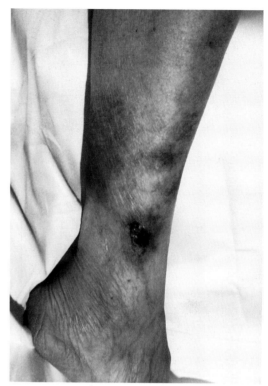

Figure 27.8
Arteriolar (hypertensive ischemic) ulcer.

the pain and promote healing. If the systemic vasodilation from the alpha-blocker does not seem adequate, then ipsilateral lumbar sympathectomy will provide vasodilation. When these ulcerations are larger than about 2 cm, a skin graft may be needed after the ulcer is cleaned up and has a base that appears healthy.

Edema of the lower extremities[13]

Swelling of the lower extremities is one of the most common problems of the elderly. It often raises concerns about cardiac disease by patients and/or relatives and as a result is usually not disregarded by them.

Basic to correct diagnosis and appropriate management is the differentiation of edema due to a systemic cause (cardiac, renal, hepatic, medication side-effect, orthostasis or nutritional) from edema due to a regional problem (venous, lymphatic or orthostatic).

Edema of systemic origin is bilateral and generally symmetrical. Even if it is long-standing, it pits readily and the overlying skin is of normal texture. Cardiac findings or abnormalities of the chest X-ray or of laboratory tests identify cardiac, renal, hepatic and nutritional types of leg edema. In the condition lipedema (symmetrical fat legs), ortho-

| Antidepressants |
| Antihypertensives |
| Anti-inflammatory drugs |
| Hormones |

Table 27.3
Drugs that may cause or aggravate edema

static edema is common since fat does not support as well as muscle.

Commonly overlooked is edema that is a side-effect of one or more medications (Table 27.3) that the patient is taking.

Management of the systemic forms of edema is basically that of the cause. In the patient with lipedema weight control, avoidance of salt and light-weight support hose (heavy support hose are not tolerated by these

persons) is usually an adequate management program.

Turning to regional edema, the differentiation is readily made on physical examination in most cases (Table 27.4).

Acute thrombosis of the deep veins of the lower extremity results in edema if the popliteal vein or more proximal deep veins are involved. In addition to the edema, the patient may complain of pain in the extremity. On physical examination the edema is soft, pits readily, and the extremity has a livid color with increased superficial venous pattern; palpation of the calf, popliteal space, Hunters canal in the thigh and of the groin may elicit pain. When suspected, deep vein thrombosis should be confirmed by an objective test, preferably duplex ultrasound since it is non-invasive, provides an image and does not depend only on physiological findings.[14] Therapy for acute deep vein thrombosis is anticoagulant therapy, if there are no contraindications to it. Initially intravenous heparin is the treatment of choice to raise the activated thromboplastin time to twice the control; when heparin is

	Venous	*Lymphatic*	*Lipedema*
Bilateral	Occasional	±	+
Symmetrical	Rarely	0	+
Stasis pigment	+	0	0
Thickened skin	0	+	0
Foot involved	+	+	0
Toes involved	0	+	0

Table 27.4
Differential features of regional types of edema

being used, a baseline prothrombin time and a platelet count and daily platelet counts during heparin therapy should be obtained. If the platelet count falls with heparin therapy, heparin should be discontinued to avoid the complications of heparin-induced thrombocytopenia.[15] The occurrence of heparin thrombocytopenia is one of the reasons to begin oral anticoagulant therapy at the same time as heparin is started. If the patient is taking a normal diet and the baseline prothrombin is normal, warfarin sodium can be administered in an initial dose of ×2.5–5 mg per day for 2 days and then an adjustment of the dose according to the prothrombin time. Heparin therapy can be discontinued after 4–5 days of warfarin therapy if the prothrombin time has been raised to the therapeutic range of INR 2.0–3.0. Oral anticoagulant therapy should be continued for at least 3 months and preferably 6 months. When the patient becomes ambulatory, good elastic support of the leg with Ace bandage or an elastic stocking with 30–40 mmHg compression at the ankle should be worn to control dependent edema and prevent the complications of postphlebitic deep venous insufficiency.

Recurrence of deep venous thrombosis in an elderly person during adequate oral anticoagulant therapy usually indicates an underlying disorder such as myeloproliferative disorders, a connective tissue disease or a neoplasm. If the patient has not been using adequate elastic support, edema due to postphlebitic deep venous insufficiency may be confused with recurrent venous thrombosis. If clinical findings and duplex ultrasound do not distinguish between these two conditions, contrast venography may be needed.

Chronic deep venous insufficiency, uncontrolled by adequate elastic support, results in dependent edema and venous stasis changes— stasis pigmentation, stasis dermatitis, lipo-

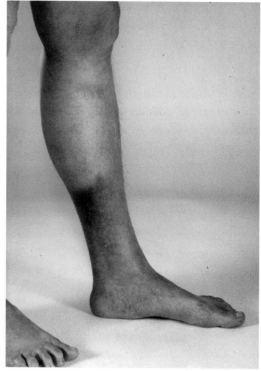

Figure 27.9
Chronic indurated cellulitis (lipodermatosclerosis) due to chronic deep venous insufficiency. (From Miller[18] with permission)

dermatosclerosis ('chronic indurated cellulitis'), and stasis ulceration—in the distal medial portion of the leg. The complication 'chronic indurated cellulitis' (Figure 27.9) is a tender reddened area of subcutaneous induration in the medial distal leg with chronic deep venous insufficiency; this complication is commonly misinterpreted as infectious but its treatment is adequate support (foam pad under Ace bandages) to control the elevated ambulatory venous pressure rather than antibiotics. Venous stasis ulceration has already been discussed.

Lipedema is the term used to describe the fatty deposition seen in some women (much more often than in men). While the patient may complain of edema, it is orthostatic in type, related to the poor support that fatty tissue provides. The diagnosis of lipedema is easy on inspection—symmetrical heavy legs with feet, and toes and skin appearing normal. Unfortunately, many persons tend to gain weight as they age and the person with lipedema has progressively larger lower extremities. Persons with lipedema tolerate elastic support poorly so elevation, weight control and salt restriction are the basic features of management.

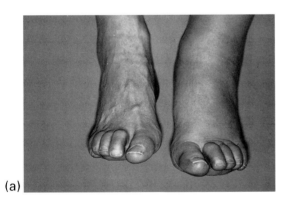

(a)

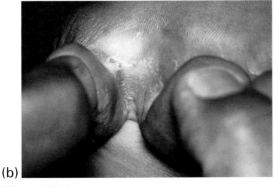

(b)

Figure 27.10
(a) Lymphedema of left foot due to recurrent lymphangitis and cellulitis from (b) chronic dermatophytosis. (Used from ACCSAP 1997–98, ACCSAP CD ROM Program, Chapter 8, Figure 54A & 54B with permission)

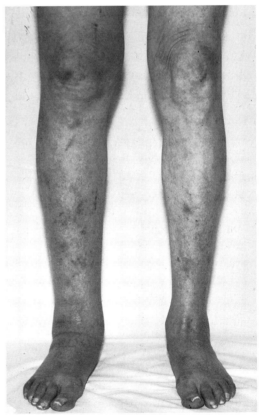

Figure 27.11
Obstructive lymphedema of right lower extremity in an elderly man with prostate cancer.

367

Lymphedema is probably the least recognized and understood type of regional edema. Idiopathic types of lymphedema have their onset before the age of 40 so are not a consideration in the octogenarian unless the problem has been life-long. The secondary types of lymphedema are 'acquired' as a result of surgical removal of nodes, damage by radiation, fibrosis from recurrent infection or involvement by neoplasm. Lymphedema as a result of surgery or radiation is an easy historical or record review diagnosis. The most common type of secondary lymphedema results from recurring lymphangitis and cellulitis secondary to dermatophytosis (Figure 27.10). Obstructive lymphedema due to neoplasm (Figure 27.11) is most often seen in persons with lymphoma or a pelvic neoplasm (ovarian or uterine in women, prostate in men). Whatever the cause, lymphedema is painless, unaccompanied by pigmentation of the skin, does not recede overnight, and involves the digits. On examination lymphedema is firm, pits poorly and the skin is thickened. The management of lymphedema includes heavy duty elastic support (40–50 mmHg compression at the ankle), intermittent pumping to reduce the edema, and measures directed at the cause.

References

1. Spittell JA Jr. Peripheral arterial disease, *Dis Mon* (1994) **40**:653–700.
2. Criqui MH, Fronek A, Klauber MR et al. The sensitivity, specificity, and predictive value of traditional clinical evaluation of peripheral arterial disease: results from noninvasive testing in a defined population. *Circulation* (1985) **71**:516–22.
3. Klein RG, Hunder GG, Stanson AW et al. Large artery involvement in giant cell (temporal) arteritis. *Ann Intern Med* (1975) **83**: 806–12.
4. Valentine RJ, Fry RE, Wheelan KR et al. Coronary-subclavian steal from reversed flow in an internal mammary artery used for coronary bypass. *Am J Cardiol* (1987) **59**:719–20.
5. McDaniel MD, Cronenwett JL. Basic data related to the natural history of intermittent claudication. *Ann Vasc Surg* (1989) **3**:273–7.
6. Ernst EEW, Matrai A. Exercise for intermittent claudication. *Cardiology Board Review* (1988) **5**:82–90.
7. Juergens JL, Barker NW, Hines EA Jr. Arteriosclerosis obliterans and review of 520 cases with special reference to pathogenic and prognostic factors. *Circulation* (1960) **21**:188–95.
8. Schadt DC, Hines EA Jr, Juergens JL et al. Chronic atherosclerotic occlusion of the femoral artery. *JAMA* (1961) **175**: 937–40.
9. Spittell JA Jr. Clinical aspects of aneurysmal disease. *Curr Prob Cardiol* (1980) **5**:6–36.
10. Marin ML, Veith EJ. Transfemoral repair of abdominal aortic aneurysm. *N Engl J Med* (1994) **331**:1751.
11. Spittell JA Jr. Diagnosis and management of leg ulcer. *Geriatrics* (1983) **38**:57–65.
12. Roenigk HH Jr, Young JR. Leg ulcers. In Young JR, Olin JW, Bartholomew JR, eds, *Peripheral Vascular Diseases* (Mosby: St Louis, 1996) 637–68.
13. Ruschhaupt WF, Fernandez BB Jr. The swollen limb. In Young JR, Olin JW, Bartholomew JR, eds, *Peripheral Vascular Diseases* (Mosby: St Louis, 1996) 669–79.
14. White RH, McGahan JP, Daschbach MM, Hartling RP. Diagnosis of deep-vein thrombosis using duplex ultrasound. *Ann Intern Med* (1989) **111**:297–304.
15. Warkentin TE, Kelton JG. A 14-year study of heparin-induced thrombocytopenia. *Am J Med* (1996) **101**:502–7.
16. Spittell JA Jr. Occlusive peripheral arterial disease: guidelines for office management. *Postgrad Med* (1982) **71**:137–51.
17. Spittell JA. Vasospastic disorders. *Cardiovasc Clin* (1983) **13**:75–88.
18. Miller WL. Chronic venous insufficiency. *Cardiovasc Clin* (1992) **22**:67–80.

28

End-of-life interventions and decisions for frail older adults

Jeff D Williamson and Walter H Ettinger, Jr

Introduction

Medical care of frail older persons with multiple chronic diseases involves decisions that weigh the risks and benefits of therapeutic modalities in patients with limited life expectancy. Many therapeutic alternatives known to enhance or improve health status, physical function, and productivity in younger people or healthy older people may adversely impact these areas for frail older people while also producing economic hardship. For all individuals and diseases, medical decisions near the end of life should seek to provide comfort and dignity while maximizing an individual's ability to interact with their family and society. Success in this endeavor is predicated upon clinical expertise, compassion for the patient and a willingness to incorporate the advice of family members, the patient and a variety of individuals with expertise in systems of care for frail older people.

Unfortunately, end-of-life care for cardiovascular diseases has not received the explicit attention that other disease entities, such as cancer and dementia, have received. Limitations in the therapeutic armamentarium for these latter diseases, at any age, have fostered explicit discussions about futility and appropriate approaches to care at the end of life. However, the spectrum of potentially successful interventions and treatments for cardiovascular disease for older adults has rapidly expanded over the past three decades. This success in treating cardiovascular disease has created more difficulty in estimating the impact of many interventions on the quality of life of older people.

The purpose of this chapter is to provide a framework for reaching decisions regarding the treatment and care of older people with cardiovascular disease who are frail and have a limited life expectancy. In addition to clinical endpoints, other important variables such as health-related quality of life and physical and cognitive function will be addressed. Incorporation of these important measures can support development and implementation of a plan of care that satisfies both the patient's and the physician's goals, and introduce new dimensions to caring for older people with limited life expectancy.

Prevalence of cardiovascular disease in patients near the end of life

In addition to greater numbers of individuals living beyond the age of 65, the number of people surviving into the upper age ranges beyond 85 years is rapidly growing. While the

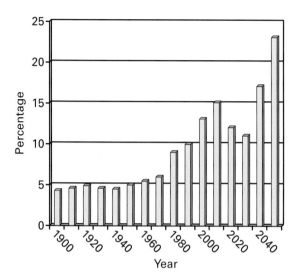

Figure 28.1
The 85 year old and older population as a percentage of the 65 year old and older population: 1900–2050. (From Spencer.[2])

number of people 65 and older will increase to 64.3 million in the year 2030, it is the oldest old, or those over the age of 85, who will be the most rapidly growing segment of the elderly population. This group of individuals, age 85 and older, has risen 281% from just over 500 000 individuals in 1950 to 2.2 million in 1990.[1] In 1990, 43% of individuals greater than the age of 65 were also in the group of individuals older than the age of 75. It is predicted that by the year 2000, nearly 48% of older individuals beyond the age of 65 will also be older than 75.[2] By the year 2050 the group of individuals over the age of 85 will constitute one-fifth of the elderly, a 10% increase over today.[3] Figure 28.1 shows the population aged 85 and over as a percentage of all those individuals older than 65 from 1900–2050.

Data from the National Center for Health Statistics in 1990 has shown that 353 out of every 1000 persons over the age of 75 have been diagnosed by a doctor as having heart disease, making this the fourth most common chronic condition in this age group.[4] Heart disease leads all conditions as a predictor of mortality and health-care use by the elderly. It is the leading diagnosis for short-stay hospital visits for people older than 65.[5] Heart disease causes more than 7000 deaths per 100 000 individuals over age 85, by far the leading cause of death in individuals this age. Cancer trails far behind with just over 1600 deaths per 100 000 individuals in this age group.[6] Therefore, treatment of individuals with cardiovascular disease and limited life expectancy will be an increasingly common situation faced by physicians.

The economic impact of cardiovascular disease is also significantly greater for individuals with advanced age, comorbid conditions, and high risk for dependency. In 1987, hospital discharge rates per 1000 people for those over the age of 85 were 90% higher than for those people age 65–74. In addition, the average hospital stay for age 65–74 was 8.2 days compared with 9.5 days for the age over 85 group.[7] Although the advent of managed care has shortened length of stay for the majority of individuals aged over 65, differences in hospital length of stay will probably remain.

A significant factor in the cost of caring for the very old is the high burden of disability in this population. Data from the Women's Health and Aging Study,[8] a study of community-dwelling older women, have shown that 51% of women over the age of 85 have difficulty raising their arms over their head while only 29.6% of women in the 65–74 years age group reported this type of difficulty. Of women aged 85 and older, 40% reported difficulty getting in and out of a bed or chair without assistance while only 18% of women aged 65–74 reported similar difficulty. Of women over the age of 85, 24% reported difficulty using the telephone compared to only 14% of women in the age group 65–74 years and 44% of women reported difficulty shopping for personal medication compared to only 11% of those age 65–74.[8]

While the burden of disease and disability contributes to the complexity of care for frail older individuals, failure to coordinate the actions of multiple health professionals, including physicians, nurses, social workers, dietitians and rehabilitation experts result in increased utilization and cost of caring for frail older people near the end of life. Therefore, a major challenge for all physicians caring for older adults in the twenty-first century will be the development of more efficient and cost-effective approaches to managing the care of older people who are frail. The successful physician will be required to be familiar with such systems and able to work well as an integral part of systems caring for older people with complex medical and physical problems.

Characterization of individuals with cardiovascular disease and limited life expectancy

The presence of cardiovascular disease or any number of diseases in a person with advanced age is not alone sufficient to identify individuals with limited life expectancy. For example, myocardial infarction, even in the presence of other diseases such as arthritis and hypertension, is not sufficient to predict life expectancy or guide the care of an older individual. Of greater importance in identifying individuals who are frail and have a limited life expectancy is the ability to care for themselves

independently and to manage prescribed treatment regimens. Disability in old age is a strong marker for individuals at high risk for acute illness, recurrent hospitalization and death.[9–14] Therefore, the ability to quickly assess independence in daily activities is an important aspect in identifying those individuals critically in need of discussions about the approach to their care near the end of life. Physicians have been shown to have inaccurate impressions of the ability of the patients for whom they care to function independently.[15] Therefore, incorporating a standardized, screening test for functional status is an important component of cardiovascular care for individuals at advanced ages. Evaluation of functional disability is a useful complement and an important guide to treatment and management decisions and planning for services required for the care of individuals with limited life expectancy.

The Activities of Daily Living (ADL) scale is one of the original methods for measuring physical function in older adults.[16] It has gained wide use in clinical settings today because of its simplicity and its utility in accurately identifying individuals with significant functional impairment and a high risk of death.[17] The ADL scale focuses on five common tasks of daily life: bathing, dressing, toileting, the ability to rise from a bed or chair and the ability to feed oneself. An additional scale, the Instrumental Activities of Daily Living (IADL) scale focuses on tasks that are slightly more complex and require a higher level of physical and cognitive functioning. Individuals with deficits in these tasks are at high risk for poor compliance with cardiovascular disease treatment regimens and will require assistance. Items assessed in the IADL scale include the ability to follow a medication schedule, the ability to shop for personal items such as prescriptions, the ability to prepare foods and the ability to handle finances, among other tasks. Incorporating selected items (Table 28.1) from these two scales will greatly assist physicians in identifying those individuals with cardiovascular disease and limited life expectancy or difficulty with treatment compliance.

While the ADL and IADL scales are helpful in identifying individuals at risk for poor health outcomes and high use of health-care services, a critical facet of assessment is to determine cognitive function. Standardized tests for identifying persons with memory loss are readily available.[18] Tests of cognitive function identify those individuals who will require assistance with implementing treatment regimens. Table 28.2 shows a list of questions that are easily incorporated into a brief interview of any older patient. While more extensive testing is required for diagnostic purposes, answers to these questions provide a reasonable assessment of the impact of an individual's cognitive function on their ability to comply with a treatment regimen. Because individuals with dementing illness have limited life expectancy and difficulty complying with complex cardiovascular disease regimens, intensive interventions may not be medically indicated or desired by the patient and family. Even simple treatment regimens in persons unable to accurately answer the questions in Table 28.2 must be implemented using the care of family members, long-term care providers or home-health nursing. However, as will be discussed, tests of cognitive function are not to be used to determine an individual's ability to participate in decisions about their care. Their primary utility is identifying individuals who will require assistance complying with treatment and who have limited life expectancy due to dementing illness.

Arriving at decisions on intensity of treatment

One of the most difficult aspects of caring for older people with chronic diseases such as cardiovascular disease involves decisions about the level of intensity of treatment that should be provided to frail, dependent, and often cognitively impaired older adults. Complicating such decisions is the changing nature of health-care delivery and concerns over the growing cost of health care, particularly near the end of life.[7] While the involvement of physicians in the evaluation of resource use will probably lead to increased complexity and difficulty in caring for frail individuals, the primary role of physicians at the bedside is to use their expertise in clinical care to coordinate effective treatments and to provide comfort and dignity for all their patients.

The physician caring for frail patients is in an excellent position both to initiate discussions about care at the end of life, and also to ensure that individual rights are maximized. Table 28.3 lists key factors that should be considered when discussing the level of intensity

Do you have difficulty:
  Walking across the room?
  Getting out of a bed or chair?
  Using or getting to and from the toilet?
  Using the telephone?
  Obtaining transportation to the doctor?
  Shopping for medications?
  Remembering to take medications?
  Cooking your own meals?

Table 28.1
Brief questionnaire for identifying clinically important functional decrements.

| PATIENT'S NAME: _____ | | DATE _____ |
| EXAMINER: _____ | | |

MAX SCORE	SCORE	ORIENTATION
5		What is the (year) (season) (date) (month) (day)
5		Where are we: (state) (county) (city) (hospital) (your home street address)
3		Name three objects (ball, flag, tree) and ask patient to repeat them now and in 5 minutes.
5		Please spell the word 'world' backwards.
3		Ask for the three objects repeated above.
Total Score	/21	

Table 28.2
Short cognitive assessment tool

of treatment to be provided to older people near the end of life. When discussing level of treatment intensity, an important challenge for physicians is the preservation of autonomy and the rights of the patient. Discussions about the intensity of therapy must avoid paternalism. It is helpful for patients, their families and their physicians to systematically review formal categories that outline the various options and levels of intensity in the treatment of cardiovascular disease. The results of such discussions, while often eliminating or reducing the use of many invasive, high risk and expensive procedures, broadens the approach to care that may allow a patient near the end of life to die at home as opposed to using the more resource-intensive and expensive inpatient hospital services.

Determining whether an older person has the capacity to make decisions about the intensity of treatment near the end of life is often discussed in terms of 'competence.' This is a legal term that often confuses the issue. Perhaps a better term is that of 'decision-making capacity.'[19] In terms of medical care, competence or decision-making capacity must be based on the specific decision at hand. In other words, individuals who may not be competent to execute a new last will and testament due to dementia or other cognitive deficits may nevertheless clearly have the decision-making capacity to determine the level of intensity of therapy they desire for a particular acute or chronic illness. There is no standardized test that determines the capacity of an individual to make such a decision. Scores on standardized tests of cognitive function have been

Informed consent requires:
- The communication of relevant, understandable, and unbiased information about the potential risks and benefits of a given intervention.
- Freedom from coercion and other factors that might unduly influence a decision
- The ability to:
  Understand the information.
  Weigh the risks and benefits.
  Make a reasoned decision based on the given information and on individual values and preferences.

Decision making should be done prospectively:
- Written documentation, via an advance directive or other format, is critical.
- Prospective decision-making should be discussed whenever feasible.
- Specificity regarding all possible medical interventions in an advance directive is often impractical. More general statements about various levels of intensity of care and common treatment decisions may be more appropriate.

Decision-making capacity relates to the ability to make specific decisions:
- Dementia and other causes of cognitive impairment do not necessarily render frail patients incapable of making decisions regarding their care.
- Legal competence (or incompetence) is not the equivalent of being incapable of participating in care decisions.

There is no standardized test to determine if frail patients are capable of making specific decisions about their care:
- Scores on standard mental function tests do not predict a patient's ability to participate in care decisions.

A variety of factors, some of which fluctuate over time and are reversible, can have an important influence on the ability to make decisions. Examples include:
- Delirium and other reversible acute confusional states
- Depression
- Pain
- Medication side-effects
- Perceived quality of life
- Perceived wishes of family and other loved ones
- Economic considerations

When a patient is found to be incapable of making a particular decision:
- His/her prior expressed wishes relevant to the decision should be taken into account whenever they are known.
- A surrogate or proxy decision maker, preferably assigned by the patient and who is known to be acting in the best interests of the patient, should be consulted.

Adapted from Ouslander et al.[19]

Table 28.3
Key principles in discussing level of treatment intensity for older adults near the end of life

shown not to be predictive of decision-making capacity and should never be used in this manner. Therefore, individuals with dementia are not automatically incapable of participating in decisions about the intensity of their care and an attempt to elicit the opinions of these patients should always be made.[20] Medical conditions which might limit the clarity of thought needed to arrive at a decision about intensity of care near the end of life should also be treated. Conditions such as delirium, pain, depression and medication side-effects must be adequately treated before the physician undertakes discussions about the intensity of care for chronic cardiovascular disease. In most situations, the primary-care physician is capable of determining the appropriateness of a patient's ability to participate in decisions about their health care. When there is disagreement about the ability of a patient to participate in such a process, then the expertise of another physician, such as a psychiatrist, may be helpful. However, input from a psychiatrist is usually unnecessary.

For those patients who have been determined to be unable to participate in decisions about the intensity of care near the end of life, a surrogate decision-maker must be identified. In situations where there is no advanced directive for a surrogate decision-maker, then close family and friends are the obvious source of guidance. Although the legal role of such individuals has not fully been established, such individuals are essential to decisions about the intensity of therapy near the end of life.

Table 28.4 lists specific examples of the level of intensity of cardiovascular care that practitioners should discuss with patients and/or their surrogate health-care decision-makers. Discussions regarding these levels are important in all patients of advanced age but are particularly important in those individuals for whom the physician has already identified

significant functional and/or cognitive deficits. It is most important that discussions about the level of care desired by a patient be completed in advance of a crisis such as an acute cardiovascular illness superimposed on chronic cardiovascular disease and disability. In addition, all care givers (family members, home health, long-term care providers) for patients with cardiovascular disease and limited life expectancy should have readily available to them the simple documentation of discussions that give guidance for treatment decisions should an acute illness or crisis arise.

It is important to briefly document discussions about intensity of care desired and the circumstances surrounding these discussions. It is also important that, although specific directives are documented, latitude is allowed so that the patient's comfort and dignity takes precedence over limitations in the setting of the care given or even the type of care given.

A.	Care in intensive care unit (ICU) including: Cardiopulmonary resuscitation (CPR) and mechanical ventilation (respirator care).
B.	Care in an acute care hospital but without CPR, respirator, or ICU care.
C.	Care in the home or nursing home only, including specific treatments when indicated (e.g. antibiotics, blood transfusion, morphine and intravenous diuretics).
D.	Comfort and supportive care only. (e.g. oxygen and morphine)

Table 28.4
Examples of levels of intensity of medical care that might be included in advance directives.

For example, individuals may request that treatment for their congestive heart failure only be provided at home. However, the necessity to establish permanent intravenous access to allow this treatment may require overnight hospitalization. A note documenting the discussion would make clear that hospitalizations for a patient who desired to stay at home are acceptable if these would facilitate making the experience at home a more comfortable one. Important principles to utilize in guiding decisions about the level of intensity in patients with cardiovascular disease near the end of life are summarized below:[18]

1. In addition to decisions about specific interventions such as cardiopulmonary resuscitation or angioplasty, general statements should include a reference to conditions such as disability and cognitive dysfunction that have significantly affected the decision to limit treatment intensity. The statement should allow for more intensive treatments when the potential benefits outweigh the risk, particularly in regards to providing comfort for the patient.

2. Decisions about specific treatments being refused must be consistent. For example, deciding to undergo CPR but declining a respirator in an intensive care unit is not a reasonable combination of decisions.

3. Decisions to forego specific treatments do not imply that the other forms of care should be withheld. For example, a no-CPR order does not preclude hospitalization for acute, severe congestive heart failure or pneumonia.

It is important that physicians caring for patients with cardiac disease explicitly address the use of cardiopulmonary resuscitation. Failure to discuss cardiopulmonary resuscitation in older people is common although almost 80% of older adults desire to have a discussion about CPR with their health-care providers.[21] Residents of long-term care facilities with cardiovascular disease are a particularly important group of individuals that should have explicit discussions about cardiopulmonary resuscitation. This is because CPR has been shown to be ineffective in all but a very few nursing home residents. Owing to poor medical condition, generally related to physical and cognitive dysfunction, residents of long-term care facilities such as nursing homes have a low survival rate for cardiopulmonary resuscitation (less than 2%).[22]

Evaluating the efficacy of therapy in patients near the end of life

It is important that physicians caring for cardiovascular disease in frail older people carefully monitor drug therapy in order to document its efficacy and minimize complications and inappropriate use of medications. There are no data from clinical trials to provide guidelines for the monitoring of drug therapy in frail older patients with cardiovascular disease. However, clinical experience indicates that reassessing the utility and efficacy of medications used in the treatment of cardiovascular disease is a commonly overlooked aspect of treating heart disease near the end of life. Because symptoms of cardiovascular disease, such as angina, often decline with declining physical function, progression of age and comorbid disease, medications previously needed to control symptoms should often be reduced in dosage or discontinued. For example, patients with stable, medically treated angina who were active and ambulatory may benefit from reduction in anti-anginal therapy if they become primarily bed or chair-bound. Physicians should routinely review the use of nitrates in older adults and a trial at lower dosages in those individuals with declining physical activity may be warranted.

Another cardiovascular medication that has been shown to be over used, particularly in institutionalized frail populations, is digitalis.[23] In addition, care givers should evaluate the need for diuretic therapy in frail older patients, particularly those who are institutionalized due to combinations of decline in physical and cognitive function. These individuals often have poor fluid intake and are highly susceptible to dehydration. Involvement of long-term care staff in monitoring vital signs allows physicians to more carefully tailor treatment for cardiovascular diseases such as congestive heart failure and hypertension and to adjust medications as a patient nears the end of life. For example, as blood pressure declines in frail older people, antihypertensive medications can be significantly reduced or eliminated. In addition to reducing the potential for side-effects, the cost of many such medications produces a significant hardship for patients who do not require them.

Alternatives to hospital inpatient care for cardiovascular disease

The acute inpatient hospital is often not the best setting for the care of older adults. The recent trends towards shorter hospitalization do not favor the formulation of comprehensive care plans that are necessary for many older individuals. In addition, hospital care is associated with delirium, depression and iatrogenic illness. Home health care is the fastest growing sector of health care in the United States today[24] and the effectiveness of home care for patients with limited life expectancy has been demonstrated in other diseases such as cancer.[24] Recent data have shown that 70% of older adults prefer to be cared for at home rather than be hospitalized.[26] Many diagnostic and treatment approaches formerly confined to the hospital setting are now available for use in the home and home care is a safe, effective and cost effective avenue for treating acute illness in this population. The home is also an ideal setting for nurses, mid-level practitioners and physicians to work with patients and families to formulate plans for care near the end of life. The range of home health care includes postacute nursing visits for several days to hospice care focused on maintaining the comfort and dignity of patients with limited life expectancy. The latter includes patients with chronic end-stage illness such as congestive heart failure and cancer.

Frail older patients with cardiovascular disease are particularly vulnerable to acute insults and rehospitalization in the (postacute) period after hospital discharge. These patients commonly receive multiple medications and the need to monitor compliance and evaluate efficacy requires a close working relationship between skilled nursing providers in the community and physicians comfortable with treating patients in their home who have difficulty in traveling to an office. The use of home services for frail older people with cardiovascular disease allows for increased emotional support, teaching about treatment schedules and medication, therapy to enhance or improve physical function related to acute exacerbations of illness, and also provides a mechanism for assistance other than a return to the emergency room or the acute inpatient setting. Most home-health agencies provide 24-hour availability and access to physicians, geriatric nurse practitioners, social workers and other care givers. Home health care for chronic disease such as coronary heart disease and other cardiovascular diseases also allows for ongoing education and communication with the family to reinforce their role in the treatment of a frail older adult as well as a greater understanding as how to cope with the patient's disease and treatment.

Although some studies have questioned the cost savings and benefits in terms of economics for home care for the elderly,[27,28] others have demonstrated improved function, lower institutionalized care, and some net savings with home care.[29] Rich et al[30] investigated older patients previously hospitalized for congestive heart failure and at high risk for admissions to nursing homes. The intervention consisted of educating the patient and family and included diet and medication review plus intensive follow-up using hospital-based home-care services. The study found lower rates of institutionalization, readmission, and lower overall cost compared to those individuals who were not enrolled in the program. Home care is clearly cost effective in the care of terminally ill patients who require minimal technology and supportive care. The benefit of posthospital home-care services for individuals requiring short-term 'transitional' care from the acute-care setting to a more stable community setting has also been shown by Townsend et al.[31] Of 903 older adults (median age 82 years) discharged from the hospital to their home, half received intense home-care service and the other half received standard care. In the intervention group, patients were provided with up to 12 hours per week, for up to 2 weeks of home care including rehabilitation, social support and instruction on medication use. For the 18 months after discharge, patients who had received home care had 2498 fewer hospital days than the control group who did not receive postacute care in-home service. This study indicates that coordinated postacute care for older patients in the home is beneficial both in terms of overall health for frail elderly adults as well as hospital use.

Once discussions about limitations in the intensity of therapy for cardiovascular disease have taken place, home care allows the patient to return to a familiar environment and the provision of care with focus on comfort and dignity, while maintaining the quality of life that older patients prefer over quantity of life.[32] Even for those patients who opt not to limit the intensity of care, high levels of skilled care in the home including intravenous administration of diuretics, antibiotics and similar agents is feasible. These resources allow patients to return home after acute exacerbations of a chronic illness in a more timely fashion while reducing hospital lengths of stay.[33]

Summary

As our population over age 80 continues to age and expand, the high prevalence of cardiovascular disease in this age group mandates the development of optimal approaches providing care for those individuals with limited life expectancy. Physicians have a responsibility to foster the comfort and dignity of older patients with advanced age and chronic illness. When cure is no longer an option, instead of believing that there is nothing else to be done for the patient and the family, there are great opportunities offering professional satisfaction that few other areas of medicine can provide. Providers of care for this population of patients are often rewarded with the gratitude of patients and their families for work that has minimized suffering and maximized participation in the affairs of family and community.

References

1. Gilford DM. Social economic, and demographic changes among the elderly. In: *The Aging Population in the Twenty-first Century: Statistics for Health Policy.* (Washington National Academy Press: Washington DC, 1988).

2. Spencer G. U.S. Bureau of the Census. Projections of the Population of the United States, by Age, Sex, and Race: 1988–2080. *Curr Pop Rep* (1989) **1018**:25.

3. Taeuber C. American in transition: an aging society. *Current Population Reports, Special Studies Series.* Bureau of the Census. Washington, DC. U.S. Department of Commerce (1983) **128**:23.

4. National Center for Health Statistics. Current Estimate from the National Health Interview Survey, 1989. *Vital and Health Statistics Series.* (1990) **176**:10.

5. National Center for Health Statistics. *Health, United States, 1989.* DHHS Pub. No. (PHS) 90-1232, Washington: Department of Health and Human Services (March 1990).

6. National Center for Health Statistics. National Hospital Discharge Survey: Annual Summary, 1987. *Vital and Health Statistics* (1989) Series 13, No. 99.

7. Lubitz JD, Riley GF. Trends in Medicare payments in the last year of life. *N Engl J Med* (1993) **328**:1092–6.

8. Guralnik JM, Fried LP, Simonsick EM et al. The Women's Health and Aging Study: Health and Social Characteristics of Older Women with Disability. (National Institute on Aging: Bethesda, MD, 1995) NIH Pub. No. 95-4009.

9. Branch LG, Haynes SG, Feinleib M et al. Functional abilities of the elderly: an update on the Massachusetts Health Care Panel Study. *Second Conference on the Epidemiology of Aging.* National Institutes of Health. (1980) DHHS Pub. No. 80-969. Bethesda, MD.

10. Branch LG, Meyers AR. Assessing physical function in the elderly. *Clin Geriatr Med* (1987) **3**:29–51.

11. Corti MC, Guralnik JM, Salive ME, Sorkin JD. Serum albumin level and physical disability as predictors of mortality in older persons. *J Am Med Assoc* (1994) **272**:1036–42.

12. Koyano W, Shibata H, Haga H, Suyama Y. Prevalence and outcome of low ADL and incontinence among the elderly: five years follow-up in a Japanese urban community. *Arch Gerontol Geriat* (1987) **5**:197–206.

13. Warren MD, Knight R. Mortality in relation to the functional capacities of people with disabilities living at home. *J Epidem Community Health* (1982) **36**:220–3.

14. Manton KG. A longitudinal study of functional change and mortality in the United States. *J Gerontol Med Sci* (1988) **43**: M5153–61.

15. Nelson E, Conger B, Douglass R et al. Functional health status levels of primary care patients. *JAMA* (1983) **249**:3331–8.

16. Katz S. Assessing self-maintainance: activities of daily living, mobility and instrumental activities of daily living. *J Am Geriatr Soc* (1983) **31**:721–7.

17. Rubenstein LV et al. Health status assessment for elderly patients: report of the Society of General Internal Medicine task force on health assessment. *J Am Geriatr Soc* (1988) **37**:562.

18. Folstein MF, Folstein SE, Mc Hugh PR. Mini-Mental State: a practical method for grading the cognitive state of patients and the clinician. *Psychiatr Res* (1975) **12**:189

19. Ouslander JG, Osterweil D, Morley J. *Medical Care in the Nursing Home.* (McGraw-Hill: New York, 1991) 358.

20. Roth LH, Meisel A, Lidz CW. Tests of competency to consent to treatment. *Am J Psychiatr* (1977) **134**:279–84.

21. Shmerling RH, Bedell SE, Lilenfeld A et al. Discussing cardiopulmonary resuscitation: a study of elderly outpatients. *J Gen Intern Med* (1988) **3**:317–21.

22. Applebaum GE, King JE, Finucane TE. The outcome of CPR initiated in nursing homes. *J Am Geriatr Soc* (1990) **38**:197–200.

23. Forman DE, Coletta D, Kenny DD et al. Clini-

cal issues related to discontinuing digoxin therapy in elderly nursing home patients. *Arch Intern Med* (1991) **151**:2194–8.

24. Steel K. Physician-directed long-term home health care for the elderly: a century long experience. *J Am Geriatr Soc* (1987) **35**:264–8.

25. Vinciguerra V, Degnan TJ, Sciortino A et al. A comparative assessment of home versus hospital comprehensive treatment for advanced cancer patients. *J Clin Oncol* (1986) **4**:1521–8.

26. Burton LC, Leff B, Harper M et al. Acceptability to patients of a home hospital. *J Am Geriatr Soc* (1988) **46**:605–9.

27. Kemper P. The evaluation of the National Long Term Care Demonstration: 10. Overview of the findings. *Health Serv Res* (1988) **23**:161–74.

28. Weissert WG. A new policy agenda for home care. *Health Aff (Millwood)* (1991) **10**:67–77.

29. Stessman J, Ginsberg G, Hammerman-Rozenberg et al. Decreased hospital utilization by older adults attributable to a home hospitalization program. *J Am Geriatr Soc* (1996) **44**:591–8.

30. Rich MW, Beckham V, Wittenberg C et al. A multidisciplinary intervention to prevent the readmission of elderly patients with congestive heart failure. *N Engl J Med* (1995) **333**:1190–5.

31. Townsend J, Piper M, Frank AO et al. Reduction in hospital readmission stay of elderly patients by a community based hospital discharge scheme: a randomized controlled trial. *BMJ* (1988) **297**:544–7.

32. McKenna RJ. Clinical aspects of cancer in the elderly: treatment decision, treatment choices and follow-up. *Cancer* (1994) **74**(Suppl 7):2107–17.

33. Goldberg AI. Technology assessment and support of life-sustaining devices in home care: The home care physician perspective. *Chest* (1994) **105**:1448–53.

29

The costs and cost effectiveness of cardiovascular care in the very elderly

Eric D Peterson and Eric L Eisenstein

Introduction

The very elderly require and receive a disproportionate amount of all cardiovascular care delivered in the US. While octogenarians make up under 5% of the general US population, they account for over 20% of all hospital admissions for acute myocardial infarction (MI) and over 30% of all MI deaths.[1-4] Furthermore, the US octogenarian population is expected to quadruple in size over the next 50 years,[5,6] challenging our society to determine what health care can and should be offered to the very aged. Beyond the effect on individuals, in aggregate, these care decisions in the aged have major economic implications for society.[7] Spurred on by changes in US demographics,[5,6] and a proliferation of expensive medical technology, the costs associated with caring for elderly cardiac patients have risen significantly. As a result, many health-care decision makers have begun to question the value of aggressive interventions in those nearing the end of life.[8-15] Before deciding to constrain therapeutic options, health-policy experts and clinicians should clearly understand the costs and cost effectiveness associated with specific cardiac treatments in the very aged.

In this chapter, we will outline the major historical forces affecting resource use in the very elderly, and define how medical health-care costs are measured. We will then examine how medical costs differ in the elderly compared with younger patients. Third, we will review cost effectiveness analysis methodologies and determine whether these studies are inherently biased against the elderly. Finally, we will review the available literature on how age influences the cost effectiveness of major cardiovascular disease treatment strategies.

Major forces influencing health-care spending in the aged

During the 1970s and through the early 1980s, medical care expenses rose exponentially in the US. As of 1994, the United States spent more than $949 billion on health care annually; double the figure which was spent just a decade earlier.[16] Much of this double-digit inflation can be attributed to the 1968 adoption of Medicare insurance coverage for all US citizens aged 65 years or older.[17] This policy change assured near full payment to hospitals and doctors for all elderly medical care, thus ushering in the 'open checkbook era' of American medicine.[18] During this period, health-care providers were paid for whatever procedures they performed ('fee-for-service'), encouraging higher use of health-care services and ·the proliferation of newer and more expensive medical technologies.[19]

In cardiovascular disease, this period witnessed a phenomenal expansion of diagnostic and therapeutic procedures. Our ability to detect and measure the extent of coronary disease was markedly broadened with the widespread availability of coronary angiography, echocardiography and nuclear perfusion imaging testing. Our therapeutic armamentarium was also augmented with new drugs (such as thrombolytic agents, angiotensin-converting-enzyme inhibitors and potent lipid lowering agents) and wider use of coronary revascularization procedures. While many of these innovations improved the outcomes of coronary disease patients, they also fueled a substantial rise in the overall societal costs of medical care.[20,21]

The end of the medical industry's golden era came during the late 1980s when spiraling costs caused the major payers (the business community and government) to reassess whether health care had assumed a disproportionate segment of society's resources. By this time, US health-care costs were nearly 2.5 times higher than those in other industrialized nations, potentially limiting the US economy's competitiveness in international markets.[22] At the same time, the emerging field of outcomes research was documenting significant differences in health-care delivery among US geographic regions. For example, in a series of studies between 1987 and 1989, Wennberg reported that citizens in Boston used twice as many hospital services as their counterparts in New Haven, yet both groups had almost identical health outcomes.[23,24] These and other studies indicated that the availability of technology (supply), rather than its true clinical need (demand), was the major factor driving health-care use. This realization led many to conclude that more medical care was not necessarily better care. The end result was that government, business and private consumers

began to challenge physicians' long-held decision-making autonomy, calling for increased accountability in medicine.

One method payers used to slow the expansion of health-care costs was to change reimbursement formulas, shifting the financial risk of patient care from the health-care insurer to the provider. For the elderly, the government switched Medicare payments from a fee-for-service (pay for all care administered) to a prospective payment system. Under the prospective payment system, hospitals receive a flat fee for treating specific presenting illnesses. Hospitals that used less than an average number of care resources (by performing fewer tests or procedures) were able to maintain a positive financial margin; those who used more resources, however, faced economic hardship.

Managed care, which became increasingly widespread in the early 1990s provided other ways of limiting and controlling costs. Large health-care organizations implemented new cost-containment methods such as capitated payment plans under which physicians received a fixed payment for taking care of a certain number of enrollees in a plan. This payment system shifted most of the financial risk from the insurers to the treating physicians and provided them with an incentive to do as little as is ethically reasonable. When cutbacks in care occur, they usually begin in the elderly.[9,11,14,15,25]

A final change in US health care that is particularly pertinent to the elderly has been the increasing acceptance that withholding care in the aged is not only ethically acceptable, but may actually be a preferable patient management strategy. Studies in the mid- to late-1980s documented that significant health-care resources were consumed during the final year of one's life.[26,27] By some estimates, as much as 30% of Medicare's entire budget is consumed by those recipients in their final year of life.[28] While a clinician's ability to identify hopeless medical situations accurately is limited, many questioned whether physicians had become too aggressive in their treatment of the very elderly.[10–14,29] For example, in a speech in 1984, then Governor Lamm of Colorado stated that 'we've got a duty to die and get out of the way with all our machines and artificial hearts and everything else like that and let the other society, our kids, build a reasonable life.'[30] In 1987, Daniel Callahan echoed this sentiment when he proposed that we need to make a 'societal decision deliberately to limit life-extending high technology care for those who have lived out a natural life-span,' which he later defined as someone in their late 70s or early 80s.[31]

These changes in health-care policy and delivery have prompted many in society to want objective assurances that expensive and aggressive procedures are worth their costs in the very elderly. Such widespread questions have brought health-care cost measurement and cost effectiveness to the forefront of this debate. As we will see, however, health-care economic analyses can often be fraught with uncertainty, particularly when applied in the very aged.[32]

Basic principles of cost measurement

In order to more fully understand the debate concerning cost and cost effectiveness of cardiovascular care in the very aged, one must have a working knowledge of how these economic outcomes are measured. The terms cost and charge are frequently used mistakenly as synonyms in many health-care studies.[33] In economic terms, the *cost* of a good or service may be defined in terms of the value of the

resources (labor, supplies, equipment and facilities) required to produce it. In a competitive marketplace, the price paid for the good or service can be used as a summary measure of these input resources. Unfortunately, health care prices (also known as *charges*) do not accurately reflect their input resources. The charges for a given medical service may vary considerably depending upon the payer. Additionally, cost shifting, or the billing practice of transferring the costs of certain high intensity health-care services to other cheaper but higher volume services, further distorts the relationship between medical charges and costs. Because of these distortions, medical charges cannot be used to accurately measure the actual monetary value of the resources that are required to deliver a given medical service.[18,33]

Methods of measuring medical costs

Given these limitations of charge data, three methods of cost measurement have been developed. A 'bottom-up' approach uses industrial engineering techniques to enumerate all input resources consumed in treating a patient (e.g. labor, consumables), determines the cost to the provider for each input, and then aggregates this information into a summary cost estimate. While the most accurate measurement method, it generally requires a sophisticated cost accounting system. Alternatively, one can use a 'top-down' approach that attempts to convert medical charges from a patient's hospital bill line items into costs using hospital-specific departmental cost-to-charge ratios (e.g. hospital specific annual Medicare Cost Report).[34] Lastly, when longer-term costs are assessed in both in- and out-patient settings, researchers often estimate overall health-care costs by aggregating 'big-ticket' resources (such as number of intensive care bed days, diagnostic cardiac catheterizations and outpatient visits). Average prices for these resources are then generated from available sources (e.g. the investigator's home institution) and assumed to apply to each patient and institution in the study. Using this method, the overall health-care costs for a patient can be estimated by counting 'big ticket' resources consumed and multiplying by the cost associated with each item.[18]

Cost components

When determining the costs associated with medical care, it is important to define which components were considered. Items used during the delivery of care (such as personnel time, IV tubing, etc.) are known as 'direct costs' and are included in all cost analyses. 'Indirect costs' (such as hospital administrative overhead) are part of the business of health-care delivery and should also be considered when computing the long-term, average costs of care. Finally, 'patient and non-medical costs' (such as a family member's lost wages resulting from caring for a sick relative) can be a considerable part of the overall cost of caring for the frail or disabled elderly patient. Unfortunately, while these nonmedical costs have been recommended for inclusion in health-care cost analyses by recently published economic guidelines,[35,36] they are often neglected because of difficulty measuring these endpoints.

An additional, and important, element of the cost analysis is its perspective.[37] With regard to perspective, most economic studies examine cost from a societal viewpoint (the total resources consumed by the care strategy) rather than from a specific insurer (Medicare), patient (out-of-pocket expenses) or hospital cost perspective.[36] The time-frame of the analyses must also be considered because comparisons of cumulative medical costs between treatment strategies can vary considerably depending on the time-frame considered. Present-day medical care decisions can have important downstream resource consequences. For example, the initial procedure cost for coronary angioplasty is considerably less than for bypass surgery. However, long-term studies have found that angioplasty patients require significantly more follow-up revascularization procedures, resulting in similar 5-year cumulative cost estimates.[38,39]

Cost drivers

Major drivers of health-care cost include patient-, treatment-, provider- and geographic-related factors.[18] Patient-related factors can influence health-care resource spending predominantly by influencing the underlying likelihood for clinical events, complications and death. Patient-related factors that have been linked to higher care costs in cardiac patients include demographic factors (such as advanced age and female gender), disease-severity-related factors (extent of coronary disease, degree of left ventricular dysfunction), and presence and severity of cormorbid illness (such as diabetes mellitus or renal insufficiency).

Treatment-related factors describe how specific patient management decisions can affect health-care costs. For example, the cost for patients hospitalized with unstable angina who undergo cardiac catheterization and revascularization therapy is nearly double that for those who are treated conservatively with medical therapy.[40] While treatment-related factors address the question of what is the 'right' strategy to use, provider-related factors address whether 'the right things were done right.' Specifically, irrespective of what clinical management decision is made, physicians often differ in the quality and the efficiency of the care they provide. Complications resulting from provider quality issues can certainly increase care costs. For example, one study found that the costs associated with bypass surgery can increase three-fold if a patient experiences postoperative complications.[41] Likewise, several studies have documented that practitioners differ in how efficiently care is delivered to similar patients. For example, patients admitted in New England with an acute MI stay, on average, 40% longer than patients admitted in the Pacific region.[42] Finally, geographic- and practice-setting-related factors can affect the cost of health-care delivery. Input costs (such as labor, fuel, rent) can vary considerably depending on the geographic location of a practice (e.g. urban versus rural, mid-west versus the west coast).[20] Additionally, large multicenter health-care organizations are often able to negotiate lower costs for consumable medical supplies, reducing their overall costs.[43]

The cost of cardiovascular care in the very elderly
Magnitude of the problem

Despite improvements in prevention and treatment, cardiovascular disease remains the leading cause of death in the United States.[1] Because the prevalence of cardiovascular disease increases exponentially with age, this is predominantly a disease of the aged. For example, those over 65 and 75 make up 13% and 5% of the US population, respectively, yet they account for approximately 55% and 30% of all admissions for myocardial infarction.[2,44] Additionally, patients aged 65 and older account for more than 75% of those admitted for major arrhythmias[1] and over two-thirds of the 2.1 million patients hospitalized with congestive heart failure were over age 65.[45] Because the elderly account for the majority of patients with cardiovascular disease, they also consume a majority of the health-care resources spent on its treatment (Table 29.1). Nearly half of the over 1.1

Treatment	Total number of cases per year in US	Percentage performed in those aged ≥65	Percentage performed in those aged ≥75	1994 cost per case ($)
Cardiac catheterization	1 122 000	48	17	10 880
Coronary angioplasty	404 000	47	16	21 760
Coronary bypass surgery	501 000	53	17	44 220
Valve surgery	66 000	58	n/a	51 000
Pacemaker implantation	139 000	84	n/a	21 000

Table 29.1
1994 US cardiovascular procedure use[1,44,129]

million diagnostic cardiac catheterizations performed annually in the US are for patients aged 65 years or older. Similarly, half of all US revascularization procedures are performed in the elderly. Over 450 000 coronary bypass and angioplasty procedures are performed annually in the United States in those over age 65. Of the 139 000 pacemakers implanted per year in this country, over 80% are placed in the elderly.[1]

The number and percentage of cardiovascular procedures performed in the elderly is also rising over time due to our increasing willingness to use these technologies in the elderly. Between 1987 and 1990, the number of catheterization and revascularization procedures performed in US Medicare patients increased by more than 45%.[46,47] Interestingly, the most dramatic rise in the use of coronary revascularization procedures has been in the

oldest old. For example, the rates of bypass surgery in octogenarians rose by 67% between 1987 and 1990.[48]

Acute cardiovascular-care costs in young and old

While the elderly as a group consume a high percentage of all cardiovascular health-care resources, it is not clear that individual cardiovascular care costs are affected by the patient's age. Studying 4000 patients admitted with coronary artery disease, Mark and colleagues (Table 29.2) found that acute care costs increased marginally with increasing patient age (1% per year older).[49] This is in contrast to a more than 300% increase in cost attributable to treatment-related factors (i.e. whether a revascularization was used).

In a separate study of 2628 Medicare patients admitted with acute myocardial

Factor	Cost increase (%)
Patient-related	
Congestive failure	12
Valvular heart disease	10
Mitral insufficiency	6
Ejection fraction <60%	0.4*
Age	1.0†
Severity of coronary disease	0.6‡
Treatment-related	
PTCA	309
CABG	440

*Per percentage change.
†Per year.
‡Per point change in coronary artery disease index.

Table 29.2
Factors affecting cost in patients with coronary artery disease: the Duke experience[49]

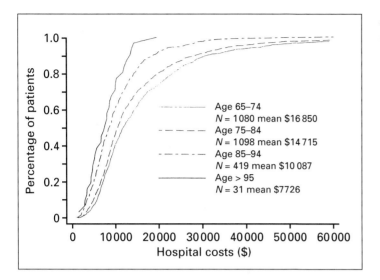

Figure 29.1
MI care costs by age group. (From Krumholtz [50])

infarction (MI), Krumholz reported that increasing patient age was actually associated with decreasing health-care costs. Specifically, using cost-to-charge ratio adjustments, the mean in-patient hospital costs were $16 850 for MI patients aged 65–74 years, $14 715 in those aged 75–84 years and $10 087 in those aged 85–94 years (Figure 29.1).[50] Finally, the SUPPORT study found that the very elderly consumed considerably fewer health-care resources than younger patients when admitted to intensive care units.[51] In this study, those over age 80 consumed only about half of the resources spent on similarly ill patients aged 50 or younger.

The two main explanations for this inverse relationship between age and health-care costs are the following. First, the use of diagnostic and interventional procedures declines markedly with increasing patient age, decreasing acute hospital costs.[47,52,53] For example, national Medicare data demonstrate that octogenarian MI patients were 2.7 times less likely to undergo noninvasive stress testing, 3.6 times less likely to receive cardiac catheterization, and 4.3 times less likely to receive coronary angioplasty or bypass surgery than similar MI patients aged 65 to 70 years.[44] Likewise, Hamel found that octogenarians were 41% less likely to receive invasive cardiac hemodynamic monitoring than patients aged under 50 years after adjusting for severity of illness.[51] A second factor leading to lower hospital costs in the elderly is the confounding influence of mortality. Patients who die following an acute cardiac admission tend to die early,[54] resulting in shorter hospital stays and lower overall acute care costs. As very elderly cardiac patients have higher early mortality rates than younger patients,[46,55] the total average hospital costs in the elderly tend to be lower than those in younger patients.[50]

Effect of age on revascularization costs

When very elderly patients undergo coronary intervention, their procedure costs are considerably higher than costs for younger patients. For example, in the Medicare population, hospital stays after bypass surgery in those aged over 80 years averaged nearly 40% longer than those aged 65–70 years (14.2 versus 10.8 days, $P < 0.001$).[48] Increased lengths of stay after bypass surgery in the very elderly result in increased overall hospital costs. The mean in-patient costs for those age 80 years or older average $27 200 (exclusive of professional fees) compared with $21 700 for those aged 65–70 years.[48]

While it is clearly more expensive to perform revascularization in the very aged than in younger patients, it should be noted that the *relative* effect of age on total costs is less than other treatment-related factors. In a detailed bypass surgery cost analysis, Smith and colleagues found that provider-related factors had a much larger impact on the final cost estimate than the patient's age or disease-related severity.[56] Cowper and colleagues reported similar results in a multicenter study, finding that patient-specific factors (including age) accounted for only 27% of the explainable variation in bypass surgery costs and provider-specific factors accounted for 63%.[57] Likewise, in percutaneous coronary revascularization cases, age only increased average PTCA costs by $790 per decade while there was over a $4000 difference between the lowest and highest cost physician.[58]

Long-term health-care costs

Advancing age appears to have both positive and negative influences on long-term cardiovascular health-care costs. On the one hand, the elderly cardiac patient is significantly more likely to require multiple hospitalizations following an incident case of coronary disease. For example, of those elderly admitted with congestive heart failure, over 50% will be readmitted within one year.[1] Similarly, up to 20% of Medicare patients who undergo bypass surgery are readmitted to hospitals within 60 days of discharge.[59] Second, elderly patients are more likely to be disabled by a cardiac event and require higher rates of long-term supportive care. Only 50% of Medicare octogenarians admitted with an acute MI were able to be discharged home compared with 78% of those MI patients aged 65–70 years.[44] When nursing-home care is required, it can average $25 000 or more per year for the rest of a patient's life span.[28]

While disease relapse and need for institutional care tend to increase long-term care costs in the very elderly, certain counterbalancing forces exist. First, as with acute care, the elderly are less likely to receive expensive interventions in follow-up care. Elderly patients undergoing coronary angioplasty are 30% less likely to require a second procedure than those under age 65 years.[60] Second, the natural life expectancy of the very elderly is shortened. Thus, they have a shorter time in which to accumulate health-care costs. The combined effect of these positive and negative effects on long-term health-care costs is unknown. Despite the importance of evaluating the long-term cost outcomes in young and old cardiac patients, such comparisons have yet to be performed.

Cost-effectiveness analysis in the elderly
Types of cost-effectiveness analyses

In medical care discussions, the term 'cost-effective' is often used to imply that a given therapy is 'worthwhile' or meets some unspecified threshold between cost and patient benefit.[61] In a more formal sense, cost-effectiveness analyses describe a specific family of analytic tools used to compare the marginal (or added) costs and health-care benefits associated with one health-care strategy relative to another strategy (usually current standard care). There are four separate types of cost-outcomes analyses: cost-minimization, cost benefit, cost-effectiveness, and cost-utility analysis.[37,62,63] In *cost-minimization* analysis, the patient benefits (outcomes) derived from each competing care strategy are assumed to be equivalent. Thus, the analytic goal is simplified to a search for the cheapest therapeutic alternative ($Cost_A - Cost_B$). Equivalent patient outcomes, however, are rare in medical care and consequences often differ between competing care strategies. In such cases, the decision-maker must weigh both the costs and potential benefits of each strategy. In *cost-benefit* analysis, health-care benefits are assigned an economic value (e.g. one life saved is worth $200 000). Once these assumptions regarding the value of health care benefits are made, the analysis again simplifies to maximizing overall net financial benefit ($ Benefit$_A$ $- Cost_A$) $-$ ($ Benefit$_B$ $- Cost_B$).

As there are considerable technical and ethical difficulties in reaching a consensus regarding the dollar value for such items as a human life,[64–67] many studies instead compare *cost-effectiveness*. Cost-effectiveness (CE) analyses directly associate the incremental costs of care with their incremental effects on health outcomes, CE ratio = ($Cost_A - Cost_B$) ÷ (Effectiveness$_A$ $-$ Effectiveness$_B$). While any patient outcome can be used as the effectiveness measure, many studies choose the 'cost per life saved' or 'cost per life years added' as a common denominator. For example, Therapy A costs $5000 more per patient treated than Therapy B. Therapy A also saves two additional lives for every 100 treated relative to Therapy B. Therefore, the cost effectiveness of Therapy A is (100 × $5000) ÷ 2 = $250 000

per life saved. If each 'saved' patient lives an average of 10 years, then another formulation of the CE ratio of Therapy A relative to Therapy B is $25 000 per additional life year.

Researchers also use cost-utility analysis to adjust for differences in quality of life since many patients value a year in perfect health more than a year lived in poor health.[68,69] Cost-utility analysis modifies the standard CE ratio noted above by devaluing time spent in less than perfect health states. For example, surveys have placed the value (or utility) of a year of life spent confined to bed as being worth approximately half of that spent in good health.[68,69] In our example above, if our two patients 'saved' by Therapy A were disabled and confined to live their 10 additional years in bed (utility = 0.5), then the comparative CE ratio of Therapy A relative to Therapy B would double to $50 000 per additional quality-adjusted life year (QALY).

To meaningfully assess a cost-effectiveness analysis, it must be compared against some external benchmarks.[70,71] Specifically, one can compare whether a new therapy with a given cost effectiveness is 'worthwhile' relative to those medical therapies currently considered standard care in medical practice. Although no universal benchmarks exist, most economists consider a therapy that adds an additional life year for $50 000 or less 'economically attractive.' In contrast, when a therapy adds a life year for over $100 000, it is generally considered economically unattractive. The middle range represents a gray zone which contains many currently used therapies.[20] Table 29.3 displays cost-effectiveness ratios that have been calculated for various cardiovascular therapies.

Two final points have to be remembered when examining the results of cost-effectiveness analyses. First, a CE ratio for a given therapy is wholly dependent on the

New therapy	Existing therapy	Patient population	Cost/ YOLS ($)*	Reference number
Beta-blockers and diuretics	No therapy	70–84-year-old hypertensive men	1 274	124
Beta-blockers	No therapy	65-year-old high risk MI survivor	4 257	109
Captopril	No therapy	80-year-old MI survivor	4 770	87
Bypass surgery	Medical therapy	55-year-old with left main coronary artery disease	6 345	125
Coronary angioplasty	Medical therapy	55-year-old men with severe angina	8 385	126
Hypertension screening	No screening	60-year-old asymptomatic men	12 464	127
Exercise stress test	No testing	60-year-old with mild pain and no LV dysfunction	14 730	128
t-PA	Streptokinase	>75-year-old with inferior acute MI	18 408	72
Lovastatin	No therapy	55–64-year-old men with heart disease and <250 mg/dl	22 661	109
Coronary care unit	Intermediate care	>75-year-old with high probability of MI	25 439	85
ICD	Amiodarone	65-year-old patients with refractory VF	57 311	89
Coronary care unit	Intermediate care	>75-year-old with moderate probability of MI	81 179	85
Bypass surgery	Medical therapy	55-year-old with two-vessel coronary artery disease	84 980	125
t-PA	Streptokinase	<40-year-old with anterior MI	123 609	72
Coronary angioplasty	Medical therapy	55-year-old men with mild angina	124 638	126

*Costs adjusted to 1996 dollars using the consumer price index.
YOLS: years of life saved.

Table 29.3
Cardiovascular CE league table

comparative therapy. For example, the CE ratio for t-PA (a thrombolytic agent) when compared with streptokinase (another thrombolytic agent) for treating acute myocardial infarction patients is considerably higher than the CE ratio for t-PA relative to a conservative treatment strategy (no reperfusion).[72] Secondly, the often reported CE ratio for a given therapy describes results for the 'average' patient and CE ratios can shift markedly in specific patient subgroups (e.g. by age group).[62]

Are CE analyses biased against the very aged?

While many consider cost-effectiveness analyses an objective, quantitative tool for determining the best use of society's fixed health-care resources, other researchers have pointed out that these methods have a number of potential theoretical and practical limitations when applied to the very elderly.[32,73–75] For example, a review of cost effectiveness research in the *New England Journal of Medicine* described these analyses as 'embodying a set of hidden value assumptions that virtually guarantee antigeriatric biases to their purportedly objective data.'[32]

From a theoretical basis, patient age may impact on cost-effectiveness ratios in a number of ways as illustrated in Figure 29.2. In terms of care costs, advancing patient age is usually associated with higher acute procedure/treatment costs (see 'The cost of cardiovascular care in the very elderly'). Age can also influence downstream health-care costs, but it remains unclear whether this cumulative impact is large for cardiovascular patients. In terms of effectiveness, the acute risks of intervention are almost always considerably higher in the elderly. Age-related changes in cardiac physiology and the accumulations of co-

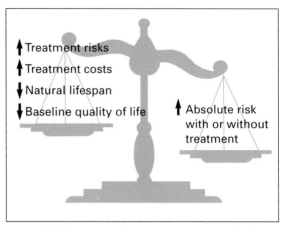

Figure 29.2
Cost effectiveness of care in the elderly: weighing the risk and benefits

morbid illness make the elderly more vulnerable for morbid or mortal events when surgical or other aggressive interventions are attempted.[76–79]

The shorter life expectancy of the very elderly can also directly impact on a therapy's CE ratio. A therapy that saves a 40 year old man (with a life-expectancy of 35 years) would appear to be five times more valuable in terms of 'added life-years' than if the therapy saved an 80 year old man (life-expectancy 7 years) in standard cost effectiveness calculations.[80] Additionally, many therapies take several years to manifest their optimal survival benefit. If the 'delay to therapeutic benefit' is sufficiently long, it may approach the life expectancy boundaries in the very aged. For example, the benefits of bypass surgery become most evident only after 5–7 years in patients with multivessel coronary disease.[81,82] This delay to benefit is equivalent to an 85 year old's life-expectancy.

Additionally, because of a higher prevalence of comorbid illness, baseline quality of life is often compromised in the very elderly cardiac patient. Therefore, therapies that add a similar number of life years in a young and an old patient may be considered more valuable in the young, healthy patient than in the very aged if a cost-utility analysis approach is used.[32] Finally, the presence of 'fixed' noncardiac disabilities (such as disabling arthritis or dementia) can also lessen the overall value (in terms of quality adjusted life years) gained by therapies that improve disease-specific symptoms.[68] For example, a cardiovascular drug or intervention that improves a patient's ischemic threshold may not alter an elderly patient's functional status if he/she is already disabled from a stroke.

While cost effectiveness analyses may appear to be age-biased, there is one major counterbalancing force, the high event rates in this patient population. The elderly cardiovascular disease patient has significantly higher baseline risk compared with younger patients, regardless of whether an aggressive or conservative therapeutic strategy is chosen. This high event rate tends to magnify even small differences in therapeutic efficacy. If a treatment offers similar relative risk reductions in young and old patients, then the absolute benefit of the therapy will be substantially greater in the elderly. For example, the relative risk reduction of thrombolytic therapy over conservative medical care in patients with an acute MI declines only slightly (from 24 to 16%) as patient age increases from under 55 years to 65–74 years of age).[83] Because baseline mortality risks increase markedly with age, the absolute benefit of thrombolytic therapy actually rises markedly with advancing age (from 11 lives saved per 1000 treated in those aged <55 years to 27 lives per 1000 in those aged 65–74).

The effect of age on cardiovascular cost-effectiveness analyses

To determine the overall effect of advancing age on cost-effectiveness analyses, we conducted a Medline search (key words: cost-effectiveness and elderly, or aged). As search algorithms, unfortunately, can often miss many cost-effectiveness articles,[61,84] we supplemented these findings with references cited in relevant review articles and those that were identified by experts in the field. The articles discussed below highlight some of the better studies that assessed the cost-effectiveness of cardiovascular technologies in both young and elderly populations. These include the cost effectiveness of: the use of intensive care units for acute coronary syndromes;[85] thrombolytics in acute MI;[72] coronary angiography in the post-MI setting;[86] angiotensin-converting enzyme (ACE) inhibitors for congestive heart failure;[87] beta-blockers for secondary prevention;[88] and automatic implantable cardioverter defibrillator (ICD) devices in patients with life-threatening arrhythmia.[89] These topics span the spectrum of cardiovascular diagnostics, pharmacological and device interventions, and demonstrate many of the promises and pitfalls of cost effectiveness analysis in the very elderly.

CE of the coronary care unit (CCU)

Although the introduction of coronary care units (CCU) in the 1950s and 1960s decreased acute MI mortality rates by more than 50%,[90,91] many practitioners have questioned whether less resource-intensive alternatives may suffice in uncomplicated patients.[92,93] With this question in mind, Tosteson and colleagues investigated the cost effectiveness of triage to a CCU versus an intermediate care unit (monitored beds) setting for uncomplicated patients with chest pain.[85] Their data came primarily from 12 139 patients enrolled in the Multicenter Chest Pain Study.[94] Resource utilization and cost data were based on 901 patients enrolled at a single hospital. Using a decision-analytic model, these authors found that the cost effectiveness of triage to a CCU (in terms of cost per year of life saved) versus an intermediate care unit varied markedly depending upon the patient's age and their underlying probability of MI. In patients with a high probability of MI (ST-segment elevation on initial electrocardiogram), the cost per year of life saved was $33 500 for 45–54 year olds but fell to $12 700 and $13 600 for patients aged 65–74 and over 75 years of age, respectively. For patients with a moderate probability of MI (chest pain for <48 hours, prior history of CAD and minor ECG changes), the cost per year of life saved was $88 400 for 45–54 year olds but only $40 200 in patients 65–74 and $43 400 for patients over 75. Thus, Tosteson reported that the CCU setting was cost-effective (i.e. cost <$50 000/YOLS) for all-aged patients with a high probability of MI, but in those patients with a moderate probability of MI, it was only cost-effective once a patient was 65 years or older. Additionally the cost effectiveness ratios for patients in all risk groups *decreased* from 45 to 74 years of age and then increased only slightly for patients over 75.

In terms of methodology, these researchers 'age-adjusted' all clinical event probabilities and non-MI life expectancies used in their decision model. This age-adjustment was based on their clinical database which demonstrated a direct association between patient age and expected mortality (ranging from 3.1% in 30–44 year olds, to 9.5% in those aged 75 years or older). However, other elements of this cost-effectiveness analysis were not adjusted for the potential impact of age. For example, Tosteson assumed that the relative efficacy of CCU care was similar in young and old patients (i.e. a 15% relative survival benefit). She also assumed that the annual excess risk of death for MI survivors in the years after discharge did not vary by patient age. In terms of cost, Tosteson assumed that index hospitalization resource use did not vary by patient age. Although this assumption was based on a previous analysis that indicated that hospital resource use was constant in young and old patients after adjusting for other clinical factors,[95] the current study did not adjust for these other important clinical characteristics. Lastly, these researchers did not consider long-term healthcare costs in their analysis.

The combined effect of these assumptions may have a powerful influence on the ultimate age-specific cost-effectiveness ratios calculated. For example, if either the relative survival benefit of CCU care declined with age or older patients 'saved' with a CCU had higher annual excess mortality associated with their MI than younger patients, then the resulting CE ratios for the very elderly would be significantly higher than those reported by Tosteson. Additionally, the assumption that index hospitalization costs will not increase in the elderly and the omission of long-term costs from the analysis will again underestimate the cost-effectiveness ratios in all patients.

Thrombolytics

There is consistent empirical evidence that thrombolytic therapy significantly reduces acute MI mortality in all aged patients.[83] The Global Utilization of Streptokinase and Tissue Plasminogen Activator for Occluded Coronary Arteries (GUSTO) trial found that a newer thrombolytic regimen, accelerated tissue plasminogen activator (t-PA), saved more lives than an older drug, streptokinase.[54] As the absolute difference in mortality between these two competing treatments was small and the cost difference was large, Mark and colleagues investigated the cost effectiveness of these two thrombolytic strategies.[72] Their study based its baseline and 1-year clinical outcomes measures on the 41 021-patient GUSTO study database and modeled long-term outcomes using the Duke Database.[96] Resource utilization data were collected for the initial hospitalization on all 23 105 US patients and up to 1-year follow-up on a random sample of 2600 US patients.

Mark found that the cost effectiveness of accelerated t-PA versus streptokinase varied greatly depending upon MI location and the patient's age (see Table 29.4). In patients with an anterior MI, the cost per year of life saved was $123 609 for patients under 40 but only $13 410 in patients over 75 years. For patients with an inferior MI, the cost per year of life saved was $203 071 for patients 40 years or under but only $16 246 in patients over 75 years of age. Like the Tosteson study, the Mark study found that CE ratios decreased with increasing patient age. However, his study did not detect an age threshold (i.e. ≥75 years) above which the CE ratios rose again. The major factor accounting for this inverse relationship between advancing age and declining CE ratios was the incremental effectiveness of t-PA versus streptokinase. The incremental life years added by t-PA over streptokinase increased with increasing patient age (from 0.04 years in anterior MI patients under age 40 years to 0.29 in those aged ≥75 years).

While all major event data were age-adjusted (and based on actual event data), health-care costs were only partially age-adjusted. Specifically, this study used trial event data to age-adjust the frequency of economically important events (such as need for

Patient subgroup	Cost-effectiveness RATIO ($)
Inferior MI, ≤40 years	203 071
Anterior MI, ≤40 years	123 609
Inferior MI, 41–60 years	74 816
Anterior MI, 41–60 years	49 877
Inferior MI, 61–75 years	27 873
Anterior MI, 61–75 years	20 601
Inferior MI, >75 years	16 246
Anterior MI, >75 years	13 410

Table 29.4
Cost effectiveness of t-PA versus streptokinase by age groups[72]

bypass surgery), but they did not adjust the estimated costs of these events by patient age (e.g. assumed similar bypass surgery costs in young and old). Additionally, this study did not include annual follow-up costs after the first year. While these additional cost adjustments would not have changed the results of the primary treatment comparisons, they would have marginally increased the cost-effectiveness ratios for the elderly.

Finally, while Mark did not report a 'J-shaped inflection point' in the CE ratios, recently published data from this trial indicate that one may exist. Reanalyzing the GUSTO database, White and colleagues reported that the survival advantage of tPA over streptokinase may actually reverse in those aged over 80 years.[55] While the study was limited due to a low number of observations in the very aged ($N = 440$), they found that tPA treatment risks (e.g. stroke) in the very elderly were very high, and may indicate that streptokinase could be a dominant strategy (less expensive, more efficacious) in the very old.[55]

Coronary angiography

The use of coronary angiography in the post-MI period has been the subject of intense investigation because of its role as a gate-keeper for more expensive revascularization procedures and because of the extreme and unexplained geographic variation in its use.[47,97–99] These findings were the impetus for Kuntz and colleagues to investigate the cost effectiveness of coronary angiography versus conservative medical care for post-MI patients.[86] Their study used a variety of sources including pooled randomized clinical trials and observational studies. In-hospital costs were derived by subgroup analysis from the 1987 Medicare claims files. Quality of life

information came from a survey of 1051 patients with recent MI.[69]

Kuntz and colleagues found that the routine coronary angiography strategy was cost effective for patients with mild post-infarction angina and a positive stress test or for patients with a prior MI. Conversely, the routine coronary angiography strategy was decidedly cost ineffective for patients with a negative stress test and no prior MI. Within most categories of patients, Kuntz found a J-shaped effect of age on relative CE ratios. The inflection point varied considerably in their analysis depending on the subgroup studied, but it occurred at a consistently lower age in men than women.

Kuntz and colleagues appeared to have age-adjusted the decision model's probabilities for the number of diseased vessels, procedure-related mortality, long-term survival and subsequent MI and revascularization. However, they failed to age-adjust costs for patients under 65. Additionally, follow-up costs were assigned based upon the initial treatment strategy without adjusting for patient age. Finally, quality of life data were based on anginal status and were not age-adjusted (to reflect the impact of comorbid disease in the elderly). The combined impact of the above factors would most likely underestimate the cost-effective ratios in the elderly relative to the young.

Angiotensin-converting enzyme inhibitor

The use of angiotensin-converting enzyme (ACE) inhibitor therapy has been shown to increase life expectancy of patients with congestive heart failure.[100–102] However, as these medicines are relatively costly, Tsevat and colleagues investigated the cost-effectiveness of ACE inhibitor therapy versus placebo for acute MI survivors.[87] This study used data from the Survival and Ventricular Enlargement (SAVE) clinical trial (N = 2231).[103] Resource utilization and cost data came from a small single institution patient cohort (N = 123) and patient utilities were assessed in an additional 82 patients.

These authors found that the cost effectiveness of captopril therapy varied significantly depending upon the patient's age. Assuming that the survival benefit associated with captopril therapy persisted beyond the 4-year experience of the SAVE trial, the cost per year of life saved was $10 400 for 50 year olds but only $5600 in 60 year olds, $4300 in 70 year olds, and $3700 in 80 year olds. When it was assumed that the survival benefit of captopril did not persist beyond 4 years, the cost per year of life saved was increased to $60 800 for 50 year olds, $9000 for 60 year olds, $4900 for 70 year olds, and $3600 for 80 year olds. Of note, Tsevat did not find an upper age limit where the cost effectiveness ratios for ACE inhibitor therapy began to rise.

These researchers age-adjusted all-cause mortality for the first 4 years based on their clinical trial data; with mortality after 4 years being extrapolated from life-tables and the Coronary Heart Disease Policy Model.[104] These estimates demonstrate that expected 4-year survival for the placebo-treated patients was highly correlated with patient age (ranging from 81.3% in 50 year olds to only 45.4% in 80 year olds). As a result, the absolute benefit of captopril therapy also rose with increasing patient age (with captopril adding 0.3 QALYs to a 50 year old's life and 0.9 to an 80 year old's relative to placebo). Regarding costs, Tsevat did not age-adjust most of their elements. Specifically, instead of calculating actual patient costs for an encounter, these researchers used DRG reimbursement as a cost surrogate without age-adjustment. They also assumed that the costs of outpatient tests were the same for all patients. Assuming that these cost elements increase with patient age, Tsevat's results may have mildly underestimated costs in the elderly. However, given the overwhelming cost effectiveness of captopril therapy, these corrections are unlikely to alter the overall economic attractiveness of this drug in the very elderly.

Beta-adrenergic antagonists

Although the long-term use of beta-adrenergic antagonists has been shown to reduce the rates of mortality and recurrent MI in acute MI survivors,[105,106] questions have been raised about their routine use in low-risk patients.[107,108] Goldman and colleagues investigated the cost-effectiveness of routine beta-blocker therapy in MI survivors of different ages and risk groups.[109] The expected 15-year risk for cardiac mortality for various age- and risk-groups was based loosely on clinical trials data and expert opinion. Overall efficacy of beta-blockers came from a pooled analysis of randomized clinical trials. Annual drug costs were estimated from a telephone survey of 10 retail pharmacy stores.

These authors found that beta-blocker therapy was cost-effective in all MI patient categories investigated. They also found that cost effectiveness varied depending upon the patient's risk group but was generally insensitive to patient age. For example, in their base-case analysis, the cost per year of life saved was approximately $13 000 for low-risk MI patients, $3600 for medium-risk patients and $2400 in high-risk patients. Patients aged between 45 and 65 had nearly identical results. Goldman did not investigate the cost-effectiveness of this agent in patients over age 65 years.

In his model, Goldman age-adjusted non-cardiac mortality for years 1–15 of his study and all-cause mortality after 15 years using US annual mortality rates. However, they did not age-adjust cardiac mortality in years 1–15. They assumed that the survival benefit of beta-blocker therapy varied only by risk group and the number of years since infarction, but not by age. Thus, their model assumed an age-constant annual cardiac mortality rate. Similarly, their model assumed that the relative reduction in annual mortality afforded by beta-blocker administration was constant regardless of patient age and risk group. In terms of their economic analysis, the only cost considered was medication costs ($208 per year). In order to simplify their analysis, the authors assumed that other medical and surgical costs in follow-up would be the same for patients receiving beta-blockers or those receiving placebo. This assumption is highly conservative, as several studies have reported that beta-blockers can reduce nonfatal ischemic events by up to 25%.[105,106] Thus, the inclusion of the cost savings from averted cardiac events could easily change beta-blockers into a dominant strategy (both more effective and less costly) in older patients (given the higher event rates in this age-group). Thus, even though the Goldman analysis may have underestimated the economic value of beta-blocking drugs, these agents appear to be quite cost effective, if not cost saving, in the very elderly.

Implantable cardioverter-defibrillator

Although implantable cardioverter-defibrillator (ICD) devices have been shown to increase life expectancy in survivors of cardiac arrest,[110] they are quite costly. Larsen and colleagues investigated the cost-effectiveness of ICD versus amiodarone and conventional anti-arrhythmic drug therapy in patients with recurrent sustained ventricular tachycardia or fibrillation (VT/VF) refractory to conventional drug therapy.[89] This study used clinical data from pooled analyses of the literature and expert judgment with cost data collected for 21 ICD patients and 43 amiodarone patients at a single site. Costs for conventional anti-arrhythmic therapy were assumed to be similar to those for amiodarone patients. These authors found that the ICD strategy was cost effective versus the other two strategies in all patient age groups studied. However, they found that the cost-effectiveness ratios tended to rise with increasing patient age. Specifically, the cost per year of life saved for ICD versus amiodarone increased from $27 561 for 45 year olds, and $29 244 for 55 year olds, to $32 674 for 65 year olds. The analysis did not have data with which to examine CE ratios for patients beyond age 65 years.

While Larsen used age-related mortality rates from US life tables to supplement the trials-based treatment-specific mortality rates, he did not specifically age-adjust these treatment-related mortality rates. The results demonstrated a minor decline in life expectancy with advancing age. For example, the average discounted marginal gain in life expectancy offered by amiodarone versus conventional therapy ranged from 1.4 years in 45 years old to 1.2 years in 65 year olds. Similarly, the marginal gain in life expectancy for ICD versus amiodarone therapy ranged from 2.5 years in 45 year olds to 1.8 years in 65 year olds. On the resource use side, costs for each strategy were not age-adjusted. Additionally, the authors used marginal rather than total hospital costs in their analyses. This method of cost measurement may underestimate the actual differences in resource use when patients are shifted from one therapy to another.[62,111] This study appears to demonstrate that the cost effectiveness of more aggressive forms of anti-arrhythmia therapy rises marginally with advancing patient age. However, the study lacked data to determine the precise impact of age on these therapies' cost effectiveness or if the therapies were cost effective in the very elderly.

Summary of cardiovascular CE analyses in the elderly

Certain summary statements can be drawn from the available literature on the effect of age on the cost effectiveness of cardiovascular therapy. The most prominent finding may actually be most notable for what is not known rather than for what has been reported. Specifically, as the very aged are often excluded from cardiovascular clinical trials, there exists a marked paucity of information regarding the efficacy of many treatments in these patients. For example, all the major bypass surgery versus medical therapy trials[81,112–114] excluded those over age 65 years. Of the 4645 patients enrolled in the percutaneous coronary angioplasty versus bypass surgery trials, less than 5% were aged 75 years or older.[115–119] Within the field of secondary prevention, the 4S, WOSCOPS and CARE studies all excluded those over age 75 years.[120–122] In fact, Gurwitz and colleagues have found that over 65% of all published cardiovascular drug trials had specific age exclusions.[123] Even when the very elderly are included, the trials often lack sufficient numbers of these patients from which to calculate stable estimates of treatment or cost outcomes. Thus, for many current cardiovascular therapies, we lack the fundamental knowledge of whether they are effective in the very elderly, let alone whether they are cost effective.

Given this knowledge deficit, we must draw preliminary conclusions from the few studies that have had sufficient data on elderly outcomes. While multiple theoretical reasons may lead one to believe that the cost effectiveness of most therapies would worsen with age (Figure 29.2), we have found the opposite to be true. Specifically, most published cardiovascular cost-effectiveness studies actually demonstrate that most therapies' CE ratios tend to decline with advancing age (Figure 29.3). This paradoxical finding of a relative improvement in therapeutic cost effectiveness with advancing age is driven by a high baseline event rate in the aged cardiac patient. This high event rate leads to higher absolute therapeutic benefits (see 'Cost-effectiveness analysis in the elderly') and thus, declining CE ratios in the very elderly.

We have also seen that this relationship between age and cost effectiveness may often be best characterized as a J-shaped curve. Specifically, for many therapies, there exists an age beyond which the acute risks (and costs) of intervention rise more quickly than its long-term benefits. At this point, the effectiveness (and subsequently, the cost effectiveness) of the therapy begins to decline. For the limited conditions for which CE data exist (Figure 29.3), this inflection point often comes around the age of 75–80 years.

Conclusions

We are currently witnessing two major changes in health care which are on a collision course with one another: the aging of our population and the need to control health-care spending. As we have shown, the elderly make up an ever-increasing majority of all cardiac patients treated in this country. As such, they tend to consume a high percentage of all health-care resources and they have become a prime target for those looking for ways to reduce health-care spending. This situation appears to be exacerbated by the lack of

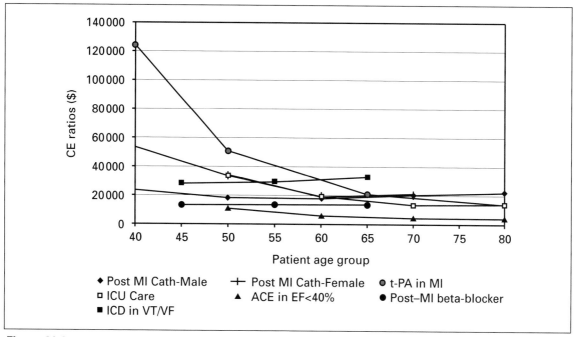

Figure 29.3
Relative cost effectiveness of CV therapies in young and old patients

empirical data ascertaining the effectiveness of cardiac care in the very aged. While many have presumed that aggressive cardiac care strategies would be less cost effective in the very aged, this presumption has not been demonstrated in the limited publications available on this topic. However, more data regarding the effectiveness of most cardiac therapies in the very aged patient are clearly needed. In the current age of financial accountability in medicine, we believe that the best method of preventing future rationing of cardiac care in the elderly is to prove its worth now.

References

1. American Heart Association: Heart and Stroke 1997 Statistical Update. *http://www.amhrt.org* (1997)

2. Roper WL, Koplan JP, Speers MA et al. Cardiovascular disease surveillance, ischemic heart disease, 1980–1989. *Centers for Disease Control and Prevention* (1993).

3. Graves EJ. Detailed diagnoses and procedures, National Hospital Discharge Survey, 1989. *Vital Health Stat 13* (1991) **108**:1–236.

4. Kapantais G, Powell-Griner E. Characteristics of persons dying of disease of heart: preliminary data from the 1986 National Mortality Followback Survey. *Vital Health Stat* (1989) **172**.

5. US Department of Commerce. Current Population Reports Special Studies P23–178. In: Anonymous, *Sixty-Five plus in America* (US Government Printing Office: Washington, DC, 1992).

6. US Senate Special Committee on Aging. *Aging America. Trend and Projections 1991* (US Government Printing Office: Washington, DC, 1991).

7. Leidl R. Effects of population aging on health care, expenditure, and financing: some illustrations. In: Callahan D, ter Meulen RHJ, Topinkova E, eds, *A World Growing Old: The Coming Health Care Challenges. Hasting Center Studies in Ethics* (Georgetown University Press: Washington, DC, 1995).

8. Callahan D. Old age and new policy. *JAMA* (1989) **261**:905–6.

9. Chelluri L, Grenvik A, Silverman M. Intensive care for critically ill elderly: mortality, costs and quality of life: review of the literature. *Arch Intern Med* (1995) **155**:1013–22.

10. Callahan D. *Setting Limits* (The Hastings Center: Briarcliff Manor, NY, 1988).

11. Callahan D. Must the old and young compete for health care resources? *Neurosurgery* (1990) **27**:160–4.

12. Callahan D. Adequate health care and an aging society: are they morally compatible? *Daedalus* (1986) **Winter**:246–7.

13. Veatch RM. Justice and the economics of terminal illness. *Hastings Cent Rep* (1988) **18**: 34–40.

14. Daniels N. Is rationing by age ever morally acceptable? *Bus Health* (1984) **1**:29–32.

15. Lewis PA, Charny M. Which of two individuals do you treat when only their ages are different and you can't treat both? *J Med Ethics* (1989) **15**:28–32.

16. Levit KR, Lazenby HC, Sivaranjan L et al. National health expenditures, 1994. *Health Care Financing Rev* (1996) **17**:205–42.

17. Gradison B. National health care and the elderly. *J Am Coll Cardiol* (1987) **10** (Suppl): 10A–13A.

18. Mark DB. Medical economics and health policy issues for interventional cardiology. In Topol EJ, ed., *Textbook of Interventional Cardiology* (W.B. Saunders: Philadelphia, 1993) 1323–53.

19. Evans RW. Health care technology and the inevitability of resource allocation and rationing decisions. *JAMA* (1983) **249**: 2047–53; 2208–19.

20. Mark DB. Economics of acute myocardial infarction. In Califf RM, ed., *Acute Myocardial Infarction and Other Ischemic Syndromes* (Current Medicine: Philadelphia, 1996) 15.1–15.15.

21. Becker ER, Morris DC. The changing socioeconomic environment for coronary artery disease. In: Talley JD, Mauldin PD, Becker ER, eds, *Cost Effective Diagnostic and Treatment of Coronary Artery Disease* (Williams & Wilkins: Baltimore, 1997).

22. US Congressional Budget Office. *Trends in Health Spending: An Update* (US Government Printing Office: Washington, DC, 1993).

23. Wennberg JE, Freeman JL, Culp WJ. Are hospital services rationed in New Haven or over-utilised in Boston? *Lancet* (1987) **i**:1185–9.

24. Wennberg JE, Freeman JL, Shelton RM, Bubolz TA. Hospital use and mortality among Medicare beneficiaries in Boston and

New Haven. *N Engl J Med* (1989) **323**:1168–73.

25. Dustan HP, Hamilton MP, McCullogh L, Page LB. Sociopolitical and ethical considerations in the treatment of cardiovascular disease in the elderly. *J Am Coll Cardiol* (1987) **10** (Suppl):14–17A.

26. Ginzberg E. The high cost of dying. *Inquiry* (1980) **17**:293–5.

27. Lubitz JD, Prihoda R. The use and costs of Medicare services in the last 2 years of life. *Health Care Financing Rev* (1984) **5**:117–31.

28. Scitovsky AA. 'The high cost of dying' revisited. *Milbank Q* (1994) **72**:561–91.

29. Furman S, Stead EA Jr, Swan HJC, Zaret BL. Application of high technology in the diagnosis and treatment of the elderly. *J Am Coll Cardiol* (1987) **10** (Suppl):22–24A.

30. Lamm RD. Speech before Colorado Health Lawyers' Association. *Denver Post* (1984) March 17.

31. Callahan D. *Setting Limits: Medical Goals in Aging Society* (Simon and Schuster, New York, 1987).

32. Avorn J. Benefit and cost analysis in geriatric care turning age discrimination into health policy. *N Engl J Med* (1984) **310**:1294–1301.

33. Finkler SA. The distinction between cost and charges. *Ann Intern Med* (1982) **96**: 102–9.

34. Lave JR, Pashos CL, Anderson GF et al. Costing medical care: using Medicare administrative data. *Medical Care* (1994) **32**:JS77–JS89.

35. Task Force on Principles for Economic Analysis of Health Care Technology. Economic analysis of health care technology. *Ann Intern Med* (1995) **122**:61–70.

36. Weinstein MC, Siegel JE, Gold MR et al for the Panel on Cost-Effectiveness in Health and Medicine. Recommendations of the panel on cost-effectiveness in health and medicine. *JAMA* (1996) **276**:1253–8.

37. Gold MR, Siegel JE, Russell LB et al. *Cost-effectiveness in Health and Medicine* (Oxford University Press: New York, 1996).

38. Hlatky MA, Rogers WJ, Johnstone I et al for the BARI Investigators. Medical care costs and quality of life after randomization to coronary angioplasty or coronary bypass surgery. *N Engl J Med* (1997) **336**:92–9.

39. Weintraub WS, Mauldin PD, Becker E et al. A comparison of the costs of and quality of life after coronary angioplasty or coronary surgery for multivessel coronary artery disease. Results from the Emory Angioplasty Versus Surgery Trial (EAST). *Circulation* (1995) **92**:2831–40.

40. Mark DB, Peterson ED. The health economics of acute coronary syndromes. *J Thrombosis Thrombolysis* (1998) **5**:S155–62.

41. Mauldin PD, Weinbtraub WS, Becker ER. Predicting hospital costs for first-time coronary artery bypass grafting from preoperative and postoperative variables. *Am J Cardiol* (1994) **74**:772–5.

42. Eisenstein EL, Newby LK, Knight JD et al. Regional variations in treatment costs and resource utilization for uncomplicated acute myocardial infarction (UMI). The 45th Annual Scientific Session of the American College of Cardiology. *J Am Coll Cardiol* (1996) **27**:330A (abst).

43. Cassak D, Columbia HCA. Why size matters. In vivo. *The Business and Medicine Report Windhover Information Inc* (1997) **15**:41–54.

44. Peterson ED, Jollis JG, Stafford JA et al. Post-MI testing in the elderly: results in 190 135 patients. *J Am Coll Cardiol* (1997) **29**: 362A.

45. Gillum RF. Epidemiology of heart failure in the United States. *Am Heart J* (1993) **126**: 1042–7.

46. Pashos CL, Newhouse JP, McNeil BJ. Temporal changes in the care and outcomes of elderly patients with acute myocardial infarction, 1987 through 1990. *JAMA* (1993) **270**: 1832–6.

47. Udvarheyli S, Gatsonis C, Epstein AM et al. Acute myocardial infarction in the Medicare population: Process of care and clinical outcomes. *JAMA* (1992) **268**:2530–6.

48. Peterson ED, Cowper PA, Jollis JG et al. Coronary artery bypass surgery in octogenarians: results in 24 461 patients. *Circulation* (1995) **92** (Suppl II):74–80.

49. Mark DB, Outcomes Research and Assessment Group. Implications of cost in treatment selection for patients with coronary heart disease. *Ann Thorac Surg* (1996) **61**:S12–15.

50. Krumholz HM, Chen J, Murillo JE et al. Clinical correlates of in-hospital costs for acute myocardial infarction in patients 65 years of age and older. *Am Heart J* (1998) **135**:523–31.

51. Hamel MB, Phillips RS, Teno JM et al for the SUPPORT Investigators. Seriously ill hospitalized adults: do you spend less on older patients? *J Am Geriatr Soc* (1996) **44**:1043–8.

52. Gurwitz JH, Osganian V, Goldberg RJ et al. Diagnostic testing in acute myocardial infarction: does patient age influence utilization patterns? The Worcester Heart Attack Study. *Am J Epidemiol* (1991) **134**:948–57.

53. Bearden DM, Allman RM, Sundarum SV et al. Age-related variability in the use of cardiovascular imaging procedures. *J Am Geriatr Soc* (1993) **41**:1075–82.

54. The GUSTO Investigators. An international randomized trial comparing four thrombolytic strategies for acute myocardial infarction. *N Engl J Med* (1993) **329**:673–82.

55. White HD, Barbash GI, Califf RM et al. Age and outcome with contemporary thrombolytic therapy. Results from the GUSTO-I Trial. *Circulation* (1996) **94**:1826–33.

56. Smith LR, Milano CA, Molter BS et al. Preoperative determinants of postoperative costs associated with coronary artery bypass graft surgery. *Circulation* (1994) **90** (Suppl II): 124–8.

57. Cowper PA, DeLong ER, Peterson ED et al. Potential for cost savings in high cost coronary artery bypass surgery patients: a New York State analysis. *J Am Coll Cardiol* (1996) **27**:371A.

58. Heidenreich PA, Chou TM, Amidon TM et al. Impact of the operating physician on costs of percutaneous transluminal coronary angioplasty. *Am J Cardiol* (1996) **77**:1169–73.

59. Cowper PA, Peterson ED, DeLong ER et al. Impact of early discharge following coronary artery bypass surgery on rates of readmission and death. *J Am Coll Cardiol* (1997) **30**: 908–13.

60. Jollis JG, Bebchuk JD, Peterson ED et al. Repeat revascularization following coronary artery bypass surgery and coronary angioplasty in patients over age 65 in the United States. *J Am Coll Cardiol* (1994) Supplement I:433A (abst).

61. Balas EA, Kretschmer RAC, Gnann W et al. Interpreting cost analyses of clinical interventions. *JAMA* (1998) **279**:54–7.

62. Drummond MF, Stoddard GL, Torrance GW: *Methods for the Economic Evaluation of Health Care Programmes* (Oxford University Press: Oxford, 1987).

63. Weinstein MC, Stason WB. Foundations of cost-effectiveness analysis for health and medical practices. *N Engl J Med* (1977) **296**: 716–24.

64. Mishan EJ. *Cost-benefit Analysis* (Praeger: New York, 1976).

65. Dunlop DW. Benefit-cost analysis: a review of its applicability in policy analysis for delivering health services. *Soc Sci Med* (1975) **9**:133–9.

66. Pliskin N, Taylor AK. General principles: cost-benefit and decision analysis. In: Bunker JP, Barnes BA, Mosteller F, eds, *Costs, Risks, and Benefits of Surgery* (Oxford University Press: New York, 1977) 5–27.

67. Landefeld JS, Seskin EP. The economic value of life: linking theory to practice. *Am J Public Health* (1982) **72**:555–66.

68. Sackett DL, Torrance GW. The utility of different health states as perceived by the general public. *J Chronic Dis* (1978) **7**: 347–58.

69. Torrance GW. Measurement of health state utilities for economic appraisal: a review. *J Health Econ* (1986) **5**:1–30.

70. Kaplan RM, Bush JW. Health-related quality of life measurement for evaluation research and policy analysis. *Health Psychol* (1981) **1**:61–80.

71. Laupacis A, Feeny D, Detsky AS, Tugwell PX. How attractive does a new technology have to be to warrant adoption and utilization? Tentative guidelines for using clinical and economic evaluations. *Can Med Assoc J* (1992) **146**:473–81.

72. Mark DB, Hlatky MA, Califf RM et al. Cost effectiveness of thrombolytic therapy with tissue plasminogen activator as compared with streptokinase for acute myocardial infarction. *N Engl J Med* (1995) **332**:1418–24.

73. Baltussen R, Leidl R, Ament A. The impact of age on cost-effectiveness ratios and its control in decision making. *Health Econ* (1996) **5**: 227–39.

74. Welch HG. Comparing apples and oranges: does cost-effectiveness analysis deal fairly with the old and young? *Gerontologist* (1991) **31**:332–6.

75. Ubel PA, Lowenstein G, Scanlon D et al. Individual utilities are inconsistent with rationing choices: a partial explanation of why Oregon's cost-effectiveness list failed. *Med Decis Making* (1996) **16**:108–116.

76. Alexander KP, Peterson ED. Coronary artery bypass grafting in the elderly. *Am Heart J* (1997) **134**:856–63.

77. Rowe JW. Health care of the elderly. *N Engl J Med* (1985) **312**:827–35.

78. Lakatta EG, Mitchell JH, Pomerance A, Rowe GG. Human aging: changes in structure and function. *J Am Coll Cardiol* (1987) **10**:42–7A.

79. Batchelor W, Peterson ED, Muhlbaier LH et al. Percutaneous interventional outcomes in octogenarians: insights from the National Cardiovascular Network. *Circulation* (1997) **29**:1–10.

80. US Bureau of the Census: 1990 Census of Population, Series CPH-L-74. In: *Modified and Actual Age, Sex, Race and Hispanic Origin Data.* (US Government Printing Office: Washington, DC, 1990).

81. Yusuf S, Zucker D, Peduzzi P et al. Effect of coronary artery bypass graft surgery on survival: overview of 10-year results from randomised trials by the Coronary Artery Bypass Graft Surgery Trialists Collaboration. *Lancet* (1994) **344**:563–70.

82. Jones RH. In search of the optimal surgical mortality. *Circulation* (1989) **79** (Suppl I): 123–36.

83. FTT (Fibrinolytic Therapy Trialists' Collaborative Group). Indications for fibrinolytic therapy in suspected acute myocardial infarction: collaborative overview of early mortality and major morbidity results from all randomised trials of more than 1000 patients. *Lancet* (1994) **343**:311–22.

84. Doubilet P, Weinstein MC, McNeil BL. Use and misuse of the term 'cost effective' in medicine. *J Clin Epidemiol* (1986) **46**:261–71.

85. Tosteson AN, Goldman L, Udvarhelyi S, Lee TH: Cost-effectiveness of a coronary care unit versus an intermediate care unit for emergency department patients with chest pain. *Circulation* (1996) **94**:143–50.

86. Kuntz KM, Tsevat J, Goldman L, Weinstein MC. Cost-effectiveness of routine coronary angiography after acute myocardial infarction. *Circulation* (1996) **94**:957–65.

87. Tsevat J, Duke D, Goldman L et al. Cost-effectiveness of captopril therapy after myocardial infarction. *J Am Coll Cardiol* (1995) **26**:914–19.

88. Goldman L, Sia B, Cook F et al. Costs and effectiveness of routine therapy with long-term beta-adrenergic antagonists after acute myocardial infarction. *N Engl J Med* (1988) **319**:152–7.

89. Larsen GC, Manolis AS, Sonnenberg FA et al. Cost-effectiveness of the implantable cardioverter-defibrillator: effect of improved battery life and comparison with amiodarone therapy. *J Am Coll Cardiol* (1992) **19**: 1323–34.

90. Day HW. An intensive coronary care area. *Dis Chest* (1963) **44**:423–7.

91. Hilberman M. Cost savings at the end of life. *N Engl J Med* (1994) **331**:477–8.

92. Koch EB, Reiser SJ: Critical care: Historical development and ethical consideration. In: Fein IA, Strosberg MA, eds, *Managing the Clinical Care Unit* (Aspen Publishers: Rockville, 1987) 3–20.

93. Reiser SJ. The intensive care unit: the unfolding and ambiguities of survival therapy. *Int J Technol Assess Health Care* (1992) **8**:382–94.

94. Lee TH, Rouan G, Weisberg MC et al. Clinical characteristics and natural history of patients with acute myocardial infaction sent home from the emergency room. *Am J Cardiol* (1987) **60**:219–24.

95. Udvarhelyi IS, Goldman L, Konaroff AL, Lee TH. Determinants of resource utilization for patients admitted for evaluation of acute chest pain. *J Gen Intern Med* (1992) **7**: 1–10.

96. Mark DB, Nelson CL, Califf RM et al. Continuing evolution of therapy for coronary artery disease: initial results from the era of coronary angioplasty. *Circulation* (1994) **89**:2015–25.

97. Pilote L, Califf RM, Sapp S et al. Regional variations across the United States in the management of acute myocardial infarction. *N Engl J Med* (1995) **333**:565–72.

98. Guadagnoli E, Hauptman PJ, Ayanian JZ et al. Variation in the use of cardiac procedures after acute myocardial infarction. *N Engl J Med* (1995) **333**:573–8.

99. Wennberg DE, Kellett MA, Dickens JD et al. The association between local diagnostic testing intensity and invasive cardiac procedures. *JAMA* (1996) **275**:1161–4.

100. The CONSENUS Trial Study Group. Effects of enalapril on mortality in severe congestive heart failure: results of the Cooperative North Scandinavia Enalapril Survival Study (CONSENSUS). *N Engl J Med* (1987) **316**:1429–35.

101. Pfeffer MA, Braunwald E, Moya LA: Effect of captopril on mortality and morbidity in patients with left ventricular dysfunction after myocardial infarction: results of the Survival and Ventricular Enlargement trial. *N Engl J Med* (1992) **327**:669–77.

102. The SOLVD Investigators. Effect of enalapril on mortality and the development of heart failure in asymptomatic patients with reduced left ventricular ejection fractions. *N Engl J Med* (1992) **327**:685–91.

103. Pfeffer MA, Braunwald E, Moye LA et al. On behalf of the SAVE Investigators. Effect of captopril on mortality and morbidity in patients with left ventricular dysfunction after myocardial infarction. *N Engl J Med* (1992) **327**:669–77.

104. Weinstein MC, Coxson PG, Williams LW et al. Forecasting coronary heart disease incidence, mortality, and cost: the Coronary Heart Disease Policy Model. *Am J Public Health* (1987) **77**:1417–26.

105. Beta-blocker Heart Attack Trial Research Group. A randomized trial of propranolol in patients with acute myocardial infarction. II. Morbidity results. *JAMA* (1983) **250**:2814–19.

106. Yusuf S, Peto R, Lewis J et al. Beta blockade during and after myocardial infarction: an overview of the randomized trials. *Prog Cardiovasc Dis* (1985) **27**:335–71.

107. Fishman WH, Furberg CD, Friedewald WT. The use of β-adrenergic blocking drugs in patients with myocardial infarction. *Curr Probl Cardiol* (1984) **9**:1–50.

108. O'Rourke RA. Clinical decisions for post-myocardial infarction patients. *Mod Concepts Cardiovasc Dis* (1986) **55**:55–60.

109. Tsevat J, Goldman L, Soukup JR. Stability of time-tradeoff utilities in survivors of myocardial infarction. *Med Decis Making* (1993) **13**:161–5.

110. Winkle RA, Thomas A. The automatic implantable cardioverter defibrillator: the US experience. In: Brugada P, Wellens HJJ, eds, *Where To Go From Here?* (Futura: Mount Kisco, NY, 1987) 663–80.

111. Eisenberg JM. Clinical economics: a guide to the economic analysis of clinical practices. *JAMA* (1989) **262**:2879–86.

112. CASS Principal Investigators and their Associates: Coronary artery surgery study (CASS): a randomized trial of coronary artery bypass surgery survival data. *Circulation* (1983) **68**:939–50.

113. Detre K, Hultgren H, Takaro T. Veterans Administration Cooperative Study of Surgery for Coronary Arterial Occlusive Disease. III. Methods and baseline characteristics, including experience with medical treatment. *Am J Cardiol* (1977) **40**:212–25.

114. Varnauskas E and the European Coronary Surgery Study Group. Twelve-year follow-up of survival in the randomized European coronary surgery study. *N Engl J Med* (1988) **319**:332–7.

115. CABRI Trial Participants. First-year results of CABRI (coronary angioplasty versus bypass revascularization investigation). *Lancet* (1995) **346**:1179–84.

116. Hamm CW, Reimers J, Ischinger T et al for the German Angioplasty Bypass Surgery Investigation. A randomized study of coronary angioplasty compared with bypass surgery in patients with symptomatic multivessel coronary disease. *N Engl J Med* (1994) **331**: 1037–43.

117. King SB, Lembo NJ, Weintraub WS et al for the Emory Angioplasty versus Surgery Trial (EAST). A randomized trial comparing coronary angioplasty with coronary bypass surgery. *N Engl J Med* (1994) **331**:1044–50.

118. RITA Trial Participants. Coronary angioplasty versus coronary artery bypass surgery: the randomized intervention treatment of angina (RITA) trial. *Lancet* (1993) **341**: 573–80.

119. The Bypass Angioplasty Revascularization Investigation (BARI) Investigators. Compari-

son of coronary bypass surgery with angioplasty in patients with multivessel disease. *N Engl J Med* (1994) **331**:496–501.

120. Miettinen TA, Pyorala K, Olsson AG et al for the Scandinavian Simvastatin Study Group. Cholesterol-lowering therapy in women and elderly patients with myocardial infarction or angina pectoris. *Circulation* (1997) **96:** 4211–18.

121. Sacks FM, Pfeffer MA, Moye LA et al for the CARE Investigators. The effect of pravastatin on coronary events after myocardial infarction in patients with average cholesterol levels. *N Engl J Med* (1996) **335**:1001–9.

122 Shepherd J, Cobbe SM, Ford I et al for the West of Scotland Coronary Prevention Study Group. Prevention of coronary heart disease with pravastatin in men with hypercholesterolemia. *N Engl J Med* (1995) **333**:1301–7.

123. Gurwitz JH, Col NF, Avorn J. The exclusion of the elderly and women from clinical trials in acute myocardial infarction. *JAMA* (1992) **268**:1417–22.

124. Johannesson M, Dahlof B, Lindholm LH et al. The cost-effectiveness of treating hypertension in elderly people: an analysis of the Swedish trial in old patients with hypertension (STOP Hypertension). *J Intern Med* (1993) **234**:317–23.

125. Weinstein MC, Stason WB. Cost-effectiveness of coronary artery bypass surgery. *Circulation* (1982) **66** (Suppl III):56–66.

126. Wong JB, Sonnenberg FA, Salem DN, Pauker SG. Myocardial revascularization for chronic stable angina. Analysis of the role of percutaneous transluminal coronary angioplasty based on data available in 1989. *Ann Intern Med* (1990) **113**:852–71.

127. Littenberg B, Garber AM, Sox HC. Screening for hypertension. *Ann Intern Med* (1990) **112**:192–202.

128. Lee TH, Fukui T, Weinstein MC et al. Cost-effectiveness of screening strategies for left main coronary artery disease in patients with stable angina. *Med Decis Making* (1988) **8:** 268–78.

129. Metropolitan Insurance Companies. Coronary artery bypass graphs: 1990 charges update. *Statistical Bull* (1972) **53**:17–24.

30

Cardiovascular care of the very aged patient in an era of managed care

Gottlieb C Friesinger and Joseph Francis

Introduction

Managed care in the United States is evolving rapidly, and presents the outside observer with a complex mosaic of administrative and clinical practices that show considerable regional variation. Octogenarians are a particularly complicated subset of the Medicare population. This chapter represents only a 'snapshot' of a huge moving picture. No attempt is made to be comprehensive but some background, general principles, and a few selected aspects pertinent to the very aged patient with cardiovascular problems will be cited. The glossary of terms provides some insight into the complexity and variability.

The recent growth of managed care has been in response to the remarkable escalation in health-care costs in all populations. Managed care as a concept has existed for a very long time but only in recent years have the practical implications been important in the Medicare population.[1-4]

For purposes of this discussion managed care will be defined as a system developed to control critical aspects of the delivery of care in a way that maintains or improves quality within a constrained resource base. Even within such a simple definition, a wide variety of features may exist (see Glossary). This definition requires implementing strategies that

provide maximum appropriate and effective care while balancing costs, access, satisfaction and quality. Early models of managed care included Kaiser Permanente in California, the Health Insurance Plan of Greater New York, and the Group Health Cooperative of Puget Sound. These plans employed physicians who provided comprehensive care for a fixed monthly fee, with the dual goals of controlling costs and providing high-quality services by coordinating all patient services including access to specialists. These early examples are staff model health maintenance organizations (HMO).

In 1965, the Federal Government guaranteed that older persons would have access to mainstream medical care by passing Medicare as an amendment to the Social Security Act. In 1973, Congress passed the Health Maintenance Organization Act that provided for the federal certification of a variety of managed-care interest entities including HMOs and independent practice associations (IPAs), that provided care to younger populations.

For its first 17 years, Medicare reimbursed only care that was provided according to its original intent, fee-for-service. In 1982, the Medicare-Risk Program was initiated under the Tax Equity and Fiscal Responsibility Act to allow older persons the option of enrolling in HMOs to receive their Medicare benefits.

This program provides a fixed capitation fee based on 95% of the local fee-for-service adjusted average per capita costs (AAPCC). In turn, the HMO has agreed to accept all financial risks associated with the care of the beneficiary. At present, 13% of the Medicare population is enrolled in HMO plans, and in mature managed-care markets (California, Arizona, Florida, Minnesota), the proportion in HMO plans may soon approach 50%. However, HMO market share falls off rapidly among Medicare beneficiaries over age 84.[5] Since the annual cost of the Medicare program now exceeds $200 billion dollars, it is clear that the current rate of increase for that program (10% annually) cannot be sustained. The 'baby boomers' will enormously accelerate all the medical issues related to aging and create further upward pressure on costs.

The Federal Balanced Budget Act (BBA) signed by President Clinton in August, 1997 was designed to slow the growth of Medicare spending particularly in hospital and home-health care, with fewer spending reductions directed toward physicians. In addition to reduced reimbursement, the BBA encourages enrolment in Medicare managed-care plans by expanding consumer options and setting a generous 'floor' capitation rate. New options include point-of-service plans (which allow out-of-network care for a higher out-of-pocket cost), private fee-for-service plans (patients can go to any physician they choose but the insurer will receive a capitated amount and must pay the difference in fee) and medical savings accounts (a government-funded high deductible insurance policy which will be used to pay for expensive care and a tax-free savings account to cover routine expenses). The effects of these changes will not be fully understood until the rules and regulations for implementation are written and a few years of data can be accumulated. Medicare funding will continue to increase substantially but the rate of spending will be slowed by an estimated $116 billion over a 5-year period.

With more than $1 trillion, 14% of the gross domestic product, committed to health care (and a large portion of that to care of the elderly), it is not surprising that many organizations, non-profit and for-profit, can qualify for the federally mandated requirements to offer a comprehensive list of benefits, comply with federal financial requirements, and still be 'profitable.'

Considerations on managed care and cardiovascular disease in octogenarians

Cardiovascular diseases are responsible for a majority of deaths in the Medicare population. More than 60% of acute myocardial infarctions occur in patients over the age of 65. Among octogenarians, mortality following acute myocardial infarction is at least 30%. The median age for patients with atrial fibrillation is 75 years. Congestive heart failure is the most common Diagnostic Related Group (DRG) in the Medicare population, with the mortality and hospitalization rates proportional to age. Systolic hypertension is common and almost exclusively found in the elderly population. Fifty percent of women will die of cardiovascular disease, most of them over the age of 65 years. Paralleling this burden of disease, there has been a dramatic increase in the use of procedures in the elderly, including octogenarians.[6–8]

The growth of the elderly population, the huge cardiovascular disease burden, and the rapidly increasing use of expensive technological procedures make it obvious that managed care is an appealing approach in the elderly. Payers who are anxious to control costs and those health-care providers and older patients who have a desire for an integrated care program, all see managed care as having the potential to provide quality service at an affordable cost.

The appeal of managed care has been blunted by concerns that quality might be compromised. The Institute of Medicine has proposed a widely accepted definition of quality 'the degree to which health services for individuals *and* populations increase the likelihood of desired health outcomes and are consistent with current professional knowledge.'[9] Including populations in the definition creates a tension for the physician. The considerations involved for treating/managing individual patients may have important implications in reference to cost and access if the treatment/management approach is extrapolated to the entire population that has the condition. Flexibility in the form of choice of physician, access to specialists, drug options and other features are matters of major importance to cardiovascular specialists and institutions delivering specialized cardiovascular care. These factors also influence patient satisfaction, but their impact on population outcomes is often unknown, and lack of standardization in clinical practices may create unnecessary increases in cost.

The overwhelming issue in many situations is the lack of data on outcomes related to a given management strategy. Discussion of quality issues is beyond the scope of this chapter but defining and measuring quality is the critical consideration. There is general agreement that mortality and morbidity are essential but insufficient measures and that the patient's perspective must be included in quality assessment.[10]

The general public and many physicians remain skeptical about the possibility of improving quality and access in managed-care arrangements, however, and believe cost containment is the only objective. Legislative and consumer actions (cited above) are producing pressures to ensure all three major objectives are served.[11-17] In 1998, the US Congress hotly debated a proposed consumer Bill of Rights for Healthcare (Table 30.1), whose provisions were applied to Medicare plans through an Executive Order signed by President Clinton.

The dramatic rate of increase in the use of highly technical expensive procedures in the Medicare population is attracting attention, in part because information concerning the incremental value beyond conventional therapy has been difficult to establish in many clinical situations. Randomized controlled trials of most therapies and procedures are not feasible in octogenarians because of the enormous heterogeneity of this older population and the circumstances under which care is given. Complex cardiovascular care is often rendered at multiple sites by multiple physicians with less than optimum coordination. In addition, quality of care must be judged more on quality of life issues rather than only mortality and complications.

A special problem exists in estimating the treatment benefits for cardiovascular disease in octogenarians because of the effect of competing risks.[18] Newly diagnosed or exacerbating cardiovascular disease may have much less effect on life expectancy because of the large number of competing risks—including advanced age per se—and increased the frequency of treatment-related adverse outcomes, including prolonged convalescence from complicated procedures such as coronary artery bypass graft surgery. Hence, the net benefit of interventions in octogenarians may be relatively small compared to younger cohorts.

Although physicians have tended to resist managed-care approaches, a recent survey of cardiovascular specialists shows a spectrum of

I. **Information disclosure.** Consumers have the right to receive accurate, easily understood information about their health plans, facilities and professionals to assist them in making informed health-care decisions.

II. **Choice of providers and plans.** Consumers have a right to a choice of health-care providers that is sufficient to assure access to appropriate high-quality health care.

III. **Access to emergency services.** Consumers have the right to access emergency health-care services when and where the need arises. Health plans should provide payment when a consumer presents to an emergency department with acute symptoms of sufficient severity – including severe pain – such that a 'prudent layperson' could reasonably expect the absence of medical attention to result in placing their health in serious jeopardy, serious impairment to bodily functions or serious dysfunction of any bodily organ or part.

IV. **Participation in treatment decisions.** Consumers have a right to fully participate in all decisions related to their medical care. Consumers who are unable to fully participate in treatment decisions have a right to be represented by parents, guardians, family members or other conservators.

V. **Respect and nondiscrimination.** Consumers have the right to considerate, respectful care from all members of the health-care industry at all times and under all circumstances. An environment of mutual respect is essential to maintain a quality health-care system.

Consumers must not be discriminated against in provision of health-care services based on race, ethnicity, national origin, religion, sex, age, current or anticipated mental or physical disability, sexual orientation, genetic information or source of payment.

VI. **Confidentiality of health information.** Consumers have the right to communicate with health-care providers in confidence and to have the confidentiality of their individually identifiable medical information protected. Consumers also have the right to review and copy their own medical records and request amendments to their records.

Source: President's Advisory Commission on Consumer Protection and Quality in the Health Care Industry, October 21, 1997.

Table 30.1
Consumer Bill of Rights and Responsibilities in Health Care

opinions about the implications of managed care.[19] Most responders voiced concern about interference with the patient–doctor relationship, constrictions on clinical decision-making, increased administrative burden and declining reimbursement as a result of involvement in managed care. There was particular objection to the role of the gatekeeper. However, nearly 90% of the cardiovascular specialty group sur-veyed had involvement with at least one managed-care organization (most had multiple) and involvement had substantially increased when compared with a similar survey in 1993. There was wide variation in the type (PPO, HMO, POS, etc.) of involvement depending on the practice group and age of the respondent. Strategies to adapt to the managed-care environment included forming networks, implementing continuous quality improvement concepts, and adopting clinical pathways especially by the larger cardiovascular specialist groups (those with nine or more physicians).

Overall, it can be assumed that managed care will increase rapidly in the Medicare population and cardiovascular specialists will be affected in important ways. Introducing standardization through clinical guidelines, provider feedback, and patient education (so-called demand management) will reduce the marked regional variation in rates of procedures and may reduce the number of cardiologists needed to deliver specialty care. The United States has an abundance of cardiologists: 6.75/100 000 population compared to 4.29/100 000 population in the industrial countries of Western Europe and Canada, which itself may be driving demand for specialized care. Physician manpower, including the ratio of primary-care providers to specialists, will be impacted by governmental as well as market-based mechanisms, although currently available information does not allow any realistic estimates in the potential decline in the use of cardiovascular services.

The US medical care delivery system is strongly focused on acute problems involving a single organ, yet octogenarians will frequently have multisystem disease and chronic complicating comorbidity. Cardiovascular specialty care provides major benefits and is essential in acute cardiovascular problems but often ignores and/or inadequately provides care that might prevent the acute crisis and/or restore optimal function after the acute episode has been effectively managed. In addition, the current and past rewards of our health-care system, in terms of both prestige and finance are disproportionately high for procedures and acute care while the goal of care in the octogenarian is frequently maintenance and restoration of function and preserving the best quality of life. Better coordination of care, simplicity of access to services (including physicians' offices and home health-care facilities) and a comprehensive range of benefits including necessary restorative and palliative care are theoretically possible under managed care and have been successfully provided in demonstration projects such as Medicare's Program of All-inclusive Care for the Elderly.[20]

Experience with managed care in the elderly population

Experience with managed care in the elderly population is limited, recent and evolving. Information obtained in managed-care systems in younger populations is not directly useful in assessing either the medical or the fiscal implications for the elderly. The heavy burden of comorbid conditions and the need for broad social and medical support make octogenarians fundamentally different from younger patients for whom the major focus is on health promotion, disease prevention or the management of a single condition.

Managed care is administratively and fiscally distinct for older Americans, for whom the Federal Government, via Medicare, is the major payer. Medicare benefits are relatively generous and, in the short term, continue to increase substantially despite recent efforts to slow the rate of rise. Medicare HMOs are more closely regulated than commercial HMOs and are not protected from corporate liability as are most employer-sponsored plans under ERISA (see Glossary). They allow disenrolment at any time rather than only at specified times as is true with commercial plans. They are 'retail marketing' rather than 'wholesale' since individual retirees, rather than employers select the plan in which they will participate. These fundamental differences make individual patient satisfaction a critical factor in the success of Medicare HMOs, and also create forces that exclude chronically ill patients from such plans.[21]

Few data are available regarding the impact of managed care on the processes and outcomes of cardiovascular services in older persons.[22–37] Existing information derives mostly from large-scale observational studies and uses imprecise and possibly inadequate measures of quality. Although randomized controlled trials comparing managed care with traditional service delivery would be preferred, such has not been done for a Medicare population nor is it practical given the enormous clinical heterogeneity found in the oldest old. Similarly, the evaluation of the same patients who transfer from an indemnity to a managed-care plan (or vice versa) can provide only limited comparative data since relatively few chronically ill patients make such a switch during any period of time. Tracking care over time is difficult and health plans are often unwilling to provide data for patients who have left the plan due to confidentiality issues and marketing concerns. Hence, studies that compare care in managed plans with that in indemnity plans are cross-sectional and limited by selection biases. Not only do patients differ in the two types of plans, but it is suspected that physicians in HMO settings may practise a less aggressive style and use fewer procedures than physicians selecting traditional FFS practice. Finally, managed care is evolving so rapidly that published data may reflect practices already abandoned by plans.

With these caveats, the available information can be summarized as follows. In younger groups of patients (excluding Medicaid recipients) there is generally equal or better satisfaction with managed-care plans compared to indemnity plans. These younger patients also

tend to be relatively healthy and have limited medical needs. Even in these groups of patients, continuity of care and choice of physician were identified problems in the managed-care group reflecting a high turnover of plans among employers. The several studies done on Medicare beneficiaries tend to give reasonably congruent results, although in this case turnover is initiated by the retiree rather than the employer.

Outcomes such as death, disability and progressive loss of function are not significantly different for managed care and indemnity care groups *except* perhaps among HMO enrollees who are older and chronically ill, attributes clarify which will be common in octogenarians.[32] However, it is important to emphasize that these groups fared poorly and were less satisfied with care regardless of the type of health insurance. Most Medicare recipients did not find managed-care plans as satisfactory in reference to access to care, waiting times and perceived thoroughness of examinations, in most studies, but these do not involve exclusively or even principally cardiovascular care.

There are many reasons to believe that managed-care plans might fail to improve the quality of care for older persons. First, capitated payment mechanisms provide much stronger incentives to select healthier patients than to improve the quality of care for the chronically ill. Indeed, no managed-care plan wants to acquire a public reputation of catering to the severely chronically ill. Despite Federal oversight of marketing, sales strategies designed specifically to attract healthy seniors (e.g. reduced membership costs at health clubs) are frequently seen.

Secondly, consumers lack information on health plan performance such as access or quality of care for chronic conditions. Medicare mandates that health plans report

HEDIS (health plan and employer data and information set) measures, but relatively few chronic disease indicators are included in that system.

Finally, despite aggressive management of costs, few health plans have truly managed clinical care or changed the practice patterns of physicians, whose approach to clinical care was developed during the fee-for-service system. New practice models that could improve quality of care will require physician leadership, management expertise, robust information systems and capital investments that are presently beyond the capability of many health plans and provider organizations.

In view of these factors, it is somewhat surprising and encouraging that studies of managed care in the elderly have shown relatively favorable comparisons. However, since data are relatively sparse, public debate has been driven by anecdote, which almost always views managed care in a negative light.

One of the 'basic units' of managed care is disease management (see Glossary). In the Medicare population, many evidence-based medical practices and treatments are underused, including β-blockers and aspirin, particularly in the oldest old.[38-40] Population and cohort-based approaches to care that utilize well-established clinical guidelines, performance measurement and feedback of performance to clinicians are viewed as positive ways to improve clinical outcomes and cost-effectiveness and reduce unnecessary practice variation.

Congestive heart failure (CHF) is the most common indication for hospitalization of older patients and has a sufficiently robust evidentiary base to implement such approaches. Disease management in a capitated or managed-care system compared favorably with conventional care for CHF.[41] In a randomized trial of a nurse-directed, multidisci-plinary approach to disease management in a high-risk group of CHF patients over the age of 70 (mean age 79), survival at 90 days without readmission and quality of life scores were better in the nurse-directed multidisciplinary group compared to the conventional treatment group. Because there was a reduction in hospital admissions, the overall costs were also less. A number of other studies with a less rigid scientific design have shown similar outcomes.[42-44] The utilization of nonphysician health-care providers in these studies suggests that the structure of the disease management process may account for the improved outcome and not the system of payment.

The Health Care Finance Administration (HCFA) demonstration project on coronary artery bypass grafting (CABG) is another illustration of 'disease management.' At seven sites of diverse character, academic as well as community hospitals, it was convincingly demonstrated that CABG could be performed with better outcomes (including mortality and patient satisfaction), with shorter lengths of stay and lower costs when an integrated, coordinated approach to care was adopted under a standardized protocol. All participating centers were selected because they had a large volume of Medicare patients and had demonstrated a low mortality rate.[45] Such studies demonstrate that the twin goals of managed care, to reduce costs and improve quality, can be achieved—at least in certain settings and with certain types of patients and for a specific procedure.

These illustrations that disease and a procedure can be managed effectively using tools such as guidelines and protocols are important. However, in the elderly, particularly octogenarians, *management* of the whole patient, rather than a single disease is the critical issue. Not only does comorbidity influence outcome but also a wide variety of nonmedical issues do; these include social support, availability of transportation, assistance with household and dietary needs and a sense of control and choice over care. Among the most important issues is addressing the complex 'end of life' decision affecting octogenarians. Patient management elements such as palliative care and home health are potentially better coordinated under a capitated reimbursement structure that does not reward high intensity acute care.

Managed care in octogenarians: possibilities and problems

Properly administered managed care provides a global integrated approach to improved care, the continuous quality improvement concept rather than the sequential evaluation of multiple elements in complex care, the randomized control model. Managed care requires a redefinition of the relationship between the cardiovascular specialist and the primary care physician. It highlights the need for a team approach with the primary-care physician who is responsible for knowing the octogenarian's values and desires in addition to the details of the medical problem and who serves as the physician advocate. This concept carries a very different connotation from the 'gatekeeper concept', which physicians invoke in a derogatory fashion when speaking of primary-care physicians involved in managed-care arrangements. A very important feature in reference to the potential for managed care in the elderly population is the fact that Medicare provides coverage of the entire elderly population and premiums are still reasonable. But under the restraints of the BBA (1997), a more collaborative arrangement involving hospital inpatient services, out-patient services, primary-care physician and cardiovascular consultant, including increasing amounts of managed care involving capitation, will evolve. The desire of managed-care organizations to avoid enrolling Medicare patients who are apt to incur larger expenses will always exist but with appropriate regulatory processes and invoking strong ethical considerations, the risk mix of Medicare patients should allow managed-care organizations to realize the goals of controlling costs and improving quality while preserving access.

The potential conflict between the goals of medicine and the goals of for-profit managed-care organizations have been emphasized. However, conflict of interest existed in fee-for-service medicine. In that setting, there was a tacit financial incentive to treat patients and/or perform procedures when the benefit may have been marginal or nonexistent. Although our society has long operated on the idea that 'more is better' and that patients appreciated having more treatment and procedures rather than fewer, it is not possible to substantiate these long-held views. The relationship between procedures and outcomes has been particularly difficult to prove in the Medicare population. Performing a greater number of procedures in the basic fee-for-service environment of the United States compared to the more managed-care arrangement in Canada has not shown benefit in reference to mortality.[8]

Another aspect of managed care which must be resolved before health-care delivery is improved is the development of better information systems. The systems to track clinical care, provide the opportunity for sophisticated evaluation of outcomes and opportunities to study cost effectiveness in the practice setting, are critical for managed care to truly succeed. Currently, multiple managed-care organizations have developed very serious problems merely in reference to 'bookkeeping,' tracking patient charges and paying health-care providers' bills, as they enrolled large numbers of patients during exuberant growth. Failure to get adequate and accurate information has resulted in serious financial problems for HMOs.

Special and specific concern in reference to managed care relates to the Academic Health Center (AHC). Although major tensions exist among the key elements of the health-care system in the US, there is agreement that the AHC is essential as a source of new knowledge, development of innovative programs and training a wide array of health-care professionals. There is a strong perception and some supporting data that managed care is eroding clinical research and possibly teaching activities of the AHC.[46,47] Clinically generated funds have become an important part of funding clinical research and protecting faculty time has been critical to carrying out research, but such cost shifting is threatened by market competition. National Institutes of Health-supported research favors laboratory-oriented research and clinical, patient-oriented research fares poorly in the grant review process further aggravating the situation.[48] Additionally, Medicare HMOs benefit when their capitated rates using the AAPCC include direct and indirect educational allotments. However, to date, few HMOs have been directly involved in the academic mission. In the current health-care climate, mechanisms must be found to fund the educational and research efforts to understand and improve care in this group of citizens with particular emphasis on patient choice and functional outcomes. Under BBA, graduate medical education dollars will be carved out from Medicare payments for managed care and provided directly to the AHC, which is a small step in the right direction.

Part of the resolution of these issues will come through physician education and altered philosophy. Health-care reform is both essential and reasonable and will include managed care, appropriate practice guidelines and population approaches. Changes in philosophy will also recognize that health policy and decisions must include some government controls and regulations since such an enormous government-supported program has been clearly shown to be subject to abuse. Despite past resistance by physicians and physician groups, the generation of physicians now being trained will enter practice with knowledge and attitudes that make many aspects of managed care acceptable, if not desirable. Physician involvement in the draft of guidelines, establishment of high ethical standards and assuming organizational leadership roles will change the practice of managed care to become more patient-centered. Such is beginning to happen in a major way. Regardless of the fiscal and structural rearrangements (there will be many) the focus must eventually be on the needs and experience of the individual patient with the recognition and acceptance of the limits of medical care in the oldest patients.[49–51]

References

1. Mayer T. HMOs: origins and development. *N Engl J Med* (1985) **312**:590–4.

2. Van Tassel RA, Pritzker MR, Pryor DB. Cardiovascular care in the managed care era. In: Topol E, ed, *Cardiovascular Medicine* (Lippincott-Raven–Philadelphia, 1998) 1135–51.

3. Ginzberg E, Ostow M. Managed care: a look back and a look ahead. *N Engl J Med* (1997) **336**:1018–29.

4. Iglehart JK. Medicare turns to HMOs. *N Engl J Med* (1985) **312**:132–6.

5. Welch WP. Growth in HMO share of the Medicare market, 1989–1994. *Health Affairs (Millwood)* (1996) **15**:201–14.

6. Peterson ED, Jollis JG, Bebchuk JD et al. Changes in mortality after myocardial revascularization in the elderly. *Ann Intern Med* (1994) **121**:919–27.

7. Peterson ED, Cowper PA, Jollis JG et al. Outcomes of coronary artery bypass graft surgery in 24 461 patients aged 80 years or older. *Circulation* (1995) **92**(Supplement 9):II85–91.

8. Tu JV, Pashos CL, Naylor CD et al. Use of cardiac procedures and outcomes in elderly patients with myocardial infarction in the United States and Canada. *N Engl J Med* (1997) **336**:1500–5.

9. Lohr KN, ed, *Medicare: A Strategy for Quality Assurance.* (National Academy Press: Washington DC, 1990).

10. Topol EJ, Califf RM. Quality of care in cardiovascular medicine. In: Topol E, ed, *Cardiovascular Medicine* (Lippincott-Raven: Philadelphia, 1998) 1119–34.

11. Bodenheimer T. The HMO backlash: righteous or reactionary? *N Engl J Med* (1996) **335**:1601–4.

12. Mirvis DM, Chang CF, Morreim EH. Protecting older people while managing their care. *J Am Geriatr Soc* (1997) **45**:645–6.

13. Lachs MS, Hirsch SR. Is managed care good or bad for geriatric medicine. *J Am Geriatr Soc* (1997) **45**:1123–7.

14. Reuben DB. Managed care: good medicine for old people? *J Am Geriatr Soc* (1997) **45**: 643–4.

15. Donelan K, Blendon RJ, Lundberg GD et al. The new medical marketplace: physicians' views. *Health Aff (Millwood)* (1997) **16**:139–48.

16. Angell M. Editorial: fixing Medicare, current reform proposals, alternative approaches. *N Engl J Med* (1997) **337**:192–5.

17. Gramm P, Rettenmaier AJ, Saving TR. Medicare policy for future generations: a search for a permanent solution. *N Engl J Med* (1998) **338**:1307–10.

18. Welch HG, Albertsen PC, Nease RF et al. Estimating treatment benefits for the elderly: the effect of competing risks. *Ann Intern Med* (1996) **124**:577–84.

19. DeMaria AN, Lee TH, Leon DF et al. Effect of managed care on cardiovascular specialists: involvement, attitudes and practice adaptations. *J Am Coll Cardiol* (1996) **28**:1884–95.

20. Eng C, Pedulla J, Eleazer GP et al. Program of All-inclusive Care for the Elderly (PACE): an innovative model of integrated geriatric care and financing. *J Am Geriatr Soc* (1997) **45**: 223–32.

21. Morgan RO, Virnig BA, DeVito CA, Persily NA. The Medicare–HMO revolving door: the healthy go in and the sick go out. *N Engl J Med* (1997) **337**:169–75.

22. Clement DG, Retchin SM, Brown RS, Stegall MH. Access and outcomes of elderly patients enrolled in managed care. *JAMA* (1994) **271**:1487–92.

23. Ware JE Jr, Bayliss MS, Rogers WH et al. Differences in 4-year health outcomes for elderly and poor, chronically ill patients treated in HMO and fee-for-service systems, results from the Medical Outcomes Study. *JAMA* (1996) **276**:1039–47.

24. Ellerbeck EF, Jencks SF, Radford MJ et al. Quality of care for Medicare patients with acute myocardial infarction. (A four-state pilot study from the Cooperative Cardiovascular Project). *JAMA* (1995) **273**:1509–14.

25. Beck T, Scott J, Williams P et al. A randomized trial of group outpatient visits for chronically

ill older HMO members: the Cooperative Health Care Clinic. *J Am Geriatr Soc* (1997) **45**:543–9.

26. Riley G, Lubitz J, Rabey E. Enrollee health status under Medicare risk contracts: an analysis of mortality rates. *Health Serv Res* (1991) **6**:137–63.

27. Lurie N, Christianson J, Finch M, Moscovice I. The effects of capitation on health and functional status of the Medicaid elderly. A randomized trial. *Ann Intern Med* (1994) **120**:506–11.

28. Preston JA, Retchin SM. The management of geriatric hypertension in health maintenance organizations. *J Am Geriatric Soc* (1991) **39**: 683–90.

29. Retchin SM, Preston J. Effects of cost containment on the care of elderly diabetics. *Arch Intern Med* (1991) **151**:2224–8.

30. Kramer AM, Fox PD, Morgenstein N. Geriatric care approaches in health maintenance organizations. *J Am Geriatr Soc* (1992) **40**: 1055–67.

31. Colenda CC, Sherman FT. Managed Medicare: an overview for the primary care physician. *Geriatrics* (1998) **53**:57–63.

32. Ware JE, Brook RH, Rogers WH et al. Comparison of health outcomes at a health maintenance organization with those of fee-for-service care. *Lancet* (1986) **i**:1017–22.

33. Miller RH, Luft HS. Managed care plan performance since 1980: a literature analysis. *JAMA* (1994) **271**:1512–19.

34. Greenfield S, Nelson EC, Zubkoff M et al. Variations in resource utilization among medical specialties and systems of care: results from the Medical Outcomes Study. *JAMA* (1992) **267**:1624–30.

35. Greenfield S, Rogers W, Mangotich M et al. Outcomes of patients with hypertension and non-insulin dependent diabetes mellitus treated by different systems and specialties: results from the Medical Outcomes Study. *JAMA* (1995) **274**:1436–44.

36. Hellinger FJ. The effect of managed care on quality: a review of recent evidence. *Arch Intern Med* (1998) **158**:833–41.

37. Carlisle DM, Siu AL, Keeler EB et al. HMO vs fee-for-service care of older persons with acute myocardial infarction. *Am J Public Health* (1992) **82**:1626–30.

38. Krumholz HM, Murillo JE, Chen J et al. Thrombolytic therapy for eligible elderly patients with acute myocardial infarction. *JAMA* (1997) **277**:1683–8.

39. Ellerbeck EF, Jencks SF, Radford MJ et al. Quality of care for Medicare patients with acute myocardial infarction. *JAMA* (1995) **273**:1509–14.

40. Krumholz HM, Philbin DM Jr, Wang Y et al. Trends in the quality of care for Medicare beneficiaries admitted to the hospital with unstable angina. *J Am Coll Cardiol* (1998) **31**:957–63.

41. Rich MW, Beckham V, Wittenberg C et al. A multidisciplinary intervention prevents the readmission of elderly patients with congestive heart failure. *N Engl J Med* (1995) **333**: 1190–5.

42. Wolinsky FD, Smith DM, Stump TE et al. The sequelae of hospitalization for congestive heart failure among older adults. *J Am Geriatr Soc* (1997) **45**:558–63.

43. Retchin SM, Brown B. Elderly patients with congestive heart failure under prepaid care. *Am J Med* (1991) **90**:36–42.

44. Kornowski R, Zeeli D, Averbuch M et al. Intensive home-care surveillance prevents hospitalization and improves morbidity rates among elderly patients severe congestive heart failure. *Am Heart J* (1995) **129**:762–6.

45. Thoumanian A. HCFA CABG demonstration protect.

46. Campbell EG, Weissman JS, Blumenthal D. Relationship between market competition and the activities and attitudes of medical school faculty. *JAMA* (1997) **278**:222–6.

47. Katz SM. Medical education and managed care: keeping pace. *J Am Geriatr Soc* (1998) **46**:381–4.

48. Williams GH, Wara DW, Carbone P. Funding for patient-oriented research. Critical strain on a fundamental linchpin. *JAMA* (1997) **278**:227–31.

49. Callahan D. Managed care and the goals of medicine. *J Am Geriatr Soc* (1998) **46**:385–8.

50. Snyder L, Tooker J. Obligations and opportunities: the role of clinical societies in the ethics of managed care. *J Am Geriatr Soc* (1998) **46**:378–80.

51. Berwick DM. Quality comes home. *Ann Intern Med* (1996) **125**:839–43.

Glossary

Managed-care terms

AAPCC: Adjusted average per capita cost. HCFA's estimate of the amount of money it costs to care for Medicare recipients in a given area under fee-for-service. Adjustment factors include age, sex, Medicaid eligibility, institutional status, working status and presence of end-stage renal disease.

Capitation: In managed-care plans, a system of prepaying doctors and hospitals a set fee to provide health care for each enrollee, without regard to the type or number of services rendered.

Coinsurance: In traditional insurance plans, the proportion the individual pays for medical services. For instance, if a plan covers 80% of a bill, the individual's coinsurance is 20%.

Copayment: A fee to patients, usually $5–$15 for doctor visits or medical services.

Deductible: In some plans, the amount paid each year for medical expenses before the insurance pays. The lower the premium, the higher the deductible.

Disease management: The process of intensively managing a particular disease across all settings of care, with a heavy emphasis on prevention, education and maintenance strategies to avoid use of more expensive options (emergency room visits, hospitalizations).

Emergency care: Medical care needed immediately because of sudden or suddenly worsening illness or injury, the time needed to reach your managed-care organization doctor or hospital appears to you to risk permanent damage to your health.

ERISA: Employee Retirement Income Security Act. Federal legislation crafted to protect employer-sponsored pension plans that unintentionally allow self-funded health plans to avoid state-mandated plans from being sued under state law for malpractice.

Fee-for-service: Traditional health coverage in which the individual or their insurer pays doctors and hospitals for each visit or service provided.

Formulary: A list of medications that plans will pay for without prior approval.

Gatekeeper: At HMOs, the primary-care doctor, usually family practitioner, internist, pediatrician or obstetrician/gynecologist, who coordinates basic care and recommends tests, treatment and referral to specialists.

Health maintenance organization (HMO): A prepaid health-care plan that provides or arranges comprehensive health services for its enrolled members.

Integrated delivery system (IDS): A group of hospitals, physicians and ancillary providers that have joined to create a system that provides comprehensive health-care services through a coordinated, client-centered continuum designed to improve health-care services in specific geographic markets and within economic limits.

Indemnity insurance: Traditional insurance that pays for specific covered services (see fee-for-service)

Utilization management: A range of procedures that permit a health plan, insurer or other payer to review the choice of treatment prospectively, concurrently or retrospectively.

Utilization review: A subset of utilization management techniques that typically encompasses preservice and during-service strategies.

Major types of HMOs

Staff model: Enrollees receive the care from salaried staff doctors at the HMO's own facility.

Group or network model: The HMO contracts with one or several groups of doctors who provide care for a fixed amount per plan member. Groups often practise in one facility.

Independent practice association model (IPA): Doctors in private practice form an association that contracts with HMOs. The physicians generally work in their own offices.

Physician hospital organization (PHO): Hybrid plans that combine characteristics of indemnity insurance and HMOs. Generally, at the time service is rendered, the insured can elect to receive the service from a network provider at a discount or at no out-of-pocket cost, or from a nonnetwork provider subject to substantially higher patient cost sharing.

Preferred Provider Organization (PPO): A contractual arrangement between independent or institutionally based providers and another entity to deliver health services to a defined population at established fees. The PPO contains a panel of physicians and health-care institutions that constitute the preferred providers. Health-care services are delivered on a fee-for-service basis at established rates, usually discounted from the physician's usual and customary rates. Economic incentives encourage PPO members to use the preferred panel.

Physician networks: Large groups of doctors band together to accept the financial risk of covering their patients' health-care needs, a role traditionally played by insurers. By bypassing insurers, doctors aim to maintain their autonomy while cutting administrative and other costs.

Medicare-managed care options

Risk contracts: Medicare pays the HMO a set amount to provide an enrollee's care. That care includes all Medicare-covered services and, depending on the plan, may include additional services such as prescription drugs and eyeglasses. Enrollees may or may not pay a monthly fee for their plan; enrollees must receive all but emergency care through their plan, they are 'locked in' to using their plan's network unless they are enrolled in an out-of-network option.

Cost contracts: This allows the enrollee to use medical services outside subject to coinsurance, deductibles and charges that apply to regular Medicare.

Health care prepayment plans (HCPPs): These were originally intended to allow employers to offer a managed-care option to their retirees. These plans are similar to cost contracts but may cover only part of the Medicare benefit package; generally they cover part B expenses (doctors), while enrollees use traditional Medicare Part A (hospital and other) expenses.

Medicare SELECT: This option supplements traditional Medicare like a medigap policy. It is not managed care but it uses similar concepts. Enrollees choose providers from an approved list to get full benefits. If they do not, Medicare will pay its traditional portion of the bill.

Index